Tumors
of the
Cervix, Vagina, and Vulva

Atlas
of
Tumor Pathology

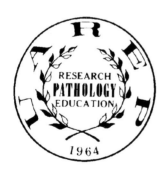

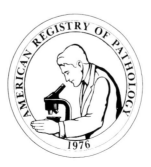

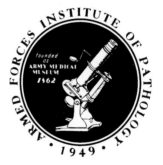

ATLAS OF TUMOR PATHOLOGY

Third Series
Fascicle 4

TUMORS OF THE
CERVIX, VAGINA, AND VULVA

by

ROBERT J. KURMAN, M.D.

Departments of Pathology and Gynecology and Obstetrics
Johns Hopkins Hospital
Baltimore, Maryland 21287

HENRY J. NORRIS, M.D.

Department of Gynecologic and Breast Pathology
Armed Forces Institute of Pathology
Washington, D.C. 20306

and

EDWARD J. WILKINSON, M.D.

Department of Pathology
University of Florida College of Medicine
Gainesville, Florida 32610

Published by the
ARMED FORCES INSTITUTE OF PATHOLOGY
Washington, D.C.

Under the Auspices of
UNIVERSITIES ASSOCIATED FOR RESEARCH AND EDUCATION IN PATHOLOGY, INC.
Bethesda, Maryland
1992

Accepted for Publication
1990

Available from the American Registry of Pathology
Armed Forces Institute of Pathology
Washington, D.C. 20306-6000
ISSN 0160-6344
ISBN 11-881041-02-6

ATLAS OF TUMOR PATHOLOGY

EDITOR
JUAN ROSAI, M.D.
Department of Pathology
Memorial Sloan-Kettering Cancer Center
New York, New York 10021-6007

ASSOCIATE EDITOR
LESLIE H. SOBIN, M.D.
Armed Forces Institute of Pathology
Washington, D.C. 20306-6000

EDITORIAL ADVISORY BOARD

EDITORS' NOTE

The Atlas of Tumor Pathology has a long and distinguished history. It was first conceived at a Cancer Research Meeting held in St. Louis in September 1947 as an attempt to standardize the nomenclature of neoplastic diseases. The first series was sponsored by the National Academy of Sciences-National Research Council. The organization of this Sisyphean effort was entrusted to the Subcommittee on Oncology of the Committee on Pathology, and Dr. Arthur Purdy Stout was the first editor-in-chief. Many of the illustrations were provided by the Medical Illustration Service of the Armed Forces Institute of Pathology, the type was set by the Government Printing Office, and the final printing was done at the Armed Forces Institute of Pathology (hence the colloquial appellation "AFIP Fascicles"). The American Registry of Pathology purchased the Fascicles from the Government Printing Office and sold them virtually at cost. Over a period of 20 years, approximately 15,000 copies each of nearly 40 Fascicles were produced. The worldwide impact that these publications have had over the years has largely surpassed the original goal. They quickly became among the most influential publications on tumor pathology ever written, primarily because of their overall high quality but also because their low cost made them easily accessible to pathologists and other students of oncology the world over.

Upon completion of the first series, the National Academy of Sciences-National Research Council handed further pursuit of the project over to the newly created Universities Associated for Research and Education in Pathology (UAREP). A second series was started, generously supported by grants from the AFIP, the National Cancer Institute, and the American Cancer Society. Dr. Harlan I. Firminger became the editor-in-chief and was succeeded by Dr. William H. Hartmann. The second series Fascicles were produced as bound volumes instead of loose leaflets. They featured a more comprehensive coverage of the subjects, to the extent that the Fascicles could no longer be regarded as "atlases" but rather as monographs describing and illustrating in detail the tumors and tumor-like conditions of the various organs and systems.

Once the second series was completed, with a success that matched that of the first, UAREP and AFIP decided to embark on a third series. A new editor-in-chief and an associate editor were selected, and a distinguished editorial board was appointed. The mandate for the third series remains the same as for the previous ones, i.e., to oversee the production of an eminently practical publication with surgical pathologists as its primary audience, but also aimed at other workers in oncology. The main purposes of this series are to promote a consistent, unified, and biologically sound nomenclature; to guide the surgical pathologist in the diagnosis of the various tumors and tumor-like lesions; and to provide relevant histogenetic, pathogenetic, and clinico-pathologic information on these entities. Just as the second series included data obtained from ultrastructural (and, in the more recent Fascicles, immunohistochemical) examination, the third series will, in addition, incorporate pertinent information obtained with the newer molecular biology techniques. As in the past, a continuous attempt will be made to correlate, whenever possible, the nomenclature used in the Fascicles with that proposed by the World Health Organization's International Histological Classification of Tumors. The format of the third series has been changed in order to incorporate additional items and to ensure a consistency of style throughout. This includes the dropping of the 's possessive in eponymic terms, in accordance with the WHO and the International Nomenclature of Diseases. Close cooperation between the various authors and their respective liaisons from the editorial board will be emphasized to minimize unnecessary repetition and discrepancies in the text and illustrations.

To its everlasting credit, the participation and commitment of the AFIP to this venture is even more substantial and encompassing than in previous series. It now extends to virtually all scientific, technical, and financial aspects of the production.

The task confronting the organizations and individuals involved in the third series is even more daunting than in the preceding efforts because of the ever-increasing complexity of the matter at hand. It is hoped that this combined effort—of which, needless to say, that represented by the authors is first and foremost—will result in a series worthy of its two illustrious predecessors and will be a suitable introduction to the tumor pathology of the twenty-first century.

Juan Rosai, M.D.
Leslie H. Sobin, M.D.

ACKNOWLEDGMENTS

The publication of this Fascicle has depended on the assistance of many individuals to whom the authors are greatly indebted. We are especially grateful to Dr. Robert E. Scully and Dr. Richard L. Kempson for their thoughtful review and comments on the entire text. In addition, we wish to thank Dr. Stanley J. Robboy for his critical review of the chapter on embryology, Dr. Peter M. Howley and Dr. Keerti V. Shah for their critique of the chapter on human papillomaviruses, and Dr. K. Kendall Pierson and Dr. F. Mack Sexton for their review of the chapter on vulvar tumors. Drs. I. Keith Stone, Nancy Sexton Hardt and David L. Dolson provided clinical support for the preparation of the vulvar chapter. We also wish to thank Mr. Raymond Lund at the Johns Hopkins Hospital and Mr. Jeffrey Knee at the University of Florida for their supervision of the photomicrography. Mrs. Sue Skierkowski, Mrs. Sandra Fortier, and Ms. Trina King typed the manuscript, and to them we are most grateful. The classification of tumors of the uterine cervix, vagina, and vulva used in this Fascicle is based on the classification proposed by the International Society of Gynecological Pathologists under the auspices of the World Health Organization. The classification of vulvar neoplasms was developed in conjunction with the International Society for the Study of Vulvar Disease. Finally, there are many other individuals who played an important role in the publication of this Fascicle who we have not specifically mentioned. To all of these people we wish to express our thanks.

Robert J. Kurman, M.D.

Henry J. Norris, M.D.

Edward J. Wilkinson, M.D.

Permission to use copyrighted illustrations has been granted by:

American College of Obstetricians and Gynecologists:
    Obstet Gynecol 44:735–48, 1974. For figures 155 and 156.
    Obstet Gynecol 45:638–46, 1975. For figure 326.
    Obstet Gynecol 48:571–8, 1976. For figure 61.
    Obstet Gynecol 62:720–7, 1983. For figure 114.

American Medical Association:
    Arch Pathol 90:473–9, 1970. For figure 236.
    Arch Pathol Lab Med 106:250–4, 1982. For figure 136.
    JAMA 202:637–9, 1967. For figure 161.

American Society for Microbiology:
    J Virol 58:225–9, 1986. For figure 27.

Blackwell Scientific Publications Ltd:
    Histopathol 12:167–76, 1988. For figures 206 and 207.

Butterworth Publishing Company:
    Principles and Techniques of Surgical Pathology, 1983. For figures 7 and 22.

Cahners Publishing Company:
    Am J Med 85 (Suppl 2A):155–8, 1988. For figure 23.

CV Mosby Company:
    Am J Obstet Gynecol 58:924–42, 1949. For figures 82 and 83.
    Clinical Gynecologic Oncology, 3rd. ed., 1989. For figure 6.

Institute for Clinical Science:
    Ann Clin Lab Sci 4:222–53, 1974. For figure 211.

JB Lippincott Company:
    Am J Clin Path 46:420–6, 1966. For figure 230.
    Cancer 54:869–75, 1984. For figures 203 and 204.
    Cancer 67:1599–1607, 1991. For figure 30.
    Clin Obstet Gynecol 34:651–61, 1991. For figure 264.

McGraw-Hill, Inc.:
    Human Embryology, 1946. For figure 1.

Raven Press Ltd. New York:
    Am J Surg Pathol 7:39–52, 1983. For figure 25.
    Histology for Pathologists, 1992. For figures 18 and 19.
    Int J Gynecol Pathol 10:107–25. For figures 261 and 276.

Royal College of Surgeons of England:
    Ann R Coll Surg Engl 3:189–209, 1948. For figures 20 and 21.

Springer-Verlag New York, Inc.:
    Blaustein's Pathology of the Female Genital Tract, 3rd ed., For figures 14, 32, 44, 45, 46, 71, 195, 227, 246.

W.B. Saunders Company:
    Human Pathol 14:831–3, 1983. For figure 4.
    Human Pathol 17:488–92, 1986. For figure 196.
    Obstet Gynecol Clin North Am 14:451–69, 1987. For figure 26.
    Semin Diagn Pathol 7:158–72, 1990. For figure 29.
    The Pathology of Incipient Neoplasia, 1986. For figure 54.

Williams and Wilkins Company:
    Langman's Medical Embryology, 5th ed., 1985. For figures 2 and 5.

TUMORS OF THE CERVIX, VAGINA, AND VULVA

Contents

TUMORS OF THE CERVIX, VAGINA, AND VULVA

EMBRYOLOGY OF THE LOWER FEMALE GENITAL TRACT

CERVIX AND VAGINA

The differential diagnosis of a number of benign and malignant lesions of the lower female genital tract is facilitated by an understanding of the embryology of these organs. In the past, our understanding of the embryology of the human cervix and vagina was based on experimental work in animals whose embryologic development differs from that of humans. These studies have been summarized by Forsberg (7), Mossman (9), and O'Rahilly (10). Studies of human fetal genital tracts implanted into athymic (nude) mice by Robboy and co-workers (4,11,13) have further modified these views. The discussion of the development of the cervix and vagina that follows is a brief account of what remains a complex and incompletely understood subject (12).

The anlage of the uterine corpus and cervix and the upper vagina is termed the uterovaginal canal. This structure develops from the fusion of the mesoderm-derived paired müllerian ducts at about day 54 postconception. The canal is initially a straight tube lined by müllerian columnar epithelium that joins the endoderm-derived urogenital sinus. The point at which the two meet is referred to as the müllerian tubercle (fig. 1). This site is destined to be the location of the vaginal orifice at the hymenal ring. At approximately day 66, the epithelium of the caudal uterovaginal canal in this location begins to stratify, either as a result of cephalad migration of cells from the urogenital sinus (1,11) or by direct squamous transformation of the columnar cells lining the uterovaginal canal (6). Clinical evidence favoring the former interpretation is provided by women born with an imperforate transverse vaginal septum (14). In these patients, the vagina lying above the septum is lined by columnar epithelium, whereas below the septum, the vagina is lined by squamous epithelium. The stratification of cells in the region of the müllerian tubercle is the first evidence of formation of the vaginal

plate, a structure unique to humans. The stratified squamous epithelial cells of the vaginal plate proliferate so that by day 77 the vagina is a nearly solid core of squamous epithelium (fig. 1). Endocervical glands and the vaginal fornices appear between 91 days (13th wk) and 15 weeks, thereby permitting the first definitive identification of the cervix (fig. 2). At this time, the vagina and cervix are highly sensitive to steroid hormones and, from about the 16th week of fetal life to birth, the cervix responds to estrogenic stimulation by marked growth. Similarly, mucin secretion in endocervical glands begins in response to estrogenic stimulation during the 7th month of gestation and decreases rapidly during the first 2 postnatal weeks, remaining at a low steady state until menarche, when increased secretion begins again.

Experimental studies in rodents provide cogent evidence that the primitive epithelium lining the uterovaginal canal is programmed to differentiate into squamous, mucinous, and tuboendometrial-like epithelia by the underlying stroma. It has been demonstrated that murine neonatal vaginal epithelium grown on uterine stroma differentiates into columnar epithelium, whereas uterine epithelium grown on vaginal stroma differentiates into squamous epithelium (2). The cytosolic proteins in the resultant epithelia reflect that of the induced rather than the original source (3).

Studies of the developing human genital tract implanted into nude mice have shown that the cervix and uterine corpus are invested by two layers of primitive mesenchyme. The inner layer is destined to become the endocervical and endometrial stroma and the outer layer the myometrium. The inner layer invests the uterine corpus and cervix gradually tapering and ending at the point where the cervix joins the vagina, possibly extending into the vagina and vulva (5). The outer layer is continuous throughout the fallopian tube, myometrium, and wall of the vagina (fig. 3). It has been postulated that the inner layer

1

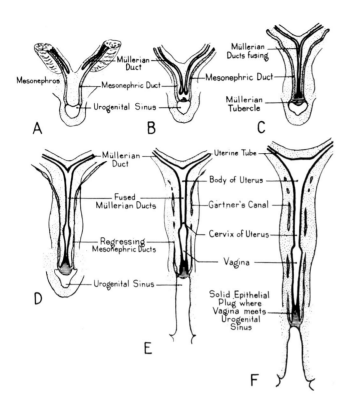

Figure 1

FUSION OF THE MÜLLERIAN DUCTS
TO FORM THE UTERUS AND VAGINA

The close relationship of the epithelia of the müllerian ducts to the urogenital sinus explains, in part, the difficulty in determining which epithelium gives rise to that of the vagina. (Fig. 363 from Patten BM. Human embryology. Philadelphia: Blakiston, 1946. Redrawn from Koff AK. Contrib Embryol, 1933; Vol 24.)

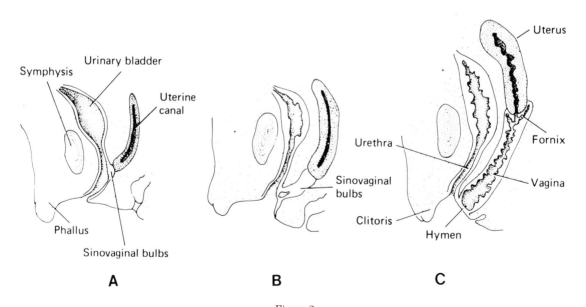

Figure 2

FORMATION OF THE UTERUS AND THE VAGINA

These sagittal sections show the formation of the uterus and vagina at various stages of development. (Fig. 15-24 from Sadler TW. Langman's medical embryology. 5th ed. Baltimore: Williams & Wilkins, 1985.)

induces differentiation of the tuboendometrial-type glandular epithelium of the fallopian tube, uterine corpus, and deep glands in the cervix (4). According to this view, the squamous epithelium of the vagina that may be derived from the urogenital sinus is not subject to the inductive stimulus of the cervicovaginal mesenchyme.

This concept of cervical and vaginal development is attractive because it offers an explanation for many of the genital tract abnormalities observed in women exposed to diethylstilbestrol (DES) and related drugs in utero. In the DES-exposed female fetus, the primary teratogenic effect of the drug may be directly on the stroma, which

in turn induces abnormalities in the overlying epithelium. In the nude mouse model, in utero DES inhibits the usual segregation of the inner and outer layers of the mesenchyme that surround the cervicovaginal canal (13). A similar mechanism may be involved in the gross structural abnormalities of the cervix (hoods, ridges, cervical hypoplasia, and vaginal fornix hypoplasia) and the abnormal contours of the endometrial cavity (uterine constriction and T-shaped uterus) that have been observed in human females exposed to DES in utero (8). In addition, enlargement of the transformation zone, evident in most DES-exposed women, may be due to a failure in the normal segregation of the underlying mesenchyme into discrete layers. As a result, the innermost layer of mesenchyme extends out laterally and cephalad beneath the ectocervix and upper vagina. This mesenchyme induces the differentiation of mucinous epithelium, i.e., the glandular component of the transformation zone, which in turn extends over the ectocervix and upper vagina. In the upper vagina, this results in mucinous-type adenosis. Failure of the upgrowth of urogenital sinus squamous epithelium results in retention of the original embryonic müllerian epithelium, and contact with the mesenchyme of the vagina results in induction of tuboendometrial-type glandular epithelium (adenosis) in the more caudal portion of the vagina (fig. 4) (11). Clear cell carcinoma in the DES-exposed woman is characteristically associated with tuboendometrial-type adenosis rather than with mucinous adenosis.

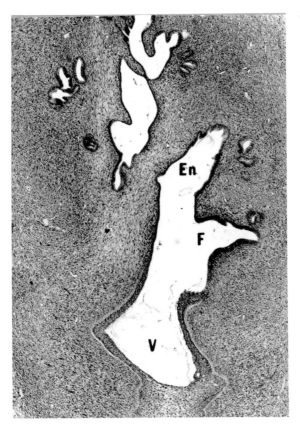

Figure 3
JUNCTION OF ENDOCERVIX AND VAGINA
WITH FORNIX-LIKE REGION
A human female genital tract aged 53 days postovulation grafted into a nude mouse exposed to progesterone for 70 days (equivalent postovulation day 123) showing the junction of endocervix (En) and vagina (V) with fornix-like region (F). Note that the inner cellular layer of stroma of the endocervix disappears near the junction of the columnar epithelium of the cervix and the squamous epithelium of the vagina. (Courtesy of Dr. S. J. Robboy, Newark, NJ.)

VULVA

The formation of the vulva becomes evident in the 4th embryonic week, when proliferation of the mesodermal stroma adjacent to the cloaca results in elevation of the overlying ectoderm. Ventrally, this results in the formation of the genital tubercle, which becomes the clitoris. Laterally, two parallel ridges, each composed of a medial and lateral fold, develop. The medial folds, or urogenital folds, develop into the labia minora. The lateral folds, or labioscrotal folds, develop into the labia majora. By the end of the 6th week of development, the urorectal septum and the cloacal plate fuse to form the urogenital membrane anteriorly and the anal membrane posteriorly. Fusion of the lower portion of the

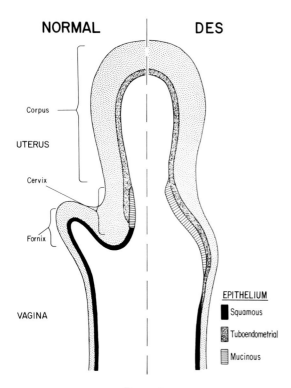

Figure 4
HYPOTHETICAL CONSEQUENCES OF PRENATAL
DIETHYLSTILBESTROL EXPOSURE TO
DEVELOPING VAGINA AND CERVIX
A normal genital tract is illustrated on the left. The genital tract in a patient exposed to diethylstilbestrol (DES) in utero is illustrated on the right. (Fig. 2 from Robboy SJ. A hypothetic mechanism of diethylstilbestrol (DES)-induced anomalies in exposed progeny. Hum Pathol 1983;14:831–3.)

labioscrotal folds anterior to the anal fold results in the formation of the perineum (fig. 5). Accordingly, the epithelia of the labia majora, the labia minora, and the clitoris are of ectodermal origin. The bilateral labioscrotal folds fuse anterior to the genital tubercle forming the mons pubis. The junction of the distal vagina with the urogenital sinus results in the development of the vulvar vestibule, which is identifiable by the 16th week. Except for a small area immediately anterior to the urethra, which may be of ectodermal origin, the vestibule is of endodermal origin. The junction of the epithelium derived from endoderm and that derived from ectoderm is seen in the adult on the inner aspects of the labia minora, marked by the junction of keratinized with non-keratinized epithelium. This line of demarkation is referred to as the vestibular line of Hart (see Anatomy of the Lower Female Genital Tract). The Bartholin gland, the major gland of the vestibule, is of endodermal origin. Homologous structures of the male and female are compared in Table 1.

The embryologic development of the lower genital tract defines the spectrum of neoplasia within broad limits. For example, adenocarcinomas of the endocervix resemble adenocarcinomas in the upper genital tract rather than adenocarcinomas of the vulva because the cervix, like the upper genital tract, is of mesodermal origin. In contrast, adenocarcinomas that arise in the ectodermally derived skin of the vulva, are mostly sweat gland carcinomas. Carcinomas arising in the Bartholin gland, which is of endodermal origin, resemble tumors of other endodermal derived tissues.

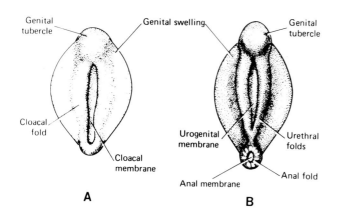

Figure 5
EMBRYOLOGY OF THE VULVA
The indifferent stage of the external genitalia is represented at approximately 4 weeks (A) and at approximately 6 weeks (B). (Fig. 15-26 from Sadler TW. Langman's medical embryology. 5th ed. Baltimore: Williams & Wilkins, 1985.)

Table 1

FEMALE AND MALE HOMOLOGUES
OF THE EXTERNAL GENITALIA OF THE HUMAN

Female	Male
Vulvar vestibule	Distal urethra
Skene glands	Prostate gland
Bartholin glands	Cowper glands (bulbourethral glands)
Minor vestibular glands	Glands of Littre
Clitoris	Corpus cavernosum of the penis
Labia minora	Corpus spongiosus of the penis
Labia majora	Scrotum

References

1. Bulmer D. The development of the human vagina. J Anat 1957;91:490–509.
2. Cunha GR. Epithelial-stromal interactions in development of the urogenital tract. Int Rev Cytol 1976;47:137–94.
3. _____ , Shannon JM, Taguchi O, Fujii H, Meloy BA. Epithelial-mesenchymal interactions in hormone-induced development. In: Sawyer RH, Fallon, JF, eds. Epithelial-mesenchymal interactions in development. New York: Praeger Publishers, 1983:51–74.
4. _____ , Taguchi O, Sugimura Y, Lawrence WD, Mahmood F, Robboy SJ. Absence of teratogenic effects of progesterone on the developing genital tract of the human female fetus. Hum Pathol 1988;19:777–83.
5. Elliot GB, Elliot JD. Superficial stromal reactions of lower genital tract. Arch Pathol 1973;95:100–1.
6. Forsberg J-G. Cervicovaginal epithelium: its origin and development. Am J Obstet Gynecol 1973;115:1025–43.
7. _____ . Development of the human vaginal epithelium. In: Hafez ESE, Evans TN, eds. The human vagina. New York: Elsevier/North-Holland, 1978:3–19. (Hafez ESE, ed. Human reproductive medicine; Vol 2.)
8. Kaufmann RH, Adam E, Binder GL, Gerthoffer E. Upper genital tract changes and pregnancy outcome in offspring exposed in utero to diethylstilbestrol. Am J Obstet Gynecol 1980;137:299–308.
9. Mossman HW. The embryology of the cervix. In: Blandau RJ, Moghissi K, eds. The biology of the cervix. Chicago: University of Chicago Press, 1973:13–22.
10. O'Rahilly R. The development of the vagina in the human. In: Blandau RJ, Bergsma D, eds. Morphogenesis and malformation of the genital system. New York: Alan R. Liss, 1977:123–36. (Bergsma D, ed. Birth defects: original article series; Vol 13, no 2.)
11. Robboy SJ. A hypothetic mechanism of diethylstilbestrol (DES)-induced anomalies in exposed progeny. Hum Pathol 1983;14:831–3.
12. _____ , Prade M, Cunha G. Vagina. In: Sternberg SS, ed. Histology for pathologists. New York: Raven Press, 1992:881–92.
13. _____ , Taguchi O, Cunha GR. Normal development of the human female reproductive tract and alterations resulting from experimental exposure to diethylstilbestrol. Hum Pathol 1982;13:190–8.
14. Ulfelder H, Robboy SJ. The embryologic development of the human vagina. Am J Obstet Gynecol 1976;126:769–76.

✧✧✧

ANATOMY OF THE LOWER FEMALE GENITAL TRACT

For a comprehensive review of the gross anatomy of the cervix, vagina, and vulva, see Krantz (10,11) and Friedrich (5), respectively. The following discussion focuses primarily on those aspects of the gross anatomy and lymphatic drainage that are pertinent to the evaluation of tumors in these locations.

CERVIX

Gross Anatomy. The cervix accounts for a half to a third of the length of the uterus, measuring 2.5 to 3.0 cm in length and 2.0 to 2.5 cm in diameter. The vaginal portion of the cervix (portio vaginalis or ectocervix) is surrounded by a reflection of the vaginal wall termed the *fornix*. A portion of the cervix that lies above the upper margin of the vagina abuts anteriorly on the bladder and is separated from it by loose connective tissue that extends into the broad ligaments laterally. Posteriorly, the upper cervix is covered by peritoneum forming the lining of the cul-de-sac. The connective tissue surrounding the cervix and vagina extends laterally and posteriorly toward the second to fourth dorsal vertebrae as the uterosacral ligaments. The chief support of the cervix, however, is from the cardinal ligaments, which are fibromuscular bands that fan out laterally from the lower uterine segment and cervix to the lateral pelvic walls (fig. 6).

Lymphatic Drainage. The cervix has a complex lymphatic drainage that is arranged in three beds. One bed underlies the epithelium of the endocervical clefts and squamous epithelium and a second bed lies deeper in the stroma. Both beds drain into perforating lymphatic vessels, which in turn empty into a serosal plexus, which drains a third bed from the outer surface of the cervix. The lymphatic channels leave the cervix via two main vessels closely related to the uterine artery that fan out anteriorly and laterally in the broad ligament, and a third vessel that progresses posterolaterally in the uterosacral ligaments toward the sacrum. The pelvic lymph nodes into which these lymphatics drain can be divided into three main groups (fig. 7). The external iliac

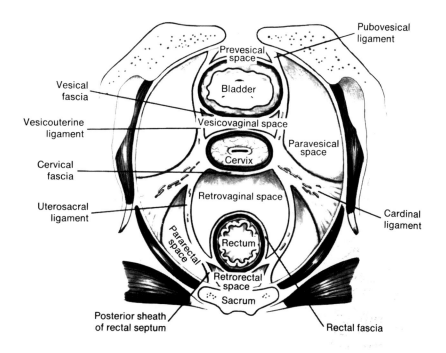

Figure 6
CROSS SECTION OF THE PELVIS AT THE LEVEL OF THE CERVIX
This schematic illustrates a cross section of the pelvis at the level of the cervix. (Fig. 3-10 from DiSaia PJ, Creasman WT. Clinical gynecologic oncology. 3rd ed. St. Louis: CV Mosby, 1989.)

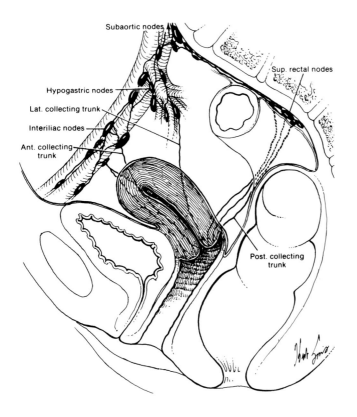

Subaortic nodes

Sup. rectal nodes

Hypogastric nodes

Lat. collecting trunk

Interiliac nodes

Ant. collecting trunk

Post. collecting trunk

Figure 7
LYMPHATIC DRAINAGE
OF THE CERVIX
The main lymphatic trunks and lymph
nodes of the uterine cervix are illustrated.
(Fig. 14-8 from Schmidt WA. Principles and
techniques of surgical pathology. Menlo Park,
CA: Addison-Wesley, 1983.)

nodes are related to the external iliac vessels, the internal iliac nodes to the internal iliac arteries, and the common iliac nodes to the common iliac arteries (7).

Colposcopic Features and Microscopic Anatomy. The bulk of the cervix is composed of fibromuscular tissue, of which fibrous tissue is the predominant component. The epithelium that lines the cervix is composed of three types: 1) native squamous epithelium, 2) glandular epithelium, and 3) metaplastic squamous epithelium. Early studies by Kaufmann and Ober (9) revealed that intraepithelial squamous lesions, i.e., dysplasia-carcinoma in situ, are almost always immediately above glandular epithelium, suggesting that neoplasia arises in squamous epithelium that is derived from glandular epithelium. The area of the cervix in which glandular epithelium undergoes metaplastic transformation to squamous epithelium is referred to as the *transformation zone*. An awareness of the colposcopic and microscopic features of both the metaplastic squamous epithelium and the transformation zone is important to appreciate the pathology of cervical neoplasia.

Squamous Epithelium

On colposcopic examination, the native squamous epithelium is smooth and pink; blood vessels are not clearly discernible. The epithelium proliferates, matures, and exfoliates under the influence of estrogenic stimulation. In contrast, progesterone inhibits maturation of squamous epithelium. Histologically, proliferation is limited to the basal and parabasal cells, which are oval with scant cytoplasm and are perpendicular to the basement membrane (fig. 8). Maturation occurs in the intermediate zone and is manifested by an increase in the amount of cytoplasm with accumulation of abundant glycogen, which is responsible for the clear vacuolated appearance of the cells in routine sections and for their uptake of iodine with the Schiller test. The superficial

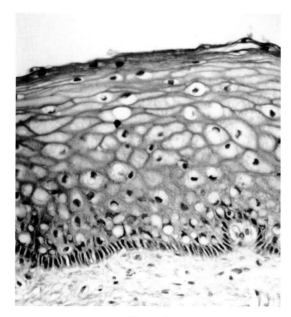

Figure 8
NATIVE SQUAMOUS EPITHELIUM
OF THE CERVIX
As illustrated in this figure, the epithelium is abundantly glycogenated. As cells approach the surface, their nuclei become progressively smaller and their cytoplasm becomes more abundant. Cells on the surface are flattened and contain eosinophilic cytoplasm.

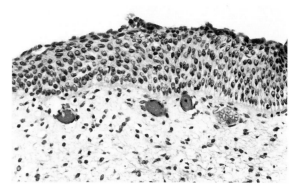

Figure 9
SQUAMOUS EPITHELIUM IN A CHILD
In this illustration, the epithelium is composed entirely of basal and parabasal cells showing no maturation.

layer contains terminally differentiated squamous cells that eventually exfoliate. These cells are flat and have abundant eosinophilic cytoplasm and pyknotic nuclei. The degree of maturation varies according to the hormonal status of the individual. In the premenarcheal girl and postmenopausal woman, the squamous epithelium undergoes little, if any, maturation and is composed almost entirely of basal and parabasal cells (fig. 9).

Endocervical Glandular Epithelium

The endocervical epithelium has been shown by three-dimensional studies to be not truly glandular but to consist of deep cleft-like infoldings of the surface epithelium into the underlying stroma (fig. 10) to a usual depth of approximately 5 mm (4). In cross section, the complex infoldings appear to be isolated glands. Colposcopic examination, after the application of 3 to 5 percent acetic acid, reveals that the glandular epithelium covers villous-like structures, each of which contains a central capillary (fig. 11). The villi are clustered together resembling

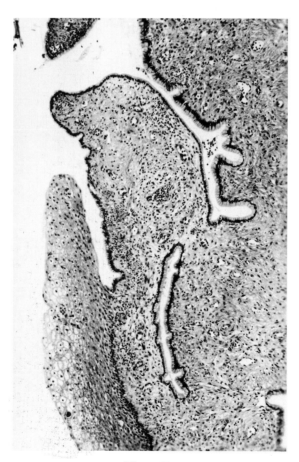

Figure 10
ENDOCERVICAL "GLANDS"
This figure illustrates cleft-like infoldings of the surface columnar epithelium extending into the underlying stroma.

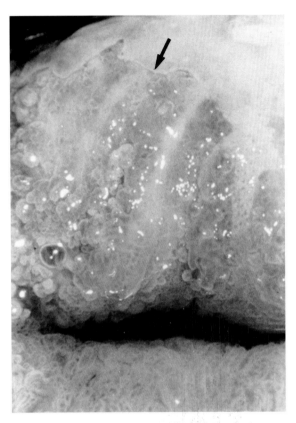

Figure 11
COLPOPHOTOGRAPH OF THE
TRANSFORMATION ZONE SHOWING
ENDOCERVICAL GLANDULAR EPITHELIUM
The upper lip of the cervix shows glandular epithelium composed of villous structures. Squamocolumnar junction is located on the ectocervix (arrow). (Courtesy of Dr. Duane Townsend, Sacramento, CA.)

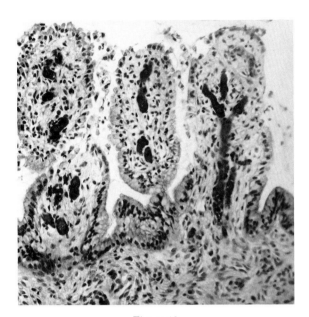

Figure 12
ENDOCERVICAL GLANDULAR EPITHELIUM
Villous structures are composed of fibrovascular cores lined by columnar mucinous epithelium.

a bunch of grapes. In 70 percent of sexually active women in the reproductive age group, the glandular epithelium extends onto the ectocervix (13). To the naked eye, the glandular epithelium appears red because of the rich subepithelial capillary network and consequently has been referred to as a cervical erosion. Because this appearance of the cervix is normal in the majority of women and is a manifestation of the normal transformation zone, the term *erosion* is erroneous. The designation *ectropion* is most widely used for this phenomenon.

Microscopically, the villous structures are rounded vascular stromal papillae lined by endocervical epithelium (fig. 12). The stroma of the papillae typically contains small numbers of chronic inflammatory cells, the presence of

which does not warrant a diagnosis of chronic cervicitis. In contrast, large numbers of lymphocytes, plasma cells, or aggregates of lymphocytes with follicular centers justify a diagnosis of chronic cervicitis. The glandular epithelium of the cervix is composed of a single layer of columnar cells with basal round to oval nuclei and finely granular cytoplasm containing abundant mucin. Argyrophilic cells can be detected in ectocervical epithelium in up to 50 percent of specimens examined. Some of the argyrophilic cells contain immunoreactive serotonin, whereas another fraction that does not display serotonin immunoreactivity is positive for chromogranin and epithelial membrane antigen (3). Mitotic activity is not observed in endocervical epithelial cells under normal circumstances, consistent with the view that these cells are derived from subcolumnar reserve cells (16).

Transformation Zone

The transformation zone is bounded by the original squamocolumnar junction and the border between the metaplastic squamous epithelium and the unaltered endocervical glandular epithelium, i.e., new squamocolumnar junction

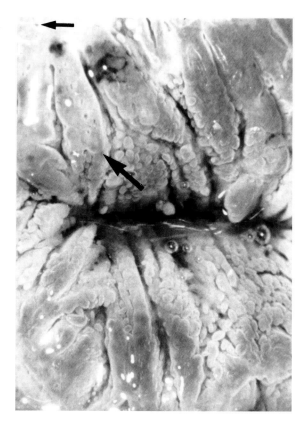

Figure 13
COLPOPHOTOGRAPH OF THE
TRANSFORMATION ZONE
The boundaries of the transformation zone are the original squamocolumnar junction identified by the most peripherally located residual gland opening (small arrow) and the border between the metaplastic squamous epithelium and the endocervical glandular epithelium (large arrow). (Courtesy of Dr. Duane Townsend, Sacramento, CA.)

(fig. 13). Although it was previously believed that the original squamocolumnar junction was at the external os, studies by Pixley (13) have shown that it is on the ectocervix in 70 percent of fetuses. The original squamocolumnar junction can be identified with the colposcope by the finding of residual gland openings surrounded by metaplastic squamous epithelium at the outer limit of the transformation zone (fig. 13). This site corresponds histologically to the most distal gland that is covered by squamous epithelium. The distal boundary of the transformation zone remains constant throughout life. In contrast, the boundary between the metaplastic squamous epithelium and the endocervical glandular epithelium

shifts. With the onset of puberty or in pregnancy, the cervix increases in volume, and the glandular epithelium is everted onto the ectocervix. After menopause, with reduction in the size of the cervix, the glandular epithelium retracts into the endocervical canal (fig. 14). Once metaplastic squamous epithelium develops, it is permanent and does not normally revert to glandular epithelium. Thus, over time, the amount of squamous epithelium increases. As it matures, metaplastic squamous epithelium becomes indistinguishable from the native squamous epithelium. Squamous metaplasia is most active during late fetal life, adolescence, and pregnancy.

The first stage of metaplasia that is recognizable with the colposcope is characterized by the development of a slightly opaque glaze over the grape-like villous structures. The tips of the villous structures fuse and then disappear as they become replaced by patches of smooth, slightly pink, metaplastic epithelium. After the application of acetic acid, the metaplastic epithelium appears white.

The initial stimulus for metaplasia is generally believed to be the lower (acid) pH of the vagina, which inactivates the buffering effect of the mucin that protects the columnar epithelium. Estrogen and progesterone may also play a role in this process.

The origin of the metaplastic squamous cells has been the subject of controversy for over 50 years. Recent immunohistochemical and two-dimensional gel electrophoresis studies have provided compelling evidence that they are derived from subcolumnar reserve cells (6,16). Using antibodies against a restricted group of cytokeratins that are consistently expressed in reserve cells, Weikel and colleagues (16) identified reserve cells in all 26 uteri that they studied. The reserve cells, which contained cytokeratins that are general markers of squamous epithelium, did not contain cytokeratins found in keratinizing squamous epithelium. In addition, subcolumnar reserve cells exhibited cytokeratins typically found in simple glandular epithelia, including endocervical epithelium. Vimentin was not identified in subcolumnar reserve cells precluding their derivation from stromal cells, as had been previously suggested. Thus, subcolumnar reserve cells appear to be facultative progenitor cells with the capacity to differentiate into either columnar or metaplastic squamous epithelium (figs. 15, 16).

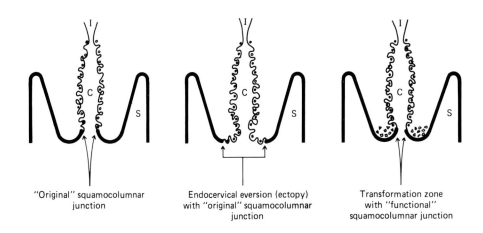

Figure 14
THREE TYPES OF SQUAMOCOLUMNAR JUNCTIONS
The portio is completely covered by native squamous epithelium, with the squamocolumnar junction at the external os (left). An ectropion has the squamocolumnar junction on the exocervix below the external os (middle). An ectropion covered by squamous epithelium forms the cervical transformation zone; the new or functional squamocolumnar junction of the transformation zone is at the external os (right). C = endocervical columnar epithelium; I = uterine isthmus; S = squamous epithelium. (Fig. 5.15 from Ferenczy A, Winkler B. Anatomy and histology of the cervix. In: Kurman RJ, ed. Blaustein's pathology of the female genital tract. 3rd ed. New York: Springer-Verlag, 1987.)

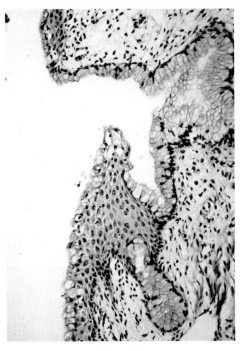

Figure 15
METAPLASTIC SQUAMOUS EPITHELIUM
Metaplastic squamous epithelium differentiates from reserve cells lifting off overlying endocervical columnar epithelium.

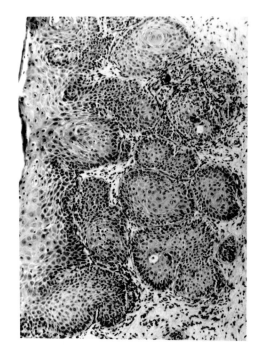

Figure 16
METAPLASTIC SQUAMOUS EPITHELIUM
The endocervical glands are completely replaced by metaplastic squamous epithelium.

VAGINA

Gross Anatomy. The vagina varies from 7 to 10 cm in length, opening into the vestibule and terminating in a circular fold around the cervix to form the vaginal fornices. The vagina lies ventral to the rectum and dorsal to the bladder, forming a 90° angle with the normal anteverted uterus so that the cervix is directly opposite the posterior wall of the vagina.

Lymphatic Drainage. The lymphatics of the vagina are closely related to those of the cervix and vulva. The superior groups of lymphatics follow the cervical vessels along the uterine artery, terminating in the external iliac lymph nodes. The middle groups, which drain most of the vagina, terminate in the hypogastric nodes. The inferior groups drain the area around the hymen and anastomose partly with the middle groups and partly with those of the vulva, terminating in the inguinal lymph nodes.

Microscopic Anatomy. The squamous epithelium of the vagina closely resembles that of the native squamous epithelium of the cervix (fig. 17); normally, keratinization does not occur. Unlike the cervix, the vagina contains no glands. Proliferation, maturation, and desquamation of the squamous epithelium are similar to those in the cervix and are influenced by estrogens and

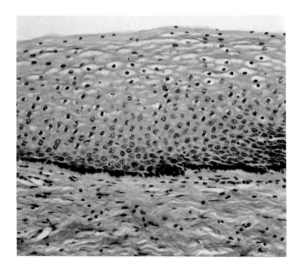

Figure 17
GLYCOGENATED SQUAMOUS EPITHELIUM
OF THE VAGINA
Glycogenated squamous epithelium of the vagina closely resembles that of the native squamous epithelium of the cervix.

progesterone. Thus, the thickness of the vaginal epithelium varies at different times during life. The hormonal status of an individual can be assessed by cytologic evaluation of exfoliated cells obtained from the lateral vaginal wall. This cellular analysis is referred to as the maturation index, in which the percentages of superficial, intermediate, and parabasal cells are recorded.

A 0.5 to 5 mm subepithelial stromal zone extends from the endocervix to the vulva (2). The stromal cells within this region are generally uniform with small spindle-shaped nuclei, but occasionally cells with bizarre nuclei, similar to those present in vaginal polyps with atypical stromal cells (pseudosarcoma botryoides), are found. It has been suggested that these polyps and sarcoma botryoides may originate in this inconspicuous stromal zone.

VULVA

Gross Anatomy. The vulva is delimited by the mons pubis anteriorly, the anus posteriorly, and the inguinal-gluteal folds laterally (fig. 18). The hymenal ring marks the medial aspect of the vulva. The major structures of the vulva include the labia majora and minora, the clitoris with its prepuce and frenulum, and the urethral meatus. The vulvar vestibule is defined as the portion of the vulva that extends from the most medial external edge of the hymenal ring laterally to the vestibular line of Hart on the medial aspects of the labia minora (fig. 19). Posteriorly, the vestibule extends to the perineal body and anteriorly, to the frenulum. Within the vestibule are the orifices of the major vestibular or Bartholin glands, as well as the urethra, the periurethral orifices of Skene glands, and the orifices of the minor vestibular glands (fig. 18).

Within the labia majora and prepuce, apocrine and sebaceous glands develop at the menarche lateral to the vestibular line of Hart (fig. 19). The labia minora are rich in blood vessels and elastic fibers but lack fat or smooth muscle, which are present in the labia majora. The epithelium of the labia minora is devoid of skin appendages or glands. Sebaceous and apocrine glands develop without hair follicles in the medial portions of the labia majora and become mixed with hair follicles in the lateral portions of the labia majora.

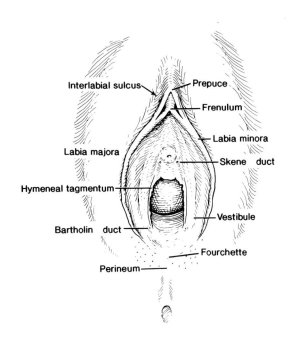

Figure 18
TOPOGRAPHY OF THE VULVA
The female external genitalia are identified in this schematic. (Fig. 1 from Wilkinson EJ, Hardt NS. Vulva. In: Sternberg SS, ed. Histology for pathologists. New York: Raven Press, 1992.)

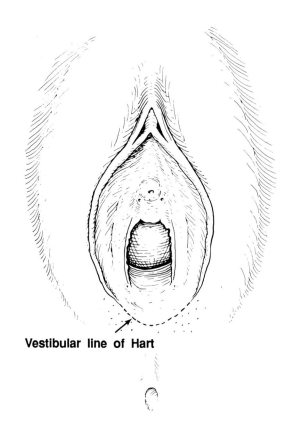

Vestibular line of Hart

Figure 19
VESTIBULAR LINE OF HART
The dotted line in this schematic defines the junction between the sebaceous gland–bearing area of the perineal body and the inferior labia majora. The lateral dark lines define the vestibular line of Hart as it extends up to the prepuce. Individual variations may occur. (Fig. 2 from Wilkinson EJ, Hardt NS. Vulva. In: Sternberg SS, ed. Histology for pathologists. New York: Raven Press, 1992.)

Lymphatic Drainage. The major lymphatic drainage of the vulva is to the femoral and inguinal lymph nodes. Lymphatic drainage from the anterior labia minora and clitoris is via channels that drain anteriorly and superiorly. These channels join the lymphatics draining the prepuce and labia majora, which then course laterally to the inguinal and femoral lymph nodes (12). The lymphatic drainage is predominantly ipsilateral, but contralateral drainage has been demonstrated in 67 percent of cases by Tc-colloid studies (8). The superficial inguinal lymph nodes receive most of the lymphatic drainage from the vulva and are the primary lymph nodes to be involved by metastatic tumor from the vulva. The superficial inguinal lymph nodes consist of 8 to 10 lymph nodes, which include superior and inferior node groups. The superior group is above the ligament of Poupart and the inferior group is between the ligament of Poupart and the junction of the saphenous vein and fascia lata.

Lymphatic drainage from both the clitoris and midline perineal area is bilateral (fig. 20). Additional lymphatic drainage from the clitoris is via the lymphatics draining the urethra and dorsal vein of the clitoris. This pathway proceeds inferiorly to the symphysis pubis through the anogenital diaphragm to join the lymphatic plexus of the anterior bladder surface, draining into the interiliac and obturator nodes, or superiorly to the femoral and internal iliac nodes (figs. 21, 22). A direct lymphatic pathway from the clitoris to the deep pelvic nodes has not been documented by in vivo colloid injection studies (8) nor have clitoral carcinomas been documented to metastasize directly to deep pelvic nodes. Like carcinomas of the vulva arising in other anterior sites, clitoral carcinomas metastasize first to superficial inguinal nodes.

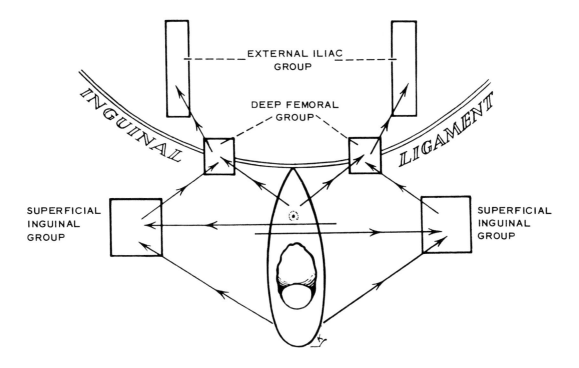

Figure 20
LYMPHATIC DRAINAGE OF THE VULVA
This schematic shows contralateral drainage due to anastomosis of lymphatic vessels across the midline. (Fig. 3 from Way S. The anatomy of the lymphatic drainage of the vulva and its influence on the radical operation for carcinoma. Ann R Coll Surg Engl 1948;3:189–209.)

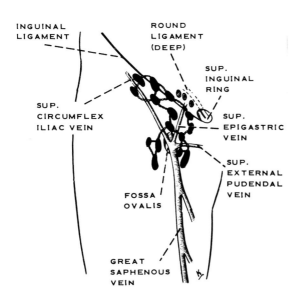

Figure 21
LYMPHATIC DRAINAGE OF THE VULVA
Lymphatic drainage of the clitoris is illustrated in this schematic. (Fig. 1 from Way S. The anatomy of the lymphatic drainage of the vulva and its influence on the radical operation for carcinoma. Ann R Coll Surg Engl 1948;3:189–209.)

Microscopic Anatomy. The vulva is covered by keratinized stratified squamous epithelium. The epithelium of the vestibule is rich in glycogen in women of reproductive age and is not keratinized. Keratinization is minimal on the frenulum, prepuce, and clitoris but progressively increases peripherally, blending with the more heavily keratinized skin of the fourchette, perineum, and surrounding skin. The stratum corneum of the glycogenated nonkeratinized areas permits transudation of fluid through the epithelium, adding to the secretion of the apocrine, eccrine, and sebaceous glands in these areas to provide a constantly moist environment. The nonkeratinized epithelium of the vestibule and vagina become rich in glycogen under the influence of estrogens.

The vestibular squamous epithelium merges with transitional-type epithelium at the tip of the urethra and at the orifices of Skene and Bartholin ducts. At the orifices of the minor vestibular glands, the transition is from stratified squamous

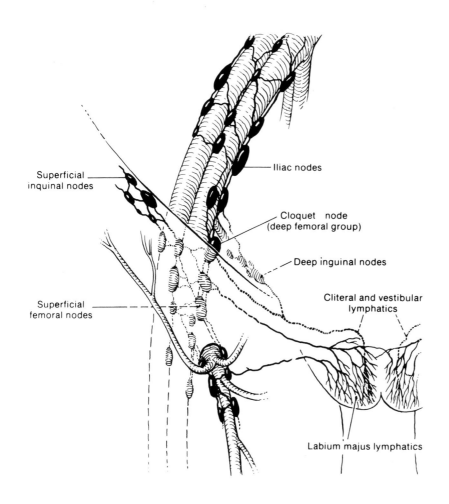

Superficial inquinal nodes

Iliac nodes

Cloquet node (deep femoral group)

Deep inguinal nodes

Cliteral and vestibular lymphatics

Superficial femoral nodes

Labium majus lymphatics

Figure 22
LYMPHATIC DRAINAGE
OF THE VULVA
This schematic illustrates a fine and diffuse network of lymphatics. (Fig. 14-4 from Schmidt WA. Principles and techniques of surgical pathology. Menlo Park, CA: Addison-Wesley, 1983.)

epithelium, to mucin-secreting columnar epithelium, with metaplastic squamous epithelium seen at the glandular-epithelial junction in adults (14).

Apocrine glands within the vulva, like the axillary apocrine glands, begin their secretory function at the menarche. The eccrine sweat glands, however, function throughout life. The paraurethral glands of Skene are distributed throughout the posterior and lateral aspects of the urethra and often have additional bilateral openings adjacent to and inferolateral to the external urethral orifice. These glands are lined by mucinous columnar epithelium.

The Bartholin glands are the major vestibular glands. They are tubuloalveolar glands with a racemose architecture. The acini are lined by simple columnar mucin-secreting epithelium. The duct is approximately 2.5 cm in length and

is lined predominantly by transitional epithelium. Near the glandular junction, the duct has mucin-secreting epithelium. The Bartholin ducts enter the vestibule bilaterally, posterolateral to the hymen.

The minor vestibular glands are simple glands lined by mucin-secreting epithelium. They are found around the urethral meatus, throughout the vestibule, and within the proximal portions of the frenulum.

The clitoris is composed predominantly of erectile tissue that is contiguous with the bilateral conjoined corpora cavernosa. The latter branch at the base of the clitoris and extend inferiorly adjacent to the pubic rami. The ischiocavernosus muscles are contained within the insertion of the crura of the corpora cavernosa. These structures, with suspensory ligaments that are found bilaterally and dorsally, provide the anatomic support for the clitoris.

REFERENCES

1. Dickinson RL. Human sex anatomy. 2nd ed. Baltimore: Williams & Wilkins, 1949.
2. Elliott GB, Elliott JD. Superficial stromal reactions of lower genital tract. Arch Pathol 1973;95:100–1.
3. Fetissof F, Serres G, Arbeille B, de Muret A, Sam-Giao M, Lansac J. Argyrophilic cells and ectocervical epithelium. Int J Gynecol Pathol 1991;10:177–90.
4. Fluhmann CF. The cervix uteri and its diseases. Philadelphia: WB Saunders, 1961:30-102.
5. Friedrich EG. Vulvar disease. 2nd ed. Philadelphia: WB Saunders, 1983. (Friedman EA, ed. Major problems in obstetrics and gynecology, Vol 9.)
6. Gigi-Leitner O, Geiger B, Levy R, Czernobilsky B. Cytokeratin expression in squamous metaplasia of the human uterine cervix. Differentiation 1986;31:191–205.
7. Gustafson RC. The vascular, lymphatic, and neural anatomy of the cervix. In: Jordan J, Singer A, eds. The cervix. London: WB Saunders, 1976:51-60.
8. Iversen T, Aas M. Lymph drainage from the vulva. Gynecol Oncol 1983;16:179–89.
9. Kaufmann C, Ober KG. The morphological changes of the cervix uteri with age and their significance in the early diagnosis of cancer. In: Wolstenholme GEW, O'Connor M, eds. Cancer of the cervix: diagnosis of early forms. London: Churchill, 1959:61. (Wolstenholme GEW, O'Connor CM, eds. Ciba Foundation Study Groups, no 3.)
10. Krantz KE. The gross and microscopic anatomy of the human vagina. Ann NY Acad Sci 1959;83:89–104.
11. . The anatomy of the human cervix, gross and microscopic. In: Blandau RJ, Moghissi K, eds. The biology of the cervix. Chicago: The University of Chicago Press, 1973:57–69.
12. Parry-Jones E. Lymphatics of the vulva. J Obstet Gynaecol Br Commonw 1963;70:751–65.
13. Pixley E. Morphology of the fetal and prepubertal cervicovaginal epithelium. In: Jordan J, Singer A, eds. The cervix. London: WB Saunders, 1976:75–87.
14. Pyka RE, Wilkinson EJ, Friedrich EG Jr, Croker BP. The histopathology of vulvar vestibulitis syndrome. Int J Gynecol Pathol 1988;7:249–57.
15. Schneppenheim P, Hamperl H, Kaufmann C, Ober KG. Die beziehungen des schleimepithels zum plattenepithel an der cervix uteri im lebenslauf der frau. Arch Gynae Kol 1958;190:303–45.
16. Weikel W, Wagner R, Moll R. Characterization of subcolumnar reserve cells and other epithelia of human uterine cervix. Demonstration of diverse cytokeratin polypeptides in reserve cells. Virchows Arch [Cell Pathol] 1987;54:98–110.

❖❖❖

HUMAN PAPILLOMAVIRUSES
AND CANCER OF THE LOWER FEMALE GENITAL TRACT

Human papillomaviruses (HPVs) have been identified in preinvasive and invasive lesions of the cervix, vagina, and vulva. The number of vaginal and vulvar cases that have been reported have been relatively small in comparison with cervical cases. This chapter focuses mainly on the relationship of HPV to cervical neoplasia; pertinent studies relating to vaginal and vulvar neoplasia are discussed briefly.

Based on epidemiologic studies, cervical cancer has been strongly linked to a sexually transmitted agent for over 100 years. A number of agents have been implicated, and in the 1960s and 1970s, attention was focused on herpes simplex virus 2 (HSV 2) based on retrospective seroepidemiologic studies showing that the prevalence of elevated antibodies to HSV 2 was higher in patients with cervical intraepithelial neoplasia (CIN) and invasive cancer than in controls. In a prospective study involving more than 10,000 women, however, the prevalence of elevated HSV antibodies in patients with CIN 2, CIN 3, and invasive cancer was similar to that of matched controls (60). This report minimizes the possible role of HSV 2 as a causative agent in cervical cancer, although it is still possible that it is a cofactor.

In the late 1970s, attention shifted to HPV, which until then had only been associated with the development of venereal warts. Although "warty" changes were identified in cervical smears from patients with cervical dysplasia and invasive cancer more than 30 years ago (25), the role of HPV in cervical neoplasia was not appreciated because of the inability to propagate HPV in tissue culture and lack of a suitable animal model. HPV was implicated in the genesis of these diseases only after the technologic advances in molecular biology and immunocytochemistry. Subsequently, our understanding of the biologic and pathologic characteristics of HPV infection has advanced so rapidly that a comprehensive review of the subject is beyond the scope of this text. For a more detailed discussion, the reader is referred to several reviews (1,6,23,32,43,49,54).

CLASSIFICATION, PROPERTIES, AND GENOMIC ORGANIZATION

Papillomavirus particles are nonenveloped and about 55 nm in diameter according to electron-microscopic measurements. The particles have an icosahedral symmetry with 72 capsomers. The viral capsid is composed of a major capsid protein with a molecular weight of about 54,000 and a minor species with a molecular weight of about 76,000. The major protein accounts for about 80 percent of the total viral protein. The viral genome exists as a double-stranded superhelical DNA molecule of approximately 8000 base pairs enclosed within the capsid.

Within a specific species, papillomaviruses are classified by DNA hybridization according to nucleotide sequence homology; for classification as a different type, there must be less than 50 percent DNA homology when tested under stringent conditions. Currently, serology plays no role in the taxonomic classification of the papillomaviruses. To date, more than 60 HPV types have been characterized, and new types continue to be identified.

The double-stranded circular DNA genomes of a number of papillomaviruses from different species have been sequenced in their entirety revealing a well-conserved genomic organization (fig. 23). The DNA sequences coding all the putative proteins are termed *open reading frames* and are located on only one DNA strand. A noncoding region also termed the *upstream regulatory region* or *long control region* is located on the same DNA strand and contains promoters for mRNA synthesis, transcriptional enhancer sequences, and the origin of DNA replication. The open reading frames are referred to as "early" or "late" by analogy with SV40 and polyoma viruses, in which particular genes become expressed in a specific chronologic sequence during the course of productive infection. The early gene products are involved in the control of viral DNA replication and viral gene expression, and individual early genes have been shown to play a role in transformation of tissue culture cell lines in

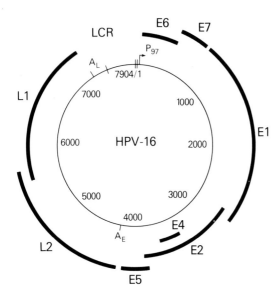

Figure 23
GENOMIC ORGANIZATION
In this genomic map of HPV 16 deduced from the DNA sequence, the nucleotide numbers are noted within the circular maps, transcription proceeds clockwise, and the major open reading frames (E1–E7, L1, and L2) are indicated. The only transcriptional promoter mapped to date for HPV 16 is designated (P_{97}). A_E and A_L represent the putative polyadenylation signals for the early and late transcripts, respectively. The viral long control region (LCR) containing the putative viral transcriptional and replication regulatory elements is noted. (Fig. 1 from Howley PM, Schlegel R. The human papillomaviruses. An overview. Am J Med 1988;85(Suppl 2A):155–8.)

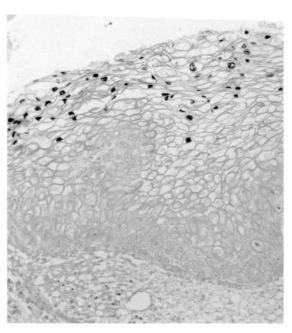

Figure 24
CAPSID PROTEIN DETECTION BY
IMMUNOHISTOCHEMISTRY
This case of CIN 1 illustrates the localization of HPV capsid antigen by immunoperoxidase in superficial and occasional intermediate cells.

the laboratory. The late genes are expressed in the final phase of infection, in accordance with their role in directing the synthesis of structural proteins involved in the assembly of viral particles, i.e., productive infection.

METHODS OF VIRAL DETECTION

Papillomavirus infection of the cervix, vagina, and vulva is associated with characteristic cellular changes in squamous epithelium, referred to as *koilocytosis* or *koilocytotic atypia*. These changes are described in detail in the section on squamous intraepithelial lesions in the chapter Tumors of the Cervix. The cellular changes, however, do not permit specific identification of the virus. Papillomaviruses can be detected in exfoliated cells or tissue biopsy specimens by electron microscopy, but specific detection depends on immunocytochemical or molecular virologic analysis (nucleic acid hybridization).

Ultrastructural analysis reveals that HPV virions are intranuclear (22) and usually in a crystalline array but occasionally associated with filaments. Viral particles are detected in only a small proportion of what are typical HPV-related lesions by light microscopy. Electron microscopy has limited value for the diagnosis of HPV because the technique is laborious and subject to considerable sampling error (15).

Papillomaviruses from diverse species have cross-reactive internal capsid antigens that can be detected with the use of antisera prepared from disrupted papillomavirus (24). With these reagents, HPV structural proteins have been detected in 50 percent of typical condylomata acuminata (30) and approximately 30 percent of preinvasive cervical lesions (figs. 24, 25) (28,30,63). This technique is relatively insensitive compared with nucleic acid hybridization tests and therefore of limited value in diagnostic surgical pathology (27). In the future, antibodies prepared to synthetic peptides or bacterial fusion

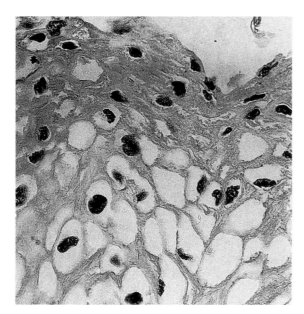

Figure 25
CAPSID PROTEIN DETECTION BY
IMMUNOHISTOCHEMISTRY

High magnification demonstrates that many of the cells in which capsid protein is localized by the immunoperoxidase method are koilocytes and flattened cells near the surface. Note the nuclear enlargement and wrinkling of the nuclear membrane. (Fig. 3 from Kurman RJ, Jenson AB, Lancaster WD. Papillomavirus infection of the cervix. II. Relationship to intraepithelial neoplasia based on the presence of specific viral structural proteins. Am J Surg Pathol 1983;7:39–52.)

proteins corresponding to the early HPV proteins may prove to be useful as diagnostic reagents.

Nucleic acid hybridization analysis for DNA is referred to as Southern blot hybridization and is a highly sensitive specific procedure that is currently considered "the gold standard" for the identification of HPV in exfoliated cells or tissue biopsy specimens (fig. 26). Nucleic acid hybridization is the association of complementary single strands of DNA or RNA to form a stable duplex, i.e., a hybrid. Duplex formation is influenced by various factors including temperature, pH, and cation concentration. By varying these factors, the hybridization reaction can be performed under stringent or relaxed conditions (fig. 27). High stringency conditions are used to characterize different HPV types, whereas low stringency conditions are performed at lower temperatures and are used to detect HPV spe-

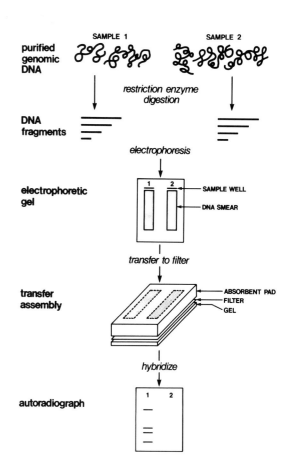

Figure 26
HPV DETECTION BY SOUTHERN BLOT ANALYSIS

Samples 1 and 2 represent high–molecular-weight DNAs purified from biopsies of two cervical lesions. The samples are cut into small fragments by restriction enzyme digestion (*Pst* I in this example) and loaded into the wells of an electrophoretic gel. An electric field is applied and the DNA fragments migrate into the gel, eventually separating according to size, with the smallest fragments at the bottom. The DNA fragments are transferred from the gel onto a filter, hybridized with ^{32}P-labeled probes (HPV 16), washed, and exposed to X-ray film. The autoradiograph at the bottom of this figure demonstrates that sample 1 contains HPV 16 DNA and exhibits the expected banding pattern produced by *Pst* I. Sample 2 does not contain HPV 16 DNA. (Fig. 4 from Lörincz AT. Detection of human papillomavirus infection by nucleic acid hybridization. Obstet Gynecol Clin North Am 1987;14:451–69.)

cific sequences of unknown type. Although a number of different methods to detect HPV nucleic acids are available, Southern blot, dot blot, in situ hybridization (fig. 28), and the polymerase chain reaction have the greatest clinical utility (33,46). The polymerase chain reaction is

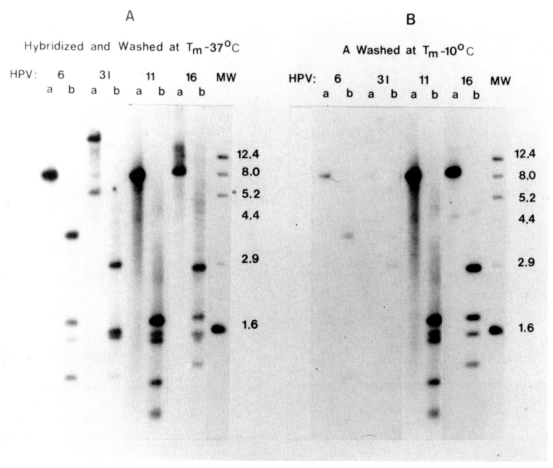

Figure 27
SOUTHERN BLOT ANALYSIS OF FOUR ANOGENITAL LESIONS
The types of HPV DNAs detected are indicated at the top of each pair of lanes: HPV 6 and HPV 11 (from two different condylomata acuminata), HPV 31 (from a mild dysplasia), and HPV 16 (from an invasive cervical carcinoma). Each sample was digested with *Bam* HI (lane a) and *Pst* I (lane b). Lane MW contains selected fragments of various HPV and pBR322 as molecular weight markers. The autoradiograph (5 days at -70°C) on the left (A) is a Southern blot hybridization at low stringency (melting temperature [Tm] -37°C) to a probe mixture of HPV 11 and HPV 16 that was washed at Tm -37°C. The same filter as shown in panel A is illustrated in panel B after a wash at high stringency (Tm -10°C). It demonstrates, as expected, a significantly greater loss of signal in lanes containing HPV 6 or HPV 31 than in lanes with HPV 11 or HPV 16, which are homologous to the probes. The probes used in this experiment were labeled with ^{32}P and had greater than 2 x 10^8 dpm/µg of DNA. (Fig. 1 from Lorincz AT, Lancaster WD, Temple GF. Cloning and characterization of the DNA of a new human papillomavirus from a woman with dysplasia of the uterine cervix. J Virol 1986;58:225–9.)

an enzymatic technique that amplifies specific target DNA sequences in the test sample to a level that permits detection by either dot blot or Southern blot hybridization. The polymerase chain reaction can amplify the target sequences at least a millionfold and has been applied to formalin-fixed paraffin-embedded tissue, thereby making it the most sensitive technique currently available (50).

HPV LIFE CYCLE

The HPV life cycle is tightly linked to squamous cell differentiation. HPV infection of the cervix is venereally transmitted and over 20 different types have been reported to preferentially infect the metaplastic squamous epithelium of the cervix. Infection begins in the basal cells and can remain dormant, i.e., so-called latent infection. At this

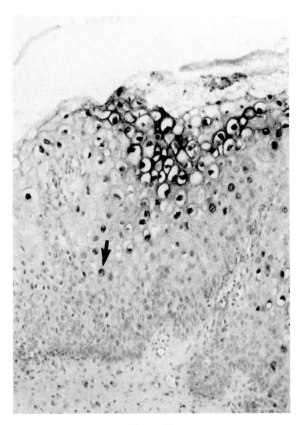

Figure 28
HPV 18 DNA DETECTED WITH
BIOTINYLATED PROBES IN A CIN 1 LESION
Although positive nuclei are clearly present in the intermediate layer (arrow), most of the positive signal is in koilocytotic cells on the surface.

stage, viral DNA can be detected by Southern blot hybridization in morphologically normal-appearing metaplastic squamous epithelium (16,36). Depending on a number of poorly understood factors, the infection may remain latent or become productive. Productive infection, resulting in the release of infectious virus, occurs in terminally differentiated squamous epithelium. Morphologically, this is manifested by a mild degree of proliferation of the basal cells and koilocytosis, i.e., a CIN 1 lesion. Koilocytosis appears to be related to expression of the viral E4 protein which disrupts the intracellular cytokeratin matrix thereby facilitating release of viral particles (11a). At this stage, viral DNA (fig. 28) and capsid protein (see figs. 24, 25) can be detected by immunohistochemistry, and viral particles can be detected by electron microscopy

in 30 to 50 percent of cases. The distribution of HPV types in CIN 1 is similar to that found in histologically normal metaplastic squamous epithelium. Whereas the prevalence of HPV DNA detection is 10 percent in normal epithelium, it is approximately 75 percent in CIN 1. In CIN 2 and 3, the prevalence of viral DNA detection is 90 percent, but viral capsid antigen and viral particles are infrequently detected, indicating a lack of productive infection. Proliferation of parabasal cells, which is a feature of CIN 2 and 3, may reflect a process of immortalization induced by HPV. HPV 16 accounts for nearly half of the viral isolates in these high-grade lesions. This more homogeneous distribution of HPVs is similar to that of invasive squamous carcinoma and differs from the heterogeneous distribution in CIN 1. HPV DNA is rarely integrated in CIN but occurs in the majority of invasive carcinomas (10), suggesting that integration may play a role in the transition from an intraepithelial to an invasive neoplasm. A hypothetical model illustrating the relationship of HPV infection to cervical neoplasia is shown in figure 29.

EVIDENCE ASSOCIATING HPV WITH NEOPLASIA

Abundant evidence in recent years has implicated HPV in the genesis of cervical neoplasia. Among the most compelling data is the detection of HPV nucleotide sequences by Southern blot hybridization in approximately 90 percent of preinvasive (fig. 28) and invasive carcinomas of the cervix (18–20,35). HPV DNA can be detected in approximately 10 percent of morphologically normal-appearing squamous epithelium of the cervix and has been detected in lymph nodes containing metastatic carcinoma. The HPV type present in the lymph nodes corresponds to that found in the primary carcinomas (31). Besides HPV DNA, mRNA usually from the E6-E7 region has been consistently found in both cervical carcinoma cell lines, such as HeLa, CaSki, and SiHa, and biopsy specimens of cervical carcinomas, indicating that the virus is being actively transcribed (48,52). Further evidence supporting a causal relationship between HPV infection and cervical neoplasia is demonstrated by the development of a lesion resembling mild dysplasia when cervical epithelium inoculated with

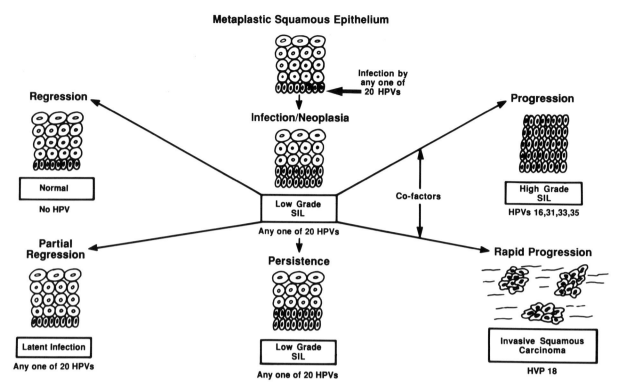

Figure 29
HYPOTHETICAL MODEL ILLUSTRATING THE RELATIONSHIP OF
HPV INFECTION TO CERVICAL NEOPLASIA

HPV infection begins in the basal cells of the metaplastic squamous epithelium. Morphologic expression of HPV infection is manifested by a low-grade squamous intraepithelial lesion (SIL) corresponding to cervical intraepithelial neoplasia (CIN) 1. If this lesion regresses completely, there is no morphologic abnormality, and DNA is not detected by Southern blot hybridization. If partial regression occurs, HPV DNA is detectable in morphologically normal epithelium, or the lesion may persist. Note that cofactors, as yet not specifically identified, are necessary for infection to progress to neoplasia. Progression to a high-grade lesion is associated most often with HPV 16, whereas rapid progression to an invasive carcinoma may be associated with HPV 18. Rapidly progressive lesions may have a rapid transit time through CIN 2 or 3 or could perhaps evolve directly into an invasive neoplasm by passing the high-grade preinvasive stage. (Fig. 11 from Ambros RA, Kurman RJ. Current concepts in the relationship of human papillomavirus infection to the pathogenesis and classification of precancerous squamous lesions of the uterine cervix. Semin Diagn Pathol 1990;7:158–72.)

HPV is grafted beneath the renal capsule of athymic mice (26). Finally, in large population-based case-controlled studies in Latin America comparing women with cervical cancer to randomly selected age-matched controls, the relative risk of cancer for women with HPV ranged up to 146 (38a,42). Relative risks of this magnitude are extremely rare in cancer epidemiology.

Besides the close association of HPV with neoplasia of the lower genital tract, there is convincing evidence from laboratory studies indicating that certain HPVs play a role in malignant transformation. Some HPV types, notably HPV 16 and HPV 18, have the ability to "transform" immortalized mouse cell lines standardly used in the laboratory, such as C127 or NIH 3T3 cells (4). The transformed cells demonstrate characteristics of a malignant phenotype such as increased saturation density, anchorage-independent growth, and tumorigenicity in athymic mice (64). In addition, it has been shown that human keratinocytes can be maintained indefinitely in vitro when transfected with the E6 and E7 genes of HPVs 16, 18, 31, and 33 but not HPVs 6 and 11. This process is referred to as *immortalization*, but these cells are not tumorigenic in nude mice and additional genetic events are required for the progression to an invasive cancer (12,21,38,41,45). Studies suggest that additional genetic events may involve the inactivation of certain cellular suppressor genes, specifically p53 and the retinoblastoma genes by the virus (14,61). These suppressor genes are thought to normally encode proteins that regulate cell growth, and therefore inactivation of these genes by the virus may therefore lead to a selective growth advantage. These data support the view that malignant transformation may be due to an inhibition of host cell control that is mediated by viral expression.

Other epidemiologic factors have also been associated with cervical cancer. For example, smoking has been associated with invasive cancer and high grade CIN but not with low grade CIN. This suggests that other factors together with particular types of HPV are involved in malignant transformation (65).

DISTRIBUTION OF HPV IN CERVICAL NEOPLASMS

HPV DNA can be detected in approximately 90 percent of invasive squamous carcinomas of the cervix (34,35). Based on the associations between specific HPV types and different grades of CIN and invasive squamous carcinoma, various HPVs can be grouped into four categories: 1) a low-risk group (HPVs 6/11, 42–44) associated principally with CIN 1 but absent from invasive carcinoma; 2) an intermediate-risk group (HPVs 31, 33, 35, 51, 52, and 58) detected principally in CIN and in a small portion of invasive carcinomas; 3) a high-risk/HPV 16 group detected equally in both CIN 2 and 3 and carcinomas; and 4) a high-risk/HPV 18 group (HPVs 18, 45, and 56) detected much more frequently in invasive carcinoma than in CIN (34).

HPVs 16 and 18 are found in approximately 70 percent of invasive squamous carcinomas, and a variety of other HPVs, including 31, 33, 35, 51, 52, and 58, account for the remainder (5,13,18,34,35). A pathologic and molecular study demonstrated further correlation between HPV type and patterns of neoplastic differentiation. Keratinizing squamous cell carcinoma is strongly associated with HPV 16 compared with nonkeratinizing squamous cell carcinoma (62), and HPV 18 is more often associated with poorly differentiated carcinomas and more frequent lymph node involvement than HPV 16–associated tumors (3). Adenocarcinomas, adenosquamous carcinomas, and small cell carci-

nomas contain a preponderance of HPV 18, although HPV 16 is also found (2,35,51,53). An in situ hybridization study demonstrated HPV 18 in adenocarcinoma of the cervix and in the adjacent invasive adenocarcinoma, providing further evidence that adenocarcinoma in situ is a precursor of invasive adenocarcinoma (56).

DISTRIBUTION OF HPV IN VAGINAL AND VULVAR NEOPLASMS

Multifocal sites of infection involving the vulva and vagina have been reported to occur in up to 70 percent of women with cervical abnormalities, and HPV DNA can be detected in the vast majority of these lesions (47). Typically, the same HPV type is present in cervical, vulvar, and vaginal lesions, but discordance may occur. In less than 10 percent of cases, more than one HPV type can be detected within the same lesion.

Typical exophytic vulvar and vaginal condylomata acuminata contain HPV 6 and 11 in approximately 80 to 90 percent of cases. In contrast, HPV DNA, nearly always type 16, has been reported in 60 to 90 percent of in situ carcinoma of the vagina and vulva (fig. 30) (7,40,54,58). The wide variety of HPVs found in preinvasive cervical lesions has not been observed in the vulvar intraepithelial lesions. In contrast, HPV, almost always HPV 16, has been found in only 20 to 40 percent of invasive vulvar carcinomas (9,11,59) and in 20 percent of vaginal squamous cell carcinomas (39). The prevalence of HPV in these tumors is substantially lower than the 90 percent detection rate in invasive squamous cell carcinoma of the cervix. A large proportion of invasive vulvar squamous carcinomas occurring in older women do not contain HPV and are not associated with vulvar intraepithelial neoplasia. On the other hand, invasive vulvar carcinoma in younger women is frequently associated with HPV and vulvar intraepithelial neoplasia (57). The histologic features of the HPV-associated and non–HPV-associated carcinomas also differ (see Tumors of the Vulva). These findings suggest that HPV is an etiologic factor for certain types of invasive vulvar cancer in young women but that other factors besides HPV are involved in squamous carcinoma of the vulva in older women (17,57).

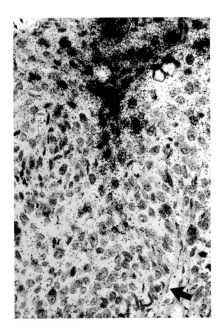

Figure 30

HPV DETECTION BY IN SITU HYBRIDIZATION

HPV 16 viral transcripts are present throughout the thickness of the epithelium in this vulvar intraepithelial lesion (VIN) 3. Although there is a high-intensity signal localized over nuclei clustered near the surface (small arrows, upper left) and in the center of the field, a positive signal is present even in cells lined just above the basement membrane (large arrow) (in situ hybridization with ^{35}S-labeled single-stranded anti-sense HPV 16 RNA probe). (Fig. 4 from Park JS, Jones RW, McLean MR, et al. Possible etiologic heterogeneity of vulvar intraepithelial neoplasia. A correlation of pathologic characteristics with human papillomavirus detection by in situ hybridization and polymerase chain reaction. Cancer 1991;67:1599–607.)

NATURAL HISTORY OF HPV INFECTION OF THE CERVIX

Currently available data on the behavior of HPV infection of the cervix are based on either retrospective studies or small prospective studies with short follow-up and should, therefore, be interpreted cautiously. In a retrospective study, Meisels and colleagues (37) reported that 9 percent of atypical flat condylomas, which correspond to moderate to severe dysplasia, progressed to carcinoma in situ or microinvasive carcinoma. Similar findings were reported by Syrjänen and colleagues (55), who found, in a prospective study, that 10 to 15 percent of HPV-related mild dysplasia progressed to higher grades of dysplasia, whereas the vast majority

persisted or regressed over a follow-up period of approximately 2 years. The authors concluded that the natural history of HPV infection of the cervix was the same as that of CIN.

Preliminary data suggest that specific HPV types play a role in the behavior of cervical neoplasia. In a prospective study of 100 patients with CIN 1, Campion and associates (8) found that 85 percent of lesions that progressed to CIN 3 contained HPV 16, whereas only 4 percent contained HPV 6. Preliminary findings from a prospective study of HPV infection in a cohort of 18,000 cytologically normal women showed that 19 women developed CIN 1 and two women developed CIN 2 or 3 over a 1-year period. Fifty-two percent of these cases of CIN contained HPV DNA in cervical lavage specimens detected by polymerase chain reaction at the time of enrollment in the study, compared to 16 percent of controls (44). These findings indicate that detection of HPV DNA in cytologically normal squamous epithelium is associated with an elevated risk for subsequent cytologic diagnosis of CIN. This study also analyzed the prevalence of HPV in women with CIN compared with those who were cytologically normal at the time of diagnosis. As estimated by the univariate odds ratio, HPV 16/18 detection was associated with a 40-fold increase in risk of CIN 1 and over a 100-fold increase in risk of prevalent CIN 2 or 3 (44). In addition, this study demonstrated that controlling for HPV infection explained most of the established epidemiologic risk factors for CIN, thus providing compelling evidence that HPV infection causes CIN. In another study, a cross-sectional analysis of 214 women showed that HPV 16 was found in 41 percent of squamous carcinoma and 37 percent of CIN, whereas HPV 18 was found in 22 percent of squamous carcinoma but only 3 percent of CIN. It was suggested that the infrequent finding of HPV 18 in CIN compared with invasive carcinoma could represent a rapid transit time of HPV 18–associated lesions through the precursor stage (29). These data, in conjunction with the reports of HPV 18 in small cell carcinomas of the cervix and the higher rate of lymph node metastasis in invasive cervical cancers containing HPV 18, suggest that tumors containing HPV 18 may be more virulent (2,3). Although HPV typing is not recommended in the routine screening or clinical management of patients at the time of this writing, these various studies strongly suggest that HPV typing will be of value in the future.

REFERENCES

1. Ambros RA, Kurman RJ. Current concepts in the relationship of human papillomavirus infection to the pathogenesis and classification of precancerous squamous lesions of the uterine cervix. Semin Diagn Pathol 1990;7:158–72.

2. _____, Park JS, Shah KV, Kurman RJ. Evaluation of histologic, morphometric, and immunohistochemical criteria in the differential diagnosis of small cell carcinomas of the cervix with particular reference to human papillomavirus types 16 and 18. Mod Pathol 1991;4:586–93.

3. Barnes W, Delgado G, Kurman RJ, et al. Possible prognostic significance of human papillomavirus type in cervical cancer. Gynecol Oncol 1988;29:267–73.

4. Bedell MA, Jones KH, Laimins LA. The E6-E7 region of human papillomavirus type 18 is sufficient for transformation of NIH 3T3 cells and rat-1 cells. J Virol 1987;61:3635–40.

5. Boshart M, Gissmann L, Ikenberg H, Kleinheinz A, Scheurlen W, zur Hausen H. A new type of papillomavirus DNA, its presence in genital cancer biopsies and in cell lines derived from cervical cancer. EMBO J 1984;3:1151–7.

6. Broker TR, Botchan M. Papillomaviruses: retrospectives and prospectives. In: Botchan M, Grodzicker T, Sharp PA, eds. DNA tumor viruses: control of gene expression and replication. Cancer cells 4. Cold Spring Harbor, NY: Cold Spring Harbor Laboratory, 1986:17–36.

7. Buscema J, Naghashfar Z, Sawada E, Daniel R, Woodruff JD, Shah K. The predominance of human papillomavirus type 16 in vulvar neoplasia. Obstet Gynecol 1988;71:601–6.

8. Campion MJ, McCance DJ, Cuzick J, Singer A. Progressive potential of mild cervical atypia: prospective, cytological, colposcopic, and virologic study. Lancet 1986;2:237–40.

9. Carson LF, Twiggs LB, Okagaki T, Clark BA, Ostrow RS, Faras AJ. Human papillomavirus DNA in adenosquamous carcinoma and squamous cell carcinoma of the vulva. Obstet Gynecol 1988;72:63–7.

10. Cullen AP, Reid R, Campion M, Lörincz AT. Analysis of the physical state of different human papillomavirus DNAs in intraepithelial and invasive cervical neoplasm. J Virol 1991;65:606–12.

11. Di Luca D, Pilotti S, Stefanon B, et al. Human papillomavirus type 16 DNA in genital tumours: a pathological and molecular analysis. J Gen Virol 1986;67:583–9.

11a. Doorbar J, Ely S, Sterling J, McClean C, Crawford L. Specific interaction between HPV-16 E1–E4 and cytokeratins results in collapse of the epithelial cell intermediate filament network. Nature 1991;352:824–7.

12. Dürst M, Dzarlieva-Petrusevska RT, Boukamp P, Fusenig NE, Gissmann L. Molecular and cytogenetic analysis of immortalized human primary keratinocytes obtained after transfection with human papillomavirus type 16 DNA. Oncogene 1987;1:251–6.

13. _____, Gissmann L, Ikenberg H, zur Hausen H. A papillomavirus DNA from a cervical carcinoma and its prevalence in cancer biopsy samples from different geographic regions. Proc Natl Acad Sci USA 1983;80:3812–5.

14. Dyson N, Howley PM, Münger K, Harlow E. The human papilloma virus-16 E7 oncoprotein is able to bind to the retinoblastoma gene product. Science 1989;243:934–7.

15. Ferenczy A, Braun L, Shah KV. Human papillomavirus (HPV) in condylomatous lesions of cervix. Am J Surg Pathol 1981;5:661–70.

16. _____, Mitao M, Nagai N, Silverstein SJ, Crum CP. Latent papillomavirus and recurring genital warts. N Engl J Med 1985;313:784–8.

17. Franquemont DW, Anderson WA, Williams J, Taylor PT, Crum CP. Vulvar carcinoma: two separate etiologies? [Abstract]. Lab Invest 1991;64:57A.

18. Fuchs PG, Girardi F, Pfister H. Human papillomavirus DNA in normal, metaplastic, preneoplastic and neoplastic epithelia of the cervix uteri. Int J Cancer 1988;41:41–5.

19. Gissmann L, deVilliers EM, zur Hausen H. Analysis of human genital warts (condylomata acuminata) and other genital tumors for human papillomavirus type 6 DNA. Int J Cancer 1982;29:143–6.

20. _____, Wolnik L, Ikenberg H, Koldovsky U, Schnürch HG, zur Hausen H. Human papillomavirus types 6 and 11 DNA sequences in genital and laryngeal papillomas and in some cervical cancers. Proc Natl Acad Sci USA 1983;80:560–3.

21. Hawley-Nelson P, Vousden KH, Hubbert NL, Lowy DR, Schiller JT. HPV 16 E6 and E7 proteins cooperate to immortalize human foreskin keratinocytes. EMBO J 1989;8:3905–10.

22. Hills E, Laverty CR. Electron microscopic detection of papilloma virus particles in selected koilocytotic cells in a routine cervical smear. Acta Cytol 1979;23:53–6.

23. Howley PM. The role of papillomaviruses in human cancer. Important Adv Oncol 1987;55–73.

24. Jenson AB, Rosenthal JD, Olson C, Pass F, Lancaster WD, Shah K. Immunologic relatedness of papillomaviruses from different species. J Natl Cancer Inst 1980;64:495–500.

25. Koss LG, Durfee GR. Unusual patterns of squamous epithelium of the uterine cervix: cytologic and pathologic study of koilocytotic atypia. Ann NY Acad Sci 1956; 63:1245–61.

26. Kreider JW, Howett MK, Wolfe SA, et al. Morphological transformation in vivo of human uterine cervix with papillomavirus from condylomata acuminata. Nature 1985;317:639–41.

27. Kurman RJ, Jenson AB, Sinclair CF, Lancaster WD. Detection of human papillomaviruses by immunocytochemistry. In: DeLellis RA, ed. Advances in immunohistochemistry. New York: Masson Publishing USA, 1984:201–21. (Sternberg SS, ed. Masson monographs in diagnostic pathology; Vol 7.)

28. _____, Jenson AB, Lancaster WD. Papillomavirus infection of the cervix. II. Relationship to intraepithelial neoplasia based on the presence of specific viral structural proteins. Am J Surg Pathol 1983;7:39–52.

29. _____, Schiffman MH, Lancaster WD, et al. Analysis of individual human papillomavirus types in cervical neoplasia: a possible role for type 18 in rapid progression. Am J Obstet Gynecol 1988;159:293–6.

30. _____, Shah KH, Lancaster WD, Jenson AB. Immunoperoxidase localization of papillomavirus antigens in cervical dysplasia and vulvar condylomas. Am J Obstet Gynecol 1981;140:931–5.

31. Lancaster WD, Castellano C, Santos C, Delgado G, Kurman RJ, Jenson AB. Human papillomavirus deoxyribonucleic acid in cervical carcinoma from primary and metastatic sites. Am J Obstet Gynecol 1986;154:115–9.

32. _____, Kurman RJ, Jenson AB. Papillomaviruses in anogenital neoplasms. In: Luderer AA, Weetall HH, eds. The human oncogenic viruses. Clifton, NJ: Humana Press, 1986:153–83.

33. Lörincz AT. Detection of human papillomavirus infection by nucleic acid hybridization. Obstet Gynecol Clin North Am 1987;14:451–69.

34. _____ , Reid R, Jenson AB, Greenberg MD, Lancaster WD, Kurman RJ. Human papillomavirus infection of the cervix: relative risk associations of fifteen common anogenital types. Obstet Gynecol 1992;79:328–37.

35. Lörincz AT, Temple GF, Kurman RJ, Jenson AB, Lancaster WD. Oncogenic association of specific human papillomavirus types with cervical neoplasia. JNCI 1987;79:671–7.

36. _____ , Temple GF, Patterson JA, Jenson AB, Kurman RJ, Lancaster WD. Correlation of cellular atypia and human papillomavirus deoxyribonucleic acid sequences in exfoliated cells of the uterine cervix. Obstet Gynecol 1986;68:508–12.

37. Meisels A, Roy M, Fortier M, et al. Human papillomavirus infection of the cervix: the atypical condyloma. Acta Cytol 1981;25:7–16.

38. Münger K, Phelps WC, Bubb V, Howley PM, Schlegel R. The E6 and E7 genes of the human papillomavirus type 16 together are necessary and sufficient for transformation of primary human keratinocytes. J Virol 1989; 63:4417–21.

38a. Muñoz N, Bosch FX, Sanjosé S, et al. The causal link between human papillomavirus and invasive cervical cancer: a population-based case control study in Colombia and Spain. Int J Cancer (in press).

39. Ostrow RS, Manias DA, Clark BA, et al. The analysis of carcinomas of the vagina for human papillomavirus DNA. Int J Gynecol Pathol 1988;7:308–14.

40. Park JS, Jones RW, McLean MR, et al. Possible etiologic heterogeneity of vulvar intraepithelial neoplasia. A correlation of pathologic characteristics with human papillomavirus detection by in situ hybridization and polymerase chain reaction. Cancer 1991;67:1599–607.

41. Pirisi L, Yasumoto S, Feller M, Doniger J, DiPaolo JA. Transformation of human fibroblasts and keratinocytes with human papillomavirus type 16 DNA. J Virol 1987; 61:1061–6.

42. Reeves WC, Brinton LA, Garcia M, et al. Human papillomavirus infection and cervical cancer in Latin America. N Engl J Med 1989;320:1437–41.

43. Reid R, ed. Human papillomavirus. Obstet Gynecol Clin North Am 1987;14:329–614.

44. Schiffman MH, Bauer HM, Glass AG, et al. Preliminary results from a prospective study of HPV infection and incident cervical neoplasia [Abstract]. Seattle: Papillomavirus Workshop, 1991.

45. Schlegel R, Phelps WC, Zhang YL, Barbosa M. Quantitative keratinocyte assay detects two biological activities of human papillomavirus DNA and identifies viral types associated with cervical carcinoma. EMBO J 1988; 7:3181–7.

46. Schneider A. Methods of identification of human papillomaviruses. In: Syrjanen K, Gissmann L, Koss LG, eds. Papillomaviruses and human disease. Berlin: Springer-Verlag, 1987:19–39.

47. Schneider A, Sawada E, Gissmann L, Shah K. Human papillomaviruses in women with a history of abnormal Papanicolaou smears and in their male partners. Obstet Gynecol 1987;69:554–62.

48. Schwarz E, Freese UK, Gissmann L, et al. Structure and transcription of human papillomavirus sequences in cervical carcinoma cells. Nature 1985;314:111–4.

49. Shah KV, Howley PM. Papillomaviruses. In: Fields BN, Knipe DM, eds. Virology. 2nd ed. New York: Raven Press, 1990:1651–76.

50. Shibata DK, Arnheim N, Martin WJ. Detection of human papilloma virus in paraffin-embedded tissue using the polymerase chain reaction. J Exp Med 1988; 167:225–30.

51. Smotkin D, Berek JS, Fu YS, Hacker NF, Major FJ, Wettstein FO. Human papillomavirus deoxyribonucleic acid in adenocarcinoma and adenosquamous carcinoma of the uterine cervix. Obstet Gynecol 1986;68:241–4.

52. Stoler MH, Broker TR. In situ hybridization detection of human papillomavirus DNAs and messenger RNAs in genital condylomas and a cervical carcinoma. Hum Pathol 1986;17:1250–8.

53. _____ , Mills SE, Gersell DJ, Walker AN. Small-cell neuroendocrine carcinoma of the cervix. A human papillomavirus type 18-associated cancer. Am J Surg Pathol 1991;15:28–32.

54. Syrjänen K, Gissmann L, Koss LG, eds. Papillomaviruses and human disease. Berlin: Springer-Verlag, 1987.

55. _____ , Vayrynen M, Saarikoski S, et al. Natural history of cervical human papillomavirus (HPV) infections based on prospective follow-up. Br J Obstet Gynaecol 1985;92:1086–92.

56. Tase T, Okagaki T, Clark BA, Twiggs LB, Ostrow RS, Faras AJ. Human papillomavirus DNA in adenocarcinoma in situ, microinvasive adenocarcinoma of the uterine cervix, and coexisting cervical squamous intraepithelial neoplasia. Int J Gynecol Pathol 1989;8:8–17.

57. Toki T, Kurman RJ, Park JS, Kessis T, Daniel RW, Shah KV. Probable nonpapillomavirus etiology of squamous cell carcinoma of the vulva in older women: a clinicopathologic study using in situ hybridization and polymerase chain reaction. Int J Gynecol Pathol 1991;10:107–25.

58. Twiggs LB, Okagaki T, Clark B, Fukushima M, Ostrow R, Faras A. A clinical, histopathologic, and molecular biologic investigation of vulvar intraepithelial neoplasia. Int J Gynecol Pathol 1988;7:48–55.

59. Venuti A, Marcante ML. Presence of human papillomavirus type 18 DNA in vulvar carcinomas and its integration into the cell genome. J Gen Virol 1989;70:1587–92.

60. Vonka V, Kanka J, Hirsch I, et al. Prospective study on the relationship between cervical neoplasia and herpes simplex type-2 virus. II. Herpes simplex type-2 antibody presence in sera taken at enrollment. Int J Cancer 1984; 33:61–6.

61. Werness BA, Levine AJ, Howley PM. Association of human papillomavirus types 16 and 18 E6 proteins with p53. Science 1990;248:76–9.

62. Wilczynski SP, Bergen S, Walker J, Liao SY, Pearlman LF. Human papillomaviruses and cervical cancer: analysis of histopathologic features associated with different viral types. Hum Pathol 1988;19:697–704.

63. Woodruff JD, Braun L, Cavalieri R, Gupta P, Pass F, Shah KV. Immunologic identification of papillomavirus antigen in condyloma tissues from the female genital tract. Obstet Gynecol 1980;56:727–32.

64. Yasumoto S, Burkhardt AL, Doniger J, DiPaolo JA. Human papillomavirus type 16 DNA-induced malignant transformation of NIH 3T3 cells. J Virol 1986; 57:572–7.

65. Zur Hausen H. Human genital cancer: synergism between two virus infections or synergism between a virus infection and initiating events? Lancet 1982; 2:1370–2.

CLASSIFICATION OF TUMORS OF THE
LOWER FEMALE GENITAL TRACT

The histologic classification of tumors of the cervix, vagina, and vulva has been revised by the International Society of Gynecological Pathologists under the auspices of the World Health Organization (WHO) (10). A new cervicovaginal cytologic nomenclature designed to replace the Papanicolaou class designations has also been developed, in accordance with the recommendations of a workshop convened by the National Cancer Institute in Bethesda, Maryland. The new cytologic classification is referred to as "The Bethesda System for Reporting Cervical/Vaginal Diagnoses" or simply the "Bethesda System" (6,8a). In the WHO histologic classification, preinvasive lesions are designated *dysplasia* and *carcinoma in situ* (CIS) or *cervical intraepithelial neoplasia* (CIN), *vaginal intraepithelial neoplasia* (VAIN), and *vulvar intraepithelial neoplasia* (VIN). In the Bethesda System, the cytologic counterparts of the cervical and vaginal lesions are designated *squamous intraepithelial lesions* (SIL), which are subdivided into low-grade and high-grade categories. In the histologic classification, lesions designated *condylomatous atypia, koilocytotic atypia,* or *flat condyloma* are grouped together with mild dysplasia (CIN 1 and VAIN 1) and classified as such. This category corresponds to low-grade SIL in the cytologic classification. The categories of moderate dysplasia (CIN 2) and severe dysplasia/CIS (CIN 3) in the histologic classification correspond to high-grade SIL in the cytologic classification. Both terminologies can be used in histologic diagnosis to facilitate correlation with the cytologic diagnosis, for example, CIN 1 (low-grade SIL), CIN 2 (high-grade SIL), or CIN 3 (high-grade SIL). In this Fascicle, the CIN terminology is used for histologic diagnosis.

In recent years, the growing awareness of the role of HPV in the genesis of cervical neoplasia and the recognition of koilocytosis introduced a new dimension into the nomenclature issue. The cytologic similarity between the typical exophytic condyloma and mild dysplasia led to the introduction of the term *flat condyloma* for the latter (4,5). Implicit in the use of the term flat condyloma is the view that it is a benign viral lesion, fundamentally different and reliably distinguishable from CIN 1, i.e., a potentially malignant lesion. More recent pathologic and molecular studies have shown, however, that the distribution of HPV types in flat condylomas is more closely related to that in CIN 1 than to condyloma acuminatum (9). In addition, the histologic distinction between flat condyloma and CIN 1 is as subjective as the distinction between severe dysplasia and CIS (2,8). For these reasons, the WHO histologic classification and the Bethesda System cytologic classification group all of the low-grade lesions, including those showing koilocytosis, as mild dysplasia or CIN 1 (low-grade SIL). In adopting this terminology, it is recognized that many lesions included within the low-grade category are viral infections that will not undergo malignant transformation and may regress spontaneously, whereas others may progress.

The division of intraepithelial lesions into low grade and high grade correlates with recent virologic data that show that within the continuum of morphologic grades of CIN, HPVs segregate into two patterns of distribution. CIN 2 and 3 (high-grade lesions) are associated for the most part with HPV 16, the virus found in the majority of invasive carcinomas. HPVs 31, 33, 35, and a few other types are found in a smaller proportion of high-grade intraepithelial lesions. In contrast, CIN 1 (low-grade lesions) may be associated with any one of the 20 HPVs that have been isolated from the cervix, including HPV 16 (3). This pattern of distribution of virus types has not been observed in the vagina and vulva. Preliminary studies reveal that most intraepithelial lesions in these sites contain HPV 16 (1,7).

Pathologic and virologic studies indicate that the ends of the morphologic spectrum of intraepithelial (preinvasive) lesions of the cervix reflect a dichotomy of an infectious and a neoplastic lesion. An appropriate classification of intraepithelial lesions should convey this concept and provide guidelines for practical management based on morphologic features that relate to prognosis. For purposes of cytology screening and triage, the Bethesda System divides the intraepithelial lesions into low-grade and high-grade categories. As previously indicated for histologic diagnosis, either the dysplasia/CIS or CIN terminologies can be used with low grade or high grade put in parentheses to facilitate correlation with the cytologic diagnosis. VIN 1,2,3 is used for vulvar intraepithelial lesions, although, as discussed in the chapter Tumors of the Vulva, there are histologic subtypes of these lesions.

HISTOLOGIC CLASSIFICATION OF TUMORS AND TUMOR-LIKE LESIONS

Uterine Cervix

1.0 Epithelial Tumors and Related Lesions
    1.1 Squamous lesions
        1.1.1 Squamous papilloma
        1.1.2 Condyloma acuminatum
        1.1.3 Squamous metaplasia
        1.1.4 Transitional metaplasia
        1.1.5 Squamous atypia
        1.1.6 Squamous intraepithelial lesions*
            1.1.6.1 Cervical intraepithelial neoplasia (CIN) 1, mild dysplasia
            1.1.6.2 CIN 2, moderate dysplasia
            1.1.6.3 CIN 3, severe dysplasia/carcinoma in situ
        1.1.7 Squamous cell carcinoma**
            1.1.7.1 Keratinizing
            1.1.7.2 Nonkeratinizing
            1.1.7.3 Verrucous
            1.1.7.4 Warty (condylomatous)
            1.1.7.5 Papillary (transitional)
            1.1.7.6 Lymphoepithelioma-like
    1.2 Glandular lesions
        1.2.1 Endocervical polyp
        1.2.2 Müllerian papilloma
        1.2.3 Glandular atypia
        1.2.4 Atypical hyperplasia (glandular dysplasia)
        1.2.5 Adenocarcinoma in situ
        1.2.6 Adenocarcinoma
            1.2.6.1 Mucinous (endocervical, intestinal, and signet-ring types)
            1.2.6.2 Endometrioid
            1.2.6.3 Clear cell

---

* In the Bethesda System for cytologic classification, squamous intraepithelial lesions are divided into low grade and high grade. CIN 1 (mild dysplasia) and lesions showing clear-cut evidence of papillomavirus effect are classified as low-grade lesions. CIN 2 (moderate dysplasia) and CIN 3 (severe dysplasia/carcinoma in situ) are classified as high grade.

**For purposes of staging and treatment the International Federation of Gynecologists and Obstetricians subdivides squamous cell carcinoma into microinvasive and frankly invasive carcinomas.

1.2.6.4   Minimal deviation (adenoma malignum)

1.2.6.5   Well-differentiated (papillary) villoglandular

1.2.6.6   Serous

1.2.6.7   Mesonephric

1.3   Other epithelial tumors

   1.3.1   Adenosquamous carcinoma

   1.3.2   Glassy cell carcinoma

   1.3.3   Adenoid cystic carcinoma

   1.3.4   Adenoid basal carcinoma

   1.3.5   Carcinoid tumor (adenocarcinoma with features of carcinoid tumor)

   1.3.6   Small cell carcinoma

   1.3.7   Undifferentiated carcinoma

2.0   Mesenchymal Tumors

   2.1   Leiomyoma

   2.2   Other benign mesenchymal tumors

   2.3   Leiomyosarcoma

   2.4   Endocervical stromal sarcoma

   2.5   Sarcoma botryoides (embryonal rhabdomyosarcoma)

   2.6   Alveolar soft-part sarcoma

   2.7   Osteosarcoma

   2.8   Other malignant mesenchymal tumors

3.0   Mixed Epithelial and Mesenchymal Tumors

   3.1   Papillary adenofibroma

   3.2   Adenosarcoma

   3.3   Malignant mixed mesodermal tumor

   3.4   Wilms tumor

4.0   Miscellaneous Tumors

   4.1   Melanocytic nevus

   4.2   Blue nevus

   4.3   Malignant melanoma

   4.4   Lymphoma and leukemia

   4.5   Tumors of germ cell type

      4.5.1   Mature teratoma

      4.5.2   Yolk sac tumor

5.0   Secondary Tumors

6.0   Tumor-Like Lesions

   6.1   Mesodermal stromal polyp (pseudosarcoma botryoides)

   6.2   Microglandular hyperplasia

   6.3   Mesonephric remnants

   6.4   Mesonephric hyperplasia

   6.5   Arias-Stella reaction

   6.6   Endometriosis

   6.7   Cysts

6.8   Decidual nodule

6.9   Placental site nodule

6.10 Amputation (traumatic) neuroma

6.11 Postoperative spindle-cell nodule

6.12 Intestinal metaplasia

6.13 Tubal metaplasia

6.14 Epidermal metaplasia

6.15 Glial polyp

6.16 Tunnel clusters

6.17 Lymphoma-like lesion

Vagina

1.0   Epithelial Tumors and Related Lesions

  1.1   Squamous lesions

    1.1.1   Squamous papilloma

    1.1.2   Condyloma acuminatum

    1.1.3   Transitional metaplasia

    1.1.4   Squamous atypia

    1.1.5   Squamous intraepithelial lesions*

      1.1.5.1   Vaginal intraepithelial neoplasia (VAIN) 1, mild dysplasia

      1.1.5.2   VAIN 2, moderate dysplasia

      1.1.5.3   VAIN 3, severe dysplasia/carcinoma in situ

    1.1.6   Squamous cell carcinoma

      1.1.6.1   Keratinizing

      1.1.6.2   Nonkeratinizing

      1.1.6.3   Verrucous

      1.1.6.4   Warty (condylomatous)

  1.2   Glandular lesions

    1.2.1   Adenosis

    1.2.2   Atypical adenosis

    1.2.3   Müllerian papilloma

    1.2.4   Adenocarcinoma

      1.2.4.1   Endometrioid

      1.2.4.2   Endocervical

      1.2.4.3   Intestinal

      1.2.4.4   Clear cell

      1.2.4.5   Mesonephric

---

* In the Bethesda System for cytologic classification, squamous intraepithelial lesions are divided into low grade and high grade. VAIN 1 (mild dysplasia) and lesions showing clear-cut evidence of papillomavirus effect are classified as low grade lesions. VAIN 2 (moderate dysplasia) and VAIN 3 (severe dysplasia/carcinoma in situ) are classified as high-grade.

1.3   Other epithelial tumors
    1.3.1   Adenosquamous carcinoma
    1.3.2   Adenoid basal carcinoma
    1.3.3   Adenoid cystic carcinoma
    1.3.4   Carcinoid tumor
    1.3.5   Small cell carcinoma
    1.3.6   Undifferentiated carcinoma

2.0   Mesenchymal Tumors
  2.1   Leiomyoma
  2.2   Rhabdomyoma
  2.3   Other benign mesenchymal tumors
  2.4   Leiomyosarcoma
  2.5   Sarcoma botryoides (embryonal rhabdomyosarcoma)
  2.6   Endometrioid stromal sarcoma
  2.7   Other malignant mesenchymal tumors

3.0   Mixed Epithelial and Mesenchymal Tumors
  3.1   Mixed tumor
  3.2   Mixed tumor resembling synovial sarcoma
  3.3   Adenosarcoma
  3.4   Malignant mixed mesodermal tumor

4.0   Miscellaneous Tumors
  4.1   Melanocytic nevus
  4.2   Blue nevus
  4.3   Malignant melanoma
  4.4   Yolk sac tumor
  4.5   Mature cystic teratoma
  4.6   Adenomatoid tumor
  4.7   Villous adenoma
  4.8   Malignant lymphoma and other lymphohistiocytic lesions

5.0   Secondary Tumors

6.0   Tumor-Like Lesions
  6.1   Vaginal polyp (mesodermal stromal polyp)
  6.2   Postoperative spindle-cell nodule
  6.3   Vault granulation tissue
  6.4   Prolapsed fallopian tube
  6.5   Endometriosis
  6.6   Decidua
  6.7   Cysts
    6.7.1   Epidermoid
    6.7.2   Müllerian
    6.7.3   Mesonephric
  6.8   Lymphoma-like lesion

Vulva

1.0   Epithelial Tumors and Related Lesions
    1.1   Squamous lesions
        1.1.1   Squamous (vestibular) papilloma
        1.1.2   Fibroepithelial polyp
        1.1.3   Condyloma acuminatum
        1.1.4   Seborrheic keratosis
        1.1.5   Keratoacanthoma
        1.1.6   Squamous intraepithelial lesions
            1.1.6.1   Vulvar intraepithelial neoplasia (VIN) 1, mild dysplasia
            1.1.6.2   VIN 2, moderate dysplasia
            1.1.6.3   VIN 3, severe dysplasia, carcinoma in situ
        1.1.7   Squamous cell carcinoma*
            1.1.7.1   Keratinizing
            1.1.7.2   Nonkeratinizing
            1.1.7.3   Basaloid
            1.1.7.4   Verrucous
            1.1.7.5   Warty (condylomatous)
            1.1.7.6   Basal cell
    1.2   Glandular lesions
        1.2.1   Papillary hidradenoma
        1.2.2   Nodular (clear cell) hidradenoma
        1.2.3   Syringoma
        1.2.4   Trichoepithelioma
        1.2.5   Trichilemmoma
        1.2.6   Adenoma of minor vestibular glands
        1.2.7   Paget disease
        1.2.8   Bartholin gland tumors
            1.2.8.1   Adenocarcinoma
            1.2.8.2   Squamous cell carcinoma
            1.2.8.3   Adenoid cystic carcinoma
            1.2.8.4   Adenosquamous carcinoma
            1.2.8.5   Transitional cell carcinoma
        1.2.9   Breast carcinoma and other tumors arising in ectopic mammary tissue
        1.2.10 Carcinomas of sweat gland origin
        1.2.11 Other adenocarcinomas
2.0   Mesenchymal Tumors
    2.1   Benign mesenchymal tumors
        2.1.1   Lipoma/fibrolipoma

---

*For purposes of clinical management squamous cell carcinoma is subdivided into superficially invasive and frankly invasive carcinomas.

  2.1.2 Hemangioma
    2.1.2.1 Capillary
    2.1.2.2 Cavernous
    2.1.2.3 Acquired
  2.1.3 Angiokeratoma
  2.1.4 Pyogenic granuloma
  2.1.5 Lymphangioma
  2.1.6 Fibroma
  2.1.7 Leiomyoma
  2.1.8 Granular cell tumor
  2.1.9 Neurofibroma
  2.1.10 Schwannoma (neurilemoma)
  2.1.11 Glomus tumor
  2.1.12 Fibrous histiocytoma
  2.1.13 Rhabdomyoma
 2.2 Malignant mesenchymal tumors
  2.2.1 Embryonal rhabdomyosarcoma (sarcoma botryoides)
  2.2.2 Aggressive angiomyxoma
  2.2.3 Leiomyosarcoma
  2.2.4 Dermatofibrosarcoma protuberans
  2.2.5 Malignant fibrous histiocytoma
  2.2.6 Epithelioid sarcoma
  2.2.7 Malignant rhabdoid tumor
  2.2.8 Malignant schwannoma
  2.2.9 Angiosarcoma
  2.2.10 Kaposi sarcoma
  2.2.11 Hemangiopericytoma
  2.2.12 Liposarcoma
  2.2.13 Alveolar soft-part sarcoma

3.0 Miscellaneous Tumors
 3.1 Melanocytic tumors
  3.1.1 Congenital melanocytic nevus
  3.1.2 Common acquired melanocytic nevus
  3.1.3 Blue nevus
  3.1.4 Dysplastic melanocytic nevus
  3.1.5 Malignant melanoma
 3.2 Malignant lymphoma
 3.3 Tumors of germ cell type
  3.3.1 Yolk sac tumor (endodermal sinus tumor)
 3.4 Neuroectodermal tumors
  3.4.1 Merkel cell tumor

4.0 Secondary Tumors

REFERENCES

1. Buscema J, Naghashfar Z, Sawada E, Daniel R, Woodruff JD, Shah KV. The predominance of human papillomavirus type 16 in vulvar neoplasia. Obstet Gynecol 1988;71:601–6.

2. Ismail SM, Colclough AB, Dinnen JS, et al. Observer variation in histopathological diagnosis and grading of cervical intraepithelial neoplasia. Br Med J 1989;298:707–10.

3. Lörincz AT, Reid R, Jenson AB, Greenberg MD, Lancaster WD, Kurman RJ. Human papillomavirus infection of the cervix: relative risk associations of fifteen common anogenital types. Obstet Gynecol 1992;79:328–37.

4. Meisels A, Fortin R. Condylomatous lesions of the cervix and vagina. I. Cytologic patterns. Acta Cytol 1976;20:505–9.

5. Meisels A, Roy M, Fortier M, et al. Human papillomavirus infection of the cervix: the atypical condyloma. Acta Cytol 1981;25:7–16.

6. National Cancer Institute Workshop. The 1988 Bethesda System for reporting cervical/vaginal cytological diagnoses. JAMA 1989;262:931–4.

6a. The Bethesda System for reporting cervical/vaginal cytologic diagnoses. Report of the 1991 Bethesda Workshop. JAMA 1992;267:1892.

7. Park JS, Jones RW, McClean MR, et al. Possible etiologic heterogeneity of vulvar intraepithelial neoplasia. A correlation of pathologic characteristics with human papillomavirus detection by in situ hybridization and polymerase chain reaction. Cancer 1991;67:1599–607.

8. Ringsted J, Amtrup F, Asklund C, et al. Reliability of histopathological diagnosis of squamous epithelial changes of the uterine cervix. Acta Pathol Microbiol Scand [A] 1978;86:273–8.

8a. The Bethesda System for reporting cervical/vaginal cytologic diseases. Report of the 1991 Bethesda Workshop. JAMA 1992;267:1892.

9. Willett GD, Kurman RJ, Reid R, Greenberg M, Jenson AB, Lorincz AT. Correlation of the histologic appearance of intraepithelial neoplasia of the cervix with human papillomavirus types. Emphasis on low grade lesions including so-called flat condyloma. Int J Gynecol Pathol 1989;8:18–25.

10. World Health Organization. Histopathologic classification of tumors and tumor-like lesions of the uterine cervix and vagina. 1992; in press.

TUMORS OF THE CERVIX

SQUAMOUS LESIONS

Squamous Papilloma

Definition. Squamous papilloma is a benign papillary lesion composed of a fibrovascular stalk covered by mature squamous epithelium. Synonyms include *fibroepithelial polyp* or *fibroepithelioma*. The fibroepithelial polyp typically contains more fibrous tissue than the squamous papilloma, but for practical purposes, this term and *ectocervical polyp* are synonymous with *squamous papilloma*.

General Features. Squamous papillomas are usually solitary, arise on the ectocervix or the squamocolumnar junction, and range in diameter from a few millimeters to 2 cm. In one study, they were found in 0.4 percent of cervical biopsy specimens (8). Squamous papillomas are less commonly encountered on the cervix than the vagina or vulva.

Microscopic Findings. Squamous papillomas have a central thick fibrovascular core with smaller branching fibrovascular papillae covered by mature squamous epithelium without cytologic atypia (fig. 31). In the older literature, squamous papillomas of the cervix were included in the category with condylomata acuminata as papillomas of the cervix (10,12). Although the venereal and viral natures of condylomas were appreciated, condylomas and squamous papillomas were considered indistinguishable morphologically. Subsequently, koilocytotic atypia, also termed *koilocytosis*, was recognized as a marker for HPV infection in the lower genital tract, and molecular virologic studies unequivocally demonstrated the presence of papillomaviruses in the condyloma acuminatum (7,15). In contrast, koilocytotic atypia is not a feature of squamous papillomas, and molecular virologic examination of similar lesions on the vulva has failed to demonstrate HPV (1,15). The different etiology of squamous papillomas and condylomas has obvious clinical significance, but the differential diagnosis may be difficult. The most useful feature is the presence of koilocytotic atypia in the condyloma; however, this finding may be absent in some condylomas, in which case the architectural features assist in the differential diagnosis. The squamous papilloma contains a central fibrovascular stalk and does not show the marked degree of arborization characteristic of the condyloma acuminatum.

Treatment. Squamous papillomas do not require specific treatment. Usually the diagnostic biopsy removes the entire lesion.

Condyloma Acuminatum

Definition. Condyloma acuminatum is a papillary, exophytic, benign neoplasm caused by papillomaviruses.

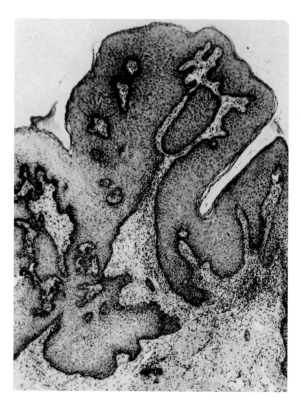

Figure 31
SQUAMOUS PAPILLOMA
A squamous papilloma containing a thick fibrovascular core and covered by mature squamous epithelium. The absence of koilocytosis and lack of arborizing papillae distinguish this from a condyloma. (Fig. 63 from Fascicle 33, Part 2, First Series.)

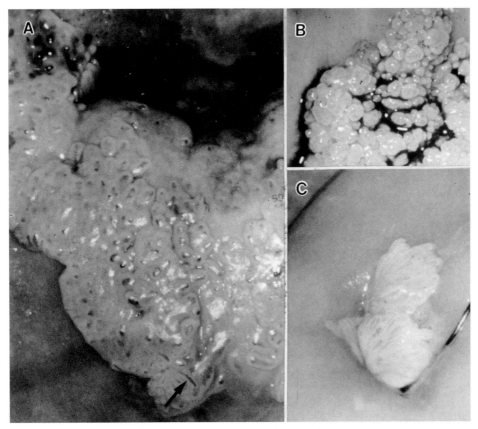

Figure 32
COLPOPHOTOGRAPH OF AN EXOPHYTIC CONDYLOMA
This figure shows a typical exophytic condyloma with confluent flattened papillae showing vascular loops (A); a condyloma involving the vagina (B); and two small condylomas at the external os (C). (Fig. 7.7 from Ferenczy A, Winkler B. Cervical intraepithelial neoplasia and condyloma. In: Kurman RJ, ed. Blaustein's pathology of the female genital tract. 3rd ed. New York: Springer-Verlag, 1987.) (Figures 32A and B are from the same patient.)

General Features. Human papillomavirus types 6 and 11 are found in 70 to 90 percent of these lesions, but occasionally, other types, including type 16, have been detected. HPV 16 is almost always found in condylomas with high-grade cytologic atypia.

Multiple condylomas are not common on the cervix; they are much more frequently encountered on the vulva. In one population-based study, the frequency of multiple condylomas in various parts of the female genital tract and adjacent areas was as follows: vulva 66 percent, vagina 37 percent, perineum 29 percent, anus 23 percent, cervix 8 percent, and urethra 4 percent (3). Condyloma acuminatum is discussed in greater detail in the chapter Tumors of the Vulva.

Gross Findings. Cervical lesions have an exophytic, spiked, or cauliflower-like appearance. Colposcopically, after application of 3 to 5 percent acetic acid, cervical lesions appear white and have typical vascular patterns because of the rich vascular supply that terminates near the tips of the papillary fronds (fig. 32).

Microscopic Findings. Condyloma acuminatum is characterized by acanthotic and sometimes hyperkeratotic squamous epithelium overlying delicate fibrovascular cores (fig. 33). The surface squamous epithelium often has an undulating appearance because of the presence of multiple round or blunted excrescences. Accompanying the exophytic growth is a marked papillomatosis that is characterized by a downward proliferation of

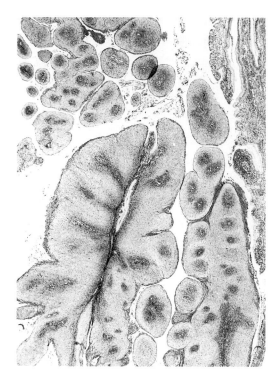

Figure 33
EXOPHYTIC CONDYLOMA
This typical exophytic condyloma shows arborizing fibrovascular cores covered by acanthotic squamous epithelium.

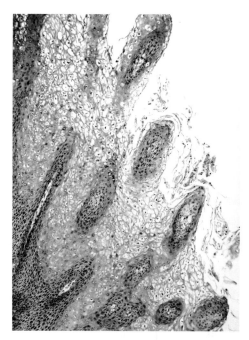

Figure 34
EXOPHYTIC CONDYLOMA
Spiked excrescences (asperities) are visible on the surface of an exophytic condyloma with extensive koilocytotic atypia. (Figures 34 and 35 are from the same patient.)

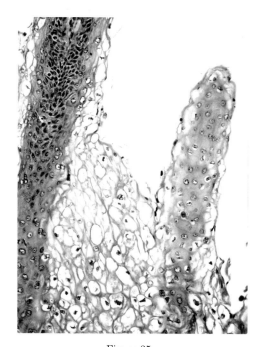

Figure 35
EXOPHYTIC CONDYLOMA
A higher magnification of figure 34 demonstrates koilocytotic atypia characterized by nuclear enlargement and wrinkling. This extensive degree of koilocytotic atypia is not seen in most condylomas.

anastomosing rete pegs. Within the papillary fronds, there is an increased number of capillaries, and as a result, there may be only a few layers of squamous epithelial cells between the capillaries and the surface. Although koilocytosis is pathognomonic for condyloma acuminatum (figs. 34, 35), it may be focal and may be absent in a single section in an otherwise typical condyloma. If uncertainty exists, deeper sections almost always demonstrate typical koilocytes. Mild cytologic atypia is typical but occasionally may be marked. Mild atypia need not be mentioned in the diagnosis, but if the atypia is marked, its presence should be specified, because the behavior of these lesions is uncertain. The degree of atypia can be graded in the same manner as that of flat lesions, i.e., condyloma with CIN 2 or 3. Mitotic activity in condylomas without CIN 2 or 3 is confined to the basal and parabasal layers but may appear close to the surface where the stromal papillae extend close to the surface. Rarely, a condyloma is sessile rather than exophytic on the cervix (figs. 36, 37).

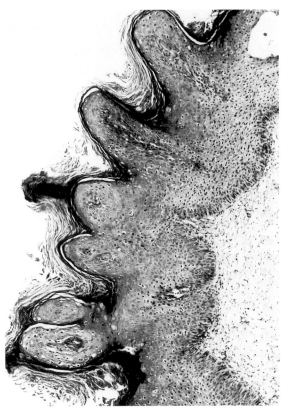

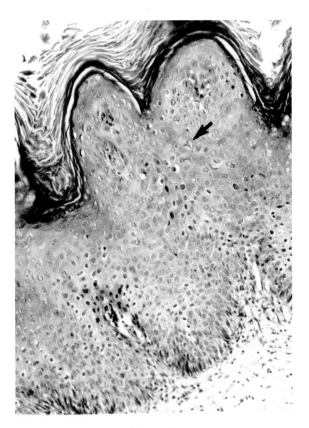

Figure 36
EXOPHYTIC CONDYLOMA
This condyloma has a broad base and shows an undulating surface with acanthotic and hyperkeratotic squamous epithelium.(Figures 36 and 37 are from the same patient.)

Figure 37
EXOPHYTIC CONDYLOMA
Higher magnification of figure 36 illustrates the absence of cytologic atypia and koilocytosis. Occasionally, abnormal mitotic figures (tripolar mitotic figure near arrow) can be seen in otherwise typical condylomas.

Prognosis and Treatment. Condylomas are benign, although occasionally a squamous cell carcinoma may develop within a condyloma (2,18). Condylomas may spontaneously regress or persist for many years. The natural history of condylomas is related in part to the immune status of the patient (9). Small lesions can be removed by excisional biopsy, and cryosurgery; laser vaporization is used for larger lesions.

Squamous Metaplasia

Definition. Squamous metaplasia refers to the replacement of endocervical epithelium by undifferentiated subcolumnar reserve cells, which differentiate into squamous epithelium. The process by which endocervical epithelium is replaced by squamous epithelium to form the transformation zone of the cervix is discussed in the chapter Anatomy of the Lower Female Gen-

ital Tract. Because of the importance of squamous metaplasia in the transformation zone as it relates to the development of cervical neoplasia, it is described in the section on squamous intraepithelial lesions.

Microscopic Findings. Squamous metaplasia is characterized early in its development by stratified undifferentiated, so-called reserve cells, which proliferate immediately beneath the columnar epithelium (see fig. 15). The reserve cells are cuboidal to low columnar with round to oval nuclei and scant cytoplasm. Reserve cells eventually acquire more abundant eosinophilic cytoplasm as they mature into squamous epithelial cells. The metaplastic squamous epithelium lacks intracytoplasmic glycogen and can usually be distinguished from the native squamous epithelium. In addition, unlike native squamous epithelium, metaplastic squamous epithelium

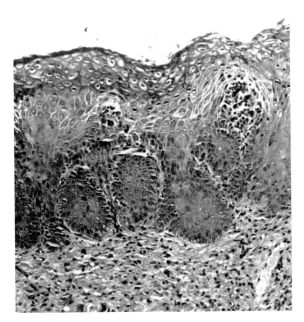

Figure 38
METAPLASTIC SQUAMOUS EPITHELIUM
This figure illustrates metaplastic squamous epithelium showing prominent cytoplasmic vacuolization on the surface. In contrast to koilocytotic atypia in which nuclei are enlarged and eccentrically located (see fig. 48), the nuclei in metaplastic squamous epithelium are not enlarged and tend to be centrally located within the cell.

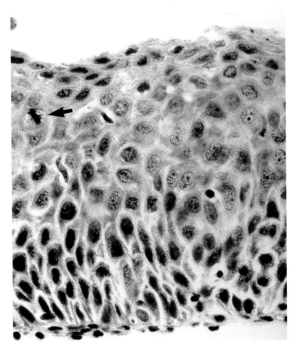

Figure 39
IMMATURE SQUAMOUS METAPLASIA
There is increased cellularity in the deep levels and increased mitotic activity (arrow) in this illustration of immature squamous metaplasia. There is retention of polarity, and the cells mature normally as they approach the surface. Chromatin is prominent, but nuclei are uniform.

overlies endocervical glands. Typically, metaplastic squamous epithelium replaces the endocervical epithelium on the surface and also extends into the endocervical glandular clefts (see fig. 16).

Differential Diagnosis. Metaplastic squamous epithelium that becomes glycogenated may be confused with CIN 1 displaying koilocytosis (fig. 38). In contrast to koilocytosis in CIN 1, the nuclei in the glycogenated metaplastic squamous epithelium are not enlarged or atypical. In addition, the nuclei in metaplastic squamous epithelium are centrally located rather than eccentrically placed.

Immature squamous metaplasia is characterized by a relatively uniform population of basal-type squamous cells with relatively scant cytoplasm and oval nuclei lacking pleomorphism. Near the surface, maturation may occur. In these instances, cells have more abundant cytoplasm and nuclei are rounder. Although there may be some coarsening of the chromatin, the nuclei are not hyperchromatic, and the nuclear membranes are smooth. There is preservation of polarity, lack of crowding, and absence of cellular disorganization

in the deeper layers. Although mitotic figures may be evident, sometimes even close to the surface, abnormal mitotic figures are rarely observed (fig. 39). Finally, the presence of a layer of mucinous epithelium on the surface, representing the last remnant of endocervical epithelium that is replaced by the metaplastic squamous epithelium, is useful in distinguishing immature metaplasia from CIN. Mucinous epithelium rarely overlies CIN.

Immature squamous metaplasia may exhibit nuclear atypia (fig. 40). This lesion has been designated *atypical immature metaplasia* (4) and may be difficult to distinguish from CIN 2 or 3. In contrast to high-grade CIN, the nuclei of atypical immature metaplasia are only slightly enlarged, round with finely granular chromatin, and have prominent nucleoli. In contrast, the nuclei in CIN are more pleomorphic and hyperchromatic, and there is more abundant mitotic activity, including the presence of abnormal mitotic figures. There is also greater cellular crowding and disorganization in CIN.

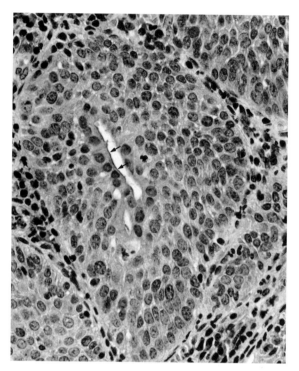

Figure 40
IMMATURE SQUAMOUS
METAPLASIA WITH ATYPIA

This figure shows immature squamous metaplasia with nuclear enlargement and mild atypia. So-called atypical immature metaplasia filling endocervical glands may simulate high-grade CIN. In contrast to CIN, the cells are not crowded or disorganized; the nuclei are uniform, round, and many have prominent nucleoli. The presence of mucinous epithelium overlying the metaplastic epithelium (arrows) is also helpful in distinguishing metaplasia from CIN. Mucinous epithelium rarely overlies CIN.

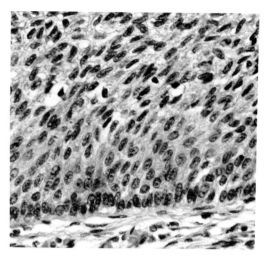

Figure 41
TRANSITIONAL METAPLASIA

Some cells have longitudinal nuclear grooves, resembling transitional epithelial cells. The lesion resembles CIN 3 because the nuclei are crowded and hyperchromatic. The lack of pleomorphism and cellular disorganization and the palisaded appearance of the basal cell layer and low mitotic activity help to distinguish this from CIN 3.

Transitional Metaplasia

Another type of metaplasia that may be seen in association with atrophy, and occasionally focally in the absence of atrophy, is so-called transitional metaplasia. The lesion usually occurs on the ectocervix but may sometimes fill endocervical glands. It is composed of basal and parabasal cells, with ovoid nuclei that are often grooved involving the full thickness of the epithelium, resembling transitional epithelium (fig. 41). Because of the full thickness involvement by basal and parabasal cells, this lesion may be confused with high-grade CIN. In contrast to CIN, however, transitional metaplasia lacks cytologic atypia and high mitotic activity.

Immunohistochemical studies reveal that the transitional-like epithelium contains serotonin-positive cells scattered in the basal layer. In addition, this type of epithelium has a distinct cytokeratin pattern that differs from both normal squamous epithelium and uroepithelium. Monoclonal antibodies specific for simple epithelial-type cytokeratins show that they are limited to the basal layer in normal squamous epithelium but are present throughout the entire epithelium in transitional metaplasia. In contrast, uroepithelium displays a pattern of immunoreactivity with cytokeratin antibodies that corresponds to superficial maturation and terminal differentiation leading to the characteristic layer of "umbrella" cells, which is not evident in transitional metaplasia (6). It therefore appears that transitional metaplasia represents a proliferation of basal cells, so-called basal cell hyperplasia.

Squamous Atypia

Definition. Squamous atypia is used to describe a lesion characterized by a relatively uniform population of cells with nuclear enlargement and prominent nucleoli. The squamous cells are not crowded and retain an orderly pattern of maturation.

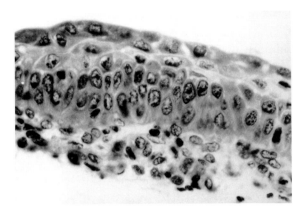

Figure 42
SQUAMOUS ATYPIA
The presence of prominent nucleoli and retention of the overall cellular organization and polarity helps to distinguish squamous atypia from CIN. In addition, the location of the lesion immediately adjacent to an ulceration indicates that it is reactive.

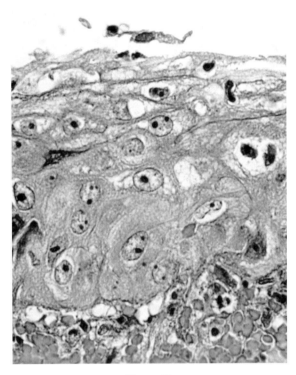

Figure 43
SQUAMOUS ATYPIA
In this illustration, squamous atypia is characterized by enlarged nuclei with prominent nucleoli in the deeper levels. The absence of coarse chromatin clumping, the smooth round nuclear membranes, and retention of polarity assist in distinguishing this lesion from CIN.

General Features. Squamous atypia usually arises in metaplastic squamous epithelium and may be seen in the absence of other abnormalities or in association with ulceration, reflecting a reparative process. Squamous atypia has been reported in 2 to 3 percent of all cervical smears (14,17).

The role of HPV in the genesis of this lesion is not entirely clear. It has been reported that between 10 and 20 percent of women with smears showing squamous atypia have HPV DNA detected by nucleic acid hybridization tests (11, 19), similar to the frequency detected in normal controls. Squamous atypia may therefore encompass a heterogeneous group of lesions, most unrelated to HPV infection and some possibly representing the earliest, but nonspecific, cellular manifestation of HPV infection.

Microscopic Findings. The squamous epithelium may be glycogenated and is only slightly thickened. The overall cellular organization and maturation is normal (fig. 42). There is no proliferation in the parabasal cell layer. Accordingly, there is minimal mitotic activity, and abnormal mitotic figures are rarely seen. The nuclei are enlarged and round. The nuclear chromatin is finely granular, and nucleoli are prominent (fig. 43). The nuclear membranes may be smooth or only slightly irregular and lack significant wrinkling. Binucleate cells are occasionally present. The squamous cells have a relatively normal nuclear-cytoplasmic ratio, and intercellular bridges are usually evident. Typically, there is an associated acute and chronic inflammatory infiltrate in the stroma, with leukocytes within the epithelium.

Differential Diagnosis. Squamous atypia should be distinguished from koilocytotic atypia and high-grade CIN. In contrast to squamous atypia, koilocytotic atypia is found in squamous epithelium in which the cellular architecture has become disorganized and maturation is abnormal. Usually, there is some degree of proliferation in the parabasal layer. The nuclear membrane is wrinkled and irregular in contour. In addition, the cell membrane of the koilocyte is thickened, and the nucleus is often eccentric within the perinuclear clear zone.

In contrast to squamous atypia, a high-grade CIN lesion shows greater proliferation and nuclear atypia. Accordingly, in high-grade CIN, there is high mitotic activity, including the presence of abnormal mitotic figures, and the nuclei show greater pleomorphism and hyperchromasia. In addition, there is marked cellular crowding and disorganization, with loss of normal squamous maturation. Finally, squamous atypia is often associated with endocervical glandular atypia characterized by a single layer of epithelial cells displaying similar abnormalities to those seen in the squamous epithelium (see fig. 92).

Although squamous atypia is often related to inflammation and repair, atypical squamous cells (atypical squamous cells of undetermined significance in the Bethesda System) in cervical smears are associated with CIN in 20 to 40 percent of cases and are also associated with invasive cancer (5,16). The diagnosis of squamous atypia can also be used for lesions with features that are suggestive but not diagnostic of HPV infection (13).

Squamous Intraepithelial Lesions

Definition. Proliferative intraepithelial squamous lesions that display abnormal maturation, nuclear enlargement, and atypia. Atypia is characterized by pleomorphism, coarse chromatin clumping, and irregular nuclear contours. Squamous intraepithelial lesions have been designated *dysplasia* (mild, moderate, severe) and *carcinoma in situ* or CIN (grades 1–3). In this Fascicle, flat lesions with strictly defined koilocytotic atypia (see Microscopic Findings) and minimal or no evidence of proliferation are included in the category of CIN 1. This category corresponds to low-grade squamous intraepithelial lesions in the Bethesda System for cytologic classification. CIN 2 and 3 correspond to high-grade squamous intraepithelial lesions in the Bethesda System (52). Higher-grade lesions with koilocytotic atypia are simply classified as CIN 2 or 3; it is not necessary to report the presence of koilocytotic atypia in either low-grade or high-grade lesions. A more detailed discussion of the terminology is presented in the chapter Classification of Tumors of the Lower Female Genital Tract.

General Features. CIN shares many of the epidemiologic characteristics of invasive carcinoma. In recent years, the age at which CIN appears has decreased, and the prevalence has increased in teenagers and women under the age

of 30 years (65). The mean age of women with CIN in one large study was 26 years (65), approximately 20 years younger than that of women with invasive carcinoma. The prevalence of these lesions in the United States has varied from 0.5 to 6.5 percent, depending on the nature of the population screened and the year the study was performed (28,72). With the introduction of mass screening programs, the prevalence of invasive carcinoma has decreased dramatically, whereas that of precursor lesions has risen as a result of an increase in cytologic detection (25).

Epidemiologic studies have shown that CIN and invasive carcinoma are related to the sexual history of both the patient and her partner (21). Rotkin (64) analyzed 17 epidemiologic studies and concluded that sexual intercourse before the age of 17 years and multiple sexual partners are the most important risk factors for the development of cervical cancer. Other factors such as coital frequency, menstrual patterns, circumcision of the partner, and number of children are covariables. The use of oral contraceptives is unrelated to the risk of squamous atypia or CIN 1 but is associated with an elevated risk of high-grade CIN that increases with longer duration of use (relative risk 4.6) (53). In a recent epidemiologic study it was found that HPV infection, detected in cervical lavages with a PCR-based method, explained most of the epidemiologic risk factors of CIN including the number of lifetime sexual partners (67a). The investigators concluded that the great majority of CIN could be attributed to HPV infection.

Numerous studies over the past decade have linked HPV infection of the cervix with CIN and invasive cancer. This subject is discussed in greater detail in the chapter Human Papillomaviruses and Cancer of the Lower Female Genital Tract. Approximately 20 HPV types can infect the metaplastic squamous epithelium of the cervix. In the majority of infected women, conservatively estimated to be 6 to 10 million a year in the United States, no lesion is detectable on colposcopic or cytologic examination (41). In an additional 1.2 million women, colposcopically detectable CIN is present. The morphologic expression of productive HPV infection, i.e., infection resulting in the release of infectious viral particles, is a CIN 1 lesion. Specific cellular manifestations of HPV infection, demonstration of HPV

DNA sequences, or both are found in approximately 80 percent of low-grade lesions. It is not known whether factors other than HPV play a role in the etiology of some low-grade lesions. A small proportion of low-grade lesions evolve into high-grade lesions, depending to some degree on both the HPV type and other as yet poorly defined risk factors, such as host immunity, genetic predisposition, and exposure to other environmental carcinogens. HPV nucleotide sequences, most often those of HPV 16, can be detected in approximately 90 percent of CIN 3 lesions.

A wide variety of studies including colpomicroscopy, electron microscopy, tissue culture, time-lapse cinematography, and autoradiography have been used to determine the point of origin and mechanism of spread of CIN (60). CIN begins in the transformation zone and spreads along the basement membrane, replacing the adjacent squamous and glandular epithelial cells. Colpomicroscopic observations and glucose-6-phosphate dehydrogenase X-chromosome marker experiments have shown that the neoplastic process begins in a single cell or in a small focus of cells. With clonal expansion, the lesion enlarges and generally becomes less differentiated as it extends into the endocervical canal.

Gross Findings. The gross appearance of CIN is best appreciated by colposcopic examination after application of 3 to 5 percent acetic acid. A variety of colposcopic patterns reflecting histologic changes in the epithelium and underlying vasculature give rise to "white epithelium," "punctation," and "mosaicism" (figs. 44, 45). These colposcopic patterns can occur in squamous metaplasia and CIN. With experience, a rough correlation between the colposcopic appearance and the grade of the CIN can be made.

The boundary of intraepithelial lesions is limited by their border with the native squamous epithelium of the ectocervix, but proximally, the

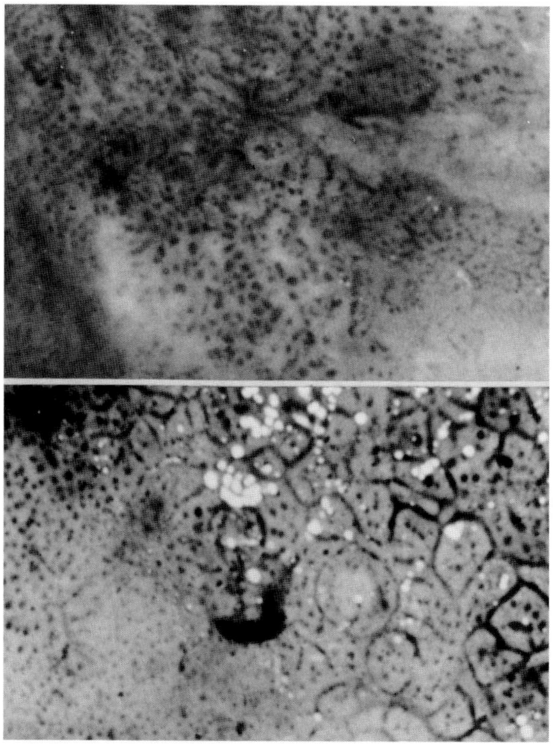

Figure 44
COLPOSCOPIC PHOTOGRAPH OF
CERVICAL INTRAEPITHELIAL NEOPLASIA
Punctation (top) and mosaicism (bottom). (Fig. 7.25 from Ferenczy A, Winkler B. Cervical intraepithelial neoplasia and condyloma. In: Kurman RJ, ed. Blaustein's pathology of the female genital tract. 3rd ed. New York: Springer-Verlag, 1987.)

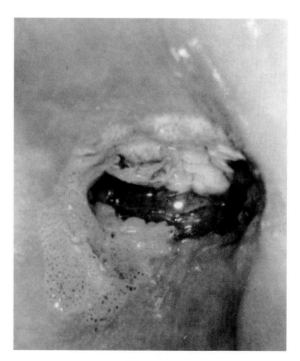

Figure 45
COLPOSCOPIC PHOTOGRAPH OF
CERVICAL INTRAEPITHELIAL NEOPLASIA
Punctation compatible with high-grade CIN. (Fig. 7.34 from Ferenczy A, Winkler B. Cervical intraepithelial neoplasia and condyloma. In: Kurman RJ, ed. Blaustein's pathology of the female genital tract. 3rd ed. New York: Springer-Verlag, 1987.)

lesion can extend for a variable distance into the endocervical canal, or even into the endometrium and fallopian tube and rarely on to the peritoneal surface. CIN occurs twice as often on the anterior lip of the cervix as on the posterior lip and is rarely observed laterally.

Microscopic Findings. CIN is characterized by abnormal cellular proliferation and maturation, and nuclear atypia. The proliferation begins in the basal and parabasal layers, with an increase in the number of immature parabasal cells that extend to a variable degree into the intermediate and superficial layers. An unusual form of papillary CIN designated *papillary squamous cell carcinoma in situ* has been reported (58), and it is described in the section Invasive Papillary Squamous Cell Carcinoma.

Mitotic activity is often increased, and abnormal mitotic figures may be present. Although abnormal mitotic figures are occasionally identified in low-grade lesions, they are found with increasing frequency in high-grade lesions. Abnormal mitotic figures may display a variety of configurations, including two-group metaphase, three-group metaphase, ring mitosis, V-shaped metaphase, tripolar mitosis, dispersed metaphase, giant mitosis, and other bizarre forms (fig. 46) (33). Although dispersed metaphase and tripolar mitotic figures may occur in diploid or polypoid lesions, the other abnormal forms are usually associated with aneuploidy.

Abnormal maturation as manifested by loss of polarity and cellular disorganization is an important feature of CIN. The degree of maturation is inversely related to the severity of the lesion. Immature parabasal cells have a high nuclear-cytoplasmic ratio. As maturation occurs in the more superficial layers, these cells acquire more eosinophilic cytoplasm. Low-grade lesions show a greater degree of maturation on both an individual cell basis and the extent to which the upper levels of the epithelium contain cells with abundant cytoplasm. Despite undergoing maturation, the cells on the surface still contain abnormal nuclei, which permits their detection in cytologic smears. Rarely, the presence of normal epithelium overlying CIN precludes a cytologic diagnosis.

Nuclear atypia is the hallmark of CIN, and it takes two forms that often overlap, making distinction on a cell-by-cell basis difficult or impossible.

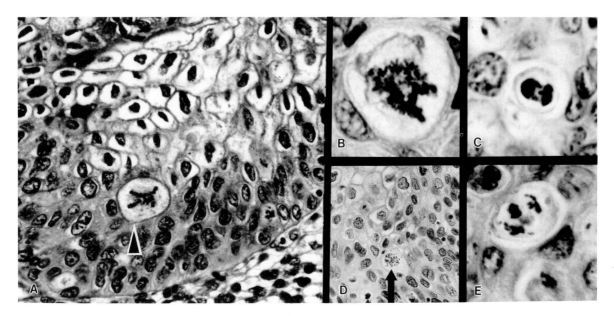

Figure 46
CERVICAL INTRAEPITHELIAL NEOPLASIA DISPLAYING ABNORMAL MITOTIC FIGURES
A variety of configurations are illustrated, including a quadripolar mitotic figure (arrowhead) in a lesion with extensive koilocytosis (A); bizarre mitotic figure with Y-shape and numerous poorly organized chromosomes (B); two-group metaphase (C); dispersed mitotic figure (arrow) with finely distributed chromosomes (D); and three-group metaphase (E). (Fig. 7.30 from Ferenczy A, Winkler B. Cervical intraepithelial neoplasia and condyloma. In: Kurman RJ, ed. Blaustein's pathology of the female genital tract. 3rd ed. New York: Springer-Verlag, 1987.)

One form, occurring mainly in the superficial levels, is a manifestation of productive HPV infection and is a feature of koilocytosis. The other form of atypia is present in the deeper levels in low-grade lesions and occupies progressively more of the epithelium in higher grade lesions. These atypical cells have an increased nuclear-cytoplasmic ratio, with coarsening of the chromatin, increased number of chromocenters, hyperchromasia, and nuclear pleomorphism (fig. 47). This form of nuclear atypia resembles the nuclear abnormalities found in malignant tumors.

Koilocytosis, or koilocytotic atypia, is a common feature of CIN and, if strictly defined, is indicative of the cytopathologic effect of HPV on squamous epithelium in the lower female genital tract. Koilocytosis may be found in any HPV-related lesion from CIN 1 to invasive squamous cell carcinoma and therefore should not be considered evidence of a "benign viral lesion." Conversely, not all HPV-related lesions exhibit koilocytosis, such as adenocarcinoma of the cervix. Virions, capsid antigen, and HPV DNA are not always detectable in koilocytes within or outside the lower female genital tract (Chapman WB, Lörincz AT, Willett G,

Kurman RJ, unpublished data). For example, the squamous component of endometrioid carcinomas of the endometrium or ovary may exhibit cytoplasmic vacuolization and nuclear atypia closely resembling koilocytosis, but HPV DNA has not been detected in these tumors.

The mature intermediate or superficial cell that displays koilocytosis has two characteristic features: 1) a clear, sharply defined perinuclear cavity associated with a peripheral rim of thickened cytoplasm, and 2) nuclear atypia (39). Nuclear atypia is characterized by enlargement, hyperchromasia, and coarsening of the chromatin. The chromatin is often dispersed along the nuclear membrane, which therefore appears thickened and irregular (figs. 48, 49). The nucleus may be central and round and may be surrounded by a clear zone. More often it is displaced to the periphery of the cell, and most of the cytoplasm is clear and the cellular membrane appears thickened. This cytoplasmic clearing has also been referred to as cavitation (fig. 49). Ultrastructural studies have shown

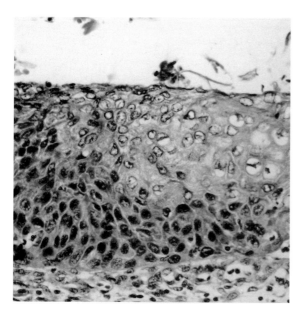

Figure 47
CIN 1 MERGING INTO CIN 3
Nuclear abnormalities compatible with koilocytotic atypia involve the intermediate and superficial cells on the right (CIN 1). Nuclear atypia of the type found in high-grade CIN involves the deeper layers of the lesion in the center and left of the field.

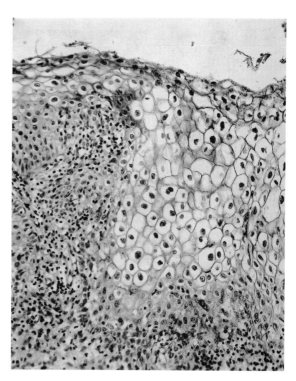

Figure 48
CIN 1
Koilocytotic atypia is manifested by enlarged cells with prominent vacuolization and enlarged hyperchromatic nuclei.

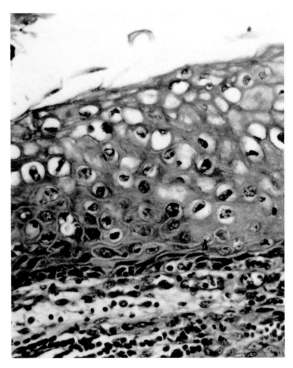

Figure 49
CIN 1
Koilocytes with enlarged nuclei show hyperchromasia and wrinkled pyknotic nuclei. The nuclei are displaced against the cell membrane. There is almost no proliferation in the parabasal cell layer.

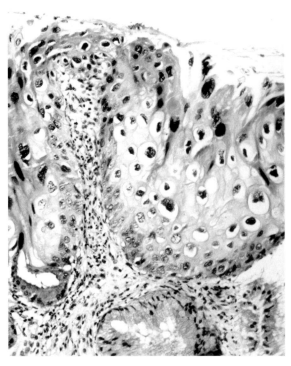

Figure 50
CIN 1
Koilocytotic atypia is characterized by markedly enlarged bizarre nuclei and prominent cytoplasmic vacuolization. These changes probably reflect degenerative changes resulting from productive viral infection. For this reason, the lesion is considered low grade.

perinuclear cytoplasmic necrosis, with the cytoplasmic fibrils condensed along the periphery of the cell (38); viral particles are present in crystalline array within the nucleus. Besides koilocytosis, there are other less specific cytologic manifestations of HPV infection, such as cells near the surface in which HPV structural protein and DNA have been identified with rounded, flattened, or raisin-shaped pyknotic nuclei and inconspicuous or absent cytoplasmic clearing (43). The nuclear-cytoplasmic ratio of these cells is typically increased, and nuclear pleomorphism may be marked. Mononucleate or multinucleate, highly pleomorphic, bizarre cells are not uncommonly observed in the superficial layers (fig. 50) (40,47,57). The nuclei frequently appear smudged, probably reflecting a degenerative change.

Koilocytosis may be confused with normal squamous epithelium with prominent cytoplasmic vacuolization (see fig. 38). Besides the abnormal nuclear features, koilocytosis is often a discrete focal lesion, whereas the vacuolated cells

in normal epithelium are present over a large ill-defined area.

Microscopic Grading. CIN is composed of a heterogeneous population of cells displaying wide diversity in their degree of maturation, proliferation, and atypia (55,59). With the CIN classification, these lesions are graded 1, 2, or 3, corresponding to mild, moderate, or severe dysplasia/carcinoma in situ. Because of the morphologic diversity, studies have shown a significant lack of intra- and interobserver reproducibility (36,62). Clinically, the most important distinction is between CIN 1 (low-grade squamous intraepithelial lesion) and CIN 2 and 3 (high-grade squamous intraepithelial lesion), because the low-grade lesions are either followed without treatment or ablated, whereas the high-grade lesions are uniformly ablated.

CIN has been traditionally graded according to the extent of replacement of the epithelium by

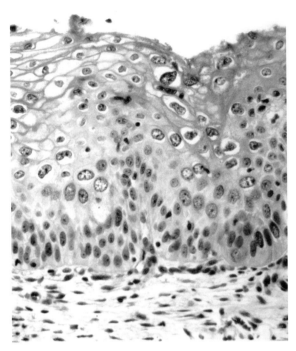

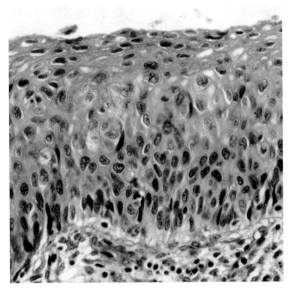

Figure 51
CIN 1

CIN 1 demonstrates thickened squamous epithelium, proliferation of parabasal cells in the lower third of the epithelium, and mild cytologic atypia characterized by slight nuclear enlargement and coarsening of the chromatin.

Figure 52
CIN 2

The cellular proliferation in this lesion involves the lower third of the epithelium, extending slightly into the middle third. The high nuclear-cytoplasmic ratio and cellular disorganization, with accompanying loss of polarity, assist in classifying this as a high-grade lesion despite surface maturation.

abnormal proliferating parabasal cells, but the degree of nuclear atypia and level to which mitotic figures are present in the epithelium must also be considered and are probably more important. If the proliferation is confined to the lower third of the epithelium, the lesion is classified as CIN 1 (low-grade SIL) (figs. 48–51). Although the upper two thirds of the epithelium contain mature cells, they are abnormal. Cells with enlarged pleomorphic nuclei typically containing hyperchromatic smudged chromatin may be present in the upper levels, but these represent degenerated cells, and such lesions are classified as CIN 1 (fig. 50). Also included in this category are lesions characterized by koilocytosis with minimal or no evidence of proliferation in the parabasal layer (fig. 49). Lesions classified as CIN 1 display a wide morphologic range. Almost all display some degree of koilocytotic atypia, which is useful in distinguishing CIN 1 from squamous atypia, which lacks this change. The nuclear atypia in CIN 1 reflects the changes

associated with productive viral infection, such as coarse chromatin clumping and greater atypia, including the presence of greater numbers of abnormal mitotic figures, in contrast to the nuclear atypia associated with malignant tumors that is present in CIN 2 and 3. In addition, there is a greater degree of cellular disorganization, crowding, and loss of polarity in high-grade CIN.

When the proliferation of atypical parabasal cells involves between one third and two thirds of the thickness of the epithelium, the lesion is classified as CIN 2 (high-grade SIL) (fig. 52) and more than two thirds as CIN 3 (high-grade SIL) (figs. 53–56). Koilocytosis may occur in CIN 2 or 3 but less often than in CIN 1. Typically, CIN 3 is composed of immature parabasal cells with oval, round, or spindle-shaped nuclei oriented in a vertical fashion (fig. 54).

Occasionally, there is discordance between the extent of maturation and the degree of nuclear atypia. In these cases there are cells with more abundant cytoplasm and well-defined cell membranes but highly atypical nuclei that are hyperchromatic and pleomorphic (fig. 55) or uniform and vesicular, with prominent coarse

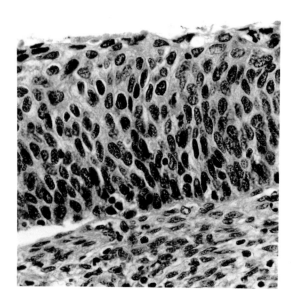

Figure 53
CIN 3
The full thickness of the epithelium is replaced by atypical immature parabasal cells. In addition, the presence of hyperchromasia, a high nuclear-cytoplasmic ratio, and marked cellular crowding and loss of polarity support the diagnosis.

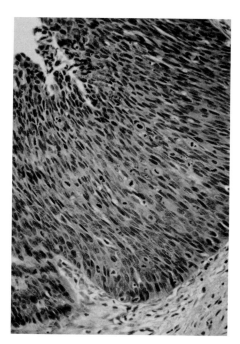

Figure 54
CIN 3
The full thickness of the epithelium is replaced by spindle-shaped cells with scant cytoplasm that results in the appearance of marked hypercellularity. (Fig. 13-11 from Jenson AB, Lancaster WD, Kurman RJ. Uterine cervix. In: Henson DE, Albores-Saavedra J, eds. The pathology of incipient neoplasia. Philadelphia: WB Saunders, 1986:249–64.)

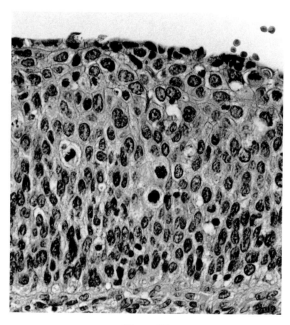

Figure 55
CIN 3
Cells with well-defined cell membranes but highly atypical nuclei and high mitotic activity replace the full thickness of the epithelium.

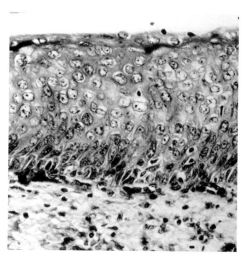

Figure 56
CIN 3
The abnormal cellular proliferation in this lesion is composed of cells with relatively uniform enlarged vesicular nuclei. Cell membranes are not clearly evident. The presence of cells with a high nuclear-cytoplasmic ratio near the surface, cellular crowding, and coarsening of the chromatin support the diagnosis.

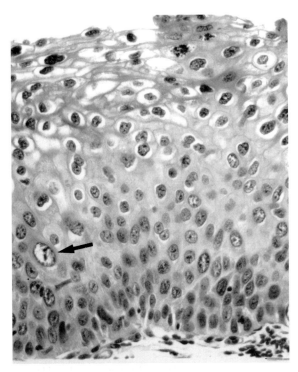

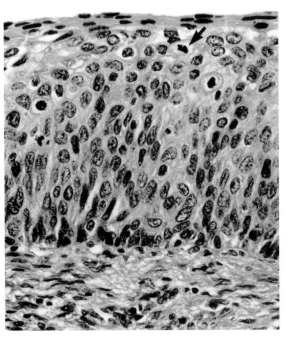

Figure 57
CIN 2
In this illustration, the proliferation involves the lower third of the epithelium, with encroachment of the middle third. There is also marked koilocytosis. Based on the extent of parabasal cell proliferation, this lesion might be graded as CIN 1, but in view of the cytologic atypia (arrow) and the mitotic figure in the superficial layers, this lesion qualifies as CIN 2.

Figure 58
CIN 3
In this illustration, the proliferation involves the lower third of the epithelium, with encroachment of the middle third. Based on the extent of proliferation of the parabasal cells, this lesion qualifies as CIN 2, but the presence of numerous mitotic figures, including one near the surface layer (arrow), elevates this lesion to CIN 3.

chromatin in the superficial levels (fig. 56). The nuclear atypia is not the type associated with productive HPV infection. In these cases, the presence of mitotic figures in the middle third of the epithelium or significant nuclear atypia in the lower third raises the grade of the lesion. Thus, a lesion in which only the lower third of the epithelium is replaced by proliferating parabasal cells but that shows marked nuclear atypia should be upgraded from CIN 1 to CIN 2 (fig. 57). Similarly, a lesion that qualifies as CIN 2 based on the extent of replacement of the epithelium by proliferating parabasal cells but has marked nuclear atypia or mitotic figures near the surface should be upgraded to CIN 3 (fig. 58). Typically, the epithelium of CIN 3 is composed of 15 to 30 layers of cells. Occasionally, a CIN 3 lesion is only 5 to 10 layers thick (fig. 59). The proliferative rate of CIN 3 is on average 12 times greater than that of CIN 1.

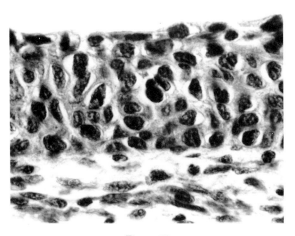

Figure 59
CIN 3
This lesion is unusual because the epithelium is relatively thin. The presence of marked nuclear atypia, pleomorphism, and loss of polarity distinguish this lesion from atrophy.

Immunohistochemistry. Although a variety of biochemical markers have been evaluated on frozen and formalin-fixed paraffin-embedded tissue, none have proven to be useful in differential diagnosis. Most CIN 1 contains high–molecular-weight but not low–molecular-weight keratins, whereas the converse is usually true of high-grade lesions (45,71). Sufficient overlap exists, however, to preclude the use of keratin antibodies in grading lesions. Similarly, studies of involucrin (66,67,77), a marker of suprabasal differentiation unrelated to keratin, and CEA, are not useful in grading CIN or distinguishing it from immature metaplasia (20,44).

Ultrastructural Findings. Ultrastructural analysis has revealed a wide range of cell surface and nuclear and cytoplasmic alterations paralleling those seen with the light microscope (29,30). These changes include a decrease in cytoplasmic glycogen and an increase in rough endoplasmic reticulum, mitochondria, and free ribosomes. The nuclei are enlarged, distorted, and have an abnormal chromatin distribution. The most striking changes, however, are those related to the cell surface. Desmosomes are easily identified in CIN 1 but markedly reduced in CIN 3. Pseudopodia on the cell membrane are reduced, and the cell surface is extremely complex (76). These changes account for the loss of intercellular cohesion in CIN 3.

Morphometric Findings. To predict the behavior of CIN more accurately, its DNA content has been measured with Feulgen microspectrophotometry. A variety of DNA ploidy patterns ranging from euploid to polyploid and aneuploid have been described. The presence of aneuploidy can be inferred in H&E sections by the presence of abnormal mitotic figures (33). In a retrospective study of 100 women with all grades of CIN, Fu and colleagues (32) reported that among 34 lesions that regressed, 29 (85 percent) were euploid and polyploid and 5 (15 percent) were aneuploid. In contrast, of 58 lesions that persisted, 55 (95 percent) were aneuploid and 3 (5 percent) were polyploid. All 8 lesions that progressed to invasive cancer were aneuploid. Hanselaar and associates (34) reported that, in a group of women over 50 years of age, 80 percent of CIN 3 lesions with or without coexistent invasive squamous carcinomas were aneuploid, but in women less than 35 years of age, 60 percent of the CIN 3 lesions were diploid. The

DNA pattern of the invasive carcinoma generally corresponded to that of the adjacent high-grade lesion, suggesting that the two were related. In addition, 20 to 40 percent of invasive squamous carcinomas are diploid (74), indicating that diploid and aneuploid lesions may progress.

HPV Studies. The immunohistochemical detection of HPV capsid antigen is of limited value clinically, although it works satisfactorily with commercially available reagents on formalin-fixed, paraffin-embedded tissue. The main shortcoming of the immunohistochemical method is lack of sensitivity. In a review of over 300 cases of CIN, HPV capsid protein was detected in 29 percent of low-grade lesions and in 7 percent of high-grade lesions (42). Similar studies with commercially available in situ hybridization reagents indicate that HPV DNA is detected in nearly 90 percent of cases of all grades of CIN (22a). This technique can be helpful in the differential diagnosis of CIN versus reactive changes since the latter rarely contains HPV as detected by this method.

Differential Diagnosis. A number of benign lesions may be confused with CIN. Immature metaplasia and atrophy are the most common lesions mistaken for high-grade CIN. In immature metaplasia, the full thickness of the epithelium is composed of immature parabasal cells with a high nuclear-cytoplasmic ratio. The cells are usually vertical, and the nuclei are only slightly hyperchromatic. The most helpful feature in distinguishing CIN from immature metaplasia is the absence of nuclear pleomorphism in the latter (see fig. 39). Immature metaplasia may have mitotic activity, but abnormal mitotic figures are not present. In addition, cellular polarity is retained, cell membranes are clearly defined, and cellular crowding is not marked. Finally, mucinous epithelium is often present on the surface of immature metaplastic squamous epithelium but rarely overlies CIN. Sometimes there may be nuclear atypia within immature metaplasia. This lesion has been designated *atypical immature metaplasia* (see fig. 40) (26).

Atrophic epithelium is occasionally difficult to distinguish from CIN because it is composed of basal and parabasal cells showing no differentiation (fig. 60). Although there is a high nuclear-cytoplasmic ratio, atrophic epithelium is thin and shows no nuclear pleomorphism, mitotic

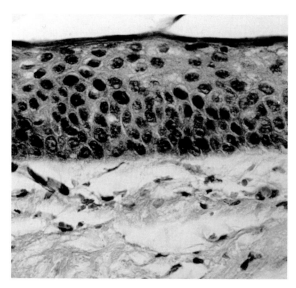

Figure 60
ATROPHY
The epithelium in this lesion is thin, and there is a high nuclear-cytoplasmic ratio in the deep levels. There is no cytologic atypia and no mitotic activity.

activity, atypia, or lack of polarity. In older women, in whom it is difficult to distinguish atrophy from a high-grade CIN, a repeat biopsy after a 2-week course of daily applied vaginal estrogen should resolve the problem by inducing maturation in atrophic epithelium. In contrast, estrogen administration does not alter the appearance of CIN.

Normal metaplastic squamous epithelium with prominent glycogen vacuolization is often confused with CIN 1 (see fig. 38). In contrast to the focal distribution of koilocytes, cells of normal squamous epithelium that have perinuclear clearing are not sharply demarcated, and the nuclei are not enlarged or atypical. Perinuclear clearing by itself may be associated with a variety of infectious microorganisms, notably *Trichomonas vaginalis* (39). In addition to the absence of nuclear atypia, normal stratification and maturation are maintained in such infections, whereas in koilocytosis, there is some degree of cellular disorganization, particularly near the surface, and there is a disturbance in the normal pattern of maturation.

Finally, CIN 3, particularly with extensive gland involvement, may be confused with microinvasive carcinoma (see Microinvasive Carcinoma).

Natural History. Table 2 summarizes some of the more recent studies that followed lesions classified as mild dysplasia or CIN 1 to determine the progression to CIN 3. The differences in the proportion of lesions undergoing progression in the various studies is due, to a large extent, to differences in study design and in the nature of the populations under investigation. For example, it has been argued that the diagnostic biopsy, by removing or destroying most of the lesion, may give a false impression of the natural history of the disease. Studies by Nasiell and associates (50,51) confirmed that, in women with CIN 2, the punch biopsy decreased the frequency of progression and increased the frequency of regression. Nonetheless, even in patients whose lesions were not biopsied, regression occurred in 50 percent of the cases, progression in 35 percent, and persistence in 15 percent. Compared with the incidence of CIN 3 in this population, the risk of progression to CIN 3 for a woman with CIN 2 was about 2000 times greater than for a woman without CIN (50). In women with CIN 1, regression occurred in 62 percent of the cases, progression to CIN 3 in 16 percent, and persistence as CIN 1 in 22 percent (51). In this study, biopsies did not alter the outcome of CIN 1. The risk of progression of CIN 1 to CIN 3 was about 560 times greater than in women without CIN. Likewise, it has been reported that CIN 3, when left untreated, has significant invasive potential, progressing to invasive cancer in approximately 20 percent of cases (37,46). Thus, the consensus is that CIN 1 may regress, persist, or progress to invasive cancer. The outcome for an individual lesion cannot be predicted with certainty but as a group, low-grade lesions are more likely to regress and high-grade lesions are more likely to persist or progress (23,24,31,54,56,68,73).

It should be noted that some investigators believe that high-grade (CIN 3) lesions do not evolve from low-grade (CIN 1) lesions, but rather, are established at the outset as high-grade lesions (21a,36a). These investigators maintain that lesion grade is influenced by location, namely that CIN developing on the ectocervix tends to be low grade whereas CIN developing in the endocervical canal tends to be high grade. According to this line of thinking, apparent progression of a low-grade lesion reflects the evolution of two concurrently established lesions

Table 2

REVIEW OF NINE PROSPECTIVE STUDIES
SHOWING THE PROGRESSION OF CIN 1 TO CIN 3

Source	Number of Patients	Progression (%)	Mean Time Interval to Progression (mo)
Campion et al. (22)	100	25	20
Robertson et al. (63)	1781	15	24
Syrjänen et al. (75)	343	14	18.7
Evans and Monaghan (27)	51	15	12
Heinzl et al. (35)	2528	10	24
Nash et al. (49)	45	33	11
Nasiell et al. (51)	555	7	24
Richart and Barron (61)	462	24	24
Meisels et al. (48)	110	9	18

with different natural histories. The majority of low-grade lesions spontaneously regress, whereas the high-grade lesions are less likely to do so. Since high-grade lesions may be small and high in the canal they may be more easily missed while a simultaneous low-grade lesion on the ectocervix is detected. This view is supported by the results of a recent natural history study. Among 241 cytologically normal women at enrollment, there were 26 women who developed biopsy confirmed CIN 2–3 within the first 12 months of follow-up (41a).

Clinical Management. The optimal management of women with CIN depends on the integration of the following procedures: 1) cytology, 2) colposcopy, 3) directed cervical biopsy, 4) endocervical curettage, and 5) cervical cone biopsy. The guiding principle is that there must be concordance between the cytologic, colposcopic, and histologic findings before treatment is instituted. The first goal is to rule out the presence of invasive disease. If this is accomplished, treatment then depends on the anatomic site and grade and extent of the CIN.

After a Papanicolaou smear showing CIN, colposcopy is performed to identify the lesion responsible for the abnormal smear and to delineate the boundaries of the cervical transformation zone. Colposcopic examination is considered satisfactory if the full extent of the lesion and the entire transformation zone are visible. Multiple biopsies of the abnormal areas and an endocervical curettage are performed to ensure that the most severe lesion has been sampled. In patients with adequate colposcopy, an endocervical curettage is performed to identify invasive squamous carcinoma, adenocarcinoma, or endocervical involvement by CIN that is not amenable to outpatient management (69). An endocervical curettage result that is positive for CIN in this circumstance should not lead immediately to a cone biopsy, however, because the majority of these positive endocervical curettage results are caused by contamination (70). Indications for a diagnostic cervical cone biopsy include 1) unsatisfactory colposcopy and an endocervical curettage that shows no more than microinvasive carcinoma; 2) biopsy or endocervical curettage suggesting invasion, revealing microinvasion, or showing CIN with deep gland involvement; 3) lack of correlation between the cytologic, colposcopic, and histologic findings; and 4) biopsy or endocervical curettage revealing adenocarcinoma in situ.

The clinical management of cervical neoplasia depends mainly on separating noninvasive from invasive disease. High-grade lesions (CIN 2 and 3) are treated, but there is no consensus in the management of low-grade lesions (CIN 1). In view of the high spontaneous regression rate of low-grade lesions, some gynecologists elect to observe such lesions, whereas other gynecologists treat them by local ablation, such as cryotherapy or by excision, notably with the use of loop electrosurgery. Patients with low-grade lesions that are not treated should have careful follow-up. High-grade lesions are treated by laser vaporization, electrocautery loop excision, cervical cone biopsy, or rarely, hysterectomy. Therapy should be based on the size and extent of the lesion, the experience of the gynecologist with various techniques, and the desires of the patient. Generally, large lesions tend to be of higher grade and involve more of the endocervical canal.

Long-term follow-up studies indicate that there is a low but significant recurrence rate of CIN after treatment. In comparing cone biopsy to hysterectomy for the treatment of CIN 3, Kolstad and Klem (37) found a 1 percent recurrence rate for patients treated by cone biopsy and a 2 percent recurrence rate for those treated by hysterectomy. These investigators found that, of 25 women with inadequately excised lesions, 4 (16 percent) had recurrences. In contrast, in a series of 948 patients with CIN 3, McIndoe and colleagues (46) found that the development of subsequent invasive disease was not influenced by whether the lesion was completely excised. The most important predictor of recurrent disease was the follow-up cytology. Among 139 women with normal cytology after incomplete excision, invasive cancer later developed in 35 percent of the cases. In contrast, invasive carcinoma developed in 22 percent of women with continuing abnormal cytology, even when the original lesion had been completely removed. Women treated for CIN must therefore undergo long-term follow-up, because these investigators found that invasive cancer was 3.2 times more likely to develop in women treated

for CIN 3 with normal follow-up by cytology than in women who had never had CIN 3.

Squamous Cell Carcinoma

Definition. All invasive neoplasms composed exclusively or almost exclusively of malignant squamous cells. These tumors are broadly divided into two categories: 1) microinvasive carcinomas, which invade the cervical stroma to a limited extent; and 2) frankly invasive carcinomas, which invade to a depth beyond the limits used to define microinvasive carcinoma.

In view of the importance of microinvasive carcinoma from the standpoint of diagnosis, treatment, and prognosis and the controversy over its definition, this category is considered separately from frankly invasive squamous carcinoma.

Microinvasive Carcinoma

Definition. The definition of microinvasive squamous cell carcinoma has evolved over the years, with the early proponents discovering that carcinomas with invasion less than 5 mm penetration of the stroma seldom metastasized. Subsequent studies relating the depth of invasion to survival or lymph node metastasis led the Society of Gynecologic Oncologists to propose a definition of microinvasion as invasion of the stroma from the point of origin to a depth of less than 3 mm; lesions with vascular/lymphatic invasion are excluded from the category. The most recent modification in the definition of microinvasive carcinoma is based on the 1985 FIGO staging (Table 3). According to the new guidelines, carcinomas showing microscopically evident minute foci of invasion, i.e., up to 1 mm, are considered stage IA1, and those that are larger but do not exceed 5 mm in depth of invasion and 7 mm in a horizontal dimension are regarded as stage IA2. Larger lesions are stage IB. The presence of vascular/lymphatic invasion does not influence the stage.

General Features. Since the recognition of small invasive carcinomas of the cervix and the introduction of the term *microcarcinoma* for this entity by Mestwerdt (132), there has been confusion in terminology, controversy over the diagnosis, and uncertainty about its treatment. A variety of terms such as *early stromal invasion, superficially invasive squamous carcinoma,*

Table 3

1985 MODIFICATION OF FIGO STAGING OF CARCINOMA OF THE CERVIX UTERI

Stage*	Description
0	Preinvasive carcinoma (intraepithelial carcinoma, carcinoma in situ).
I	Carcinoma strictly confined to the cervix (extension to the corpus should be disregarded).
IA	Preclinical carcinomas of the cervix, i.e., those diagnosed only by microscopy.
IA1	Minimal microscopically evident stromal invasion.
IA2	Lesions detected microscopically that can be measured. The upper limit of the measurement should not show a depth of invasion of more than 5 mm taken from either the base of the epithelium, either surface or glandular, from which it originates. A second dimension, the horizontal spread, must not exceed 7 mm. Larger lesions should be staged as IB.
IB	Lesions of greater dimensions than stage IA2 regardless of whether seen clinically. Preformed space involvement should not alter the staging but should be specifically recorded for possible use in future treatment decisions.
IIA	Invasive carcinoma that extends beyond the cervix, involving the upper two thirds of the vagina.
IIB	Invasive carcinoma that involves the upper two thirds of the vagina, with parametrial infiltration that has not reached the pelvic side wall.
III	Invasive carcinoma that extends to either lateral pelvic wall and/or the lower third of the vagina and/or hydronephrosis or nonfunction of kidney due to tumor.
IV	Invasive carcinoma that involves the mucosa of the urinary bladder and/or rectum or extends beyond the true pelvis.

* Stage 0 includes those cases with full thickness involvement of epithelium, with atypical cells but with no signs of invasion into the stroma.

Over the last several decades, there has been continued confusion about the stages of preclinical invasive carcinoma of the cervix. Several classification systems have been developed but have generally not been satisfactory. The addition of colposcopy in many countries has caused further confusion as to what is a clinical lesion. There has also been increased pressure to put measurements into the definition. For these reasons, a new definition is proposed.

Stage IA carcinoma should include minimal microscopically evident stromal invasion and small cancerous tumors of measurable size. Stage IA should be divided into those lesions with minute foci of invasion visible only microscopically as stage IA1, and the macroscopically measurable microcarcinomas as stage IA2, to gain further knowledge of the clinical behavior of these lesions. The term *IB occult* should be omitted.

The diagnosis of both stages IA1 and IA2 should be based on microscopic examination of removed tissue, preferably a cone, which must include the entire lesion. As noted above, the lower limit of stage IA2 disease is that it can be measured macroscopically (even if dots need to be placed on the slide before measurement), and the upper limit of IA2 is defined by measuring the two largest dimensions in any given section. The depth of invasion should not be more than 5 mm taken from the base of the epithelium, either surface or glandular, from which it originates. The second dimension, the horizontal spread, must not exceed 7 mm. Vascular space involvement, either venous or lymphatic, should not alter the staging but should be specifically recorded because it may affect treatment decisions in the future. Lesions of greater size should be staged as IB.

As a rule, it is impossible to estimate clinically whether a cancer of the cervix has extended to the corpus. Extension to the corpus should therefore be disregarded.

Table 4

CORRELATION OF DEPTH OF INVASION WITH
LYMPH NODE METASTASIS AND RECURRENCE OR DEATH

Depth of Invasion	No. of Patients	Positive Lymph Nodes	Recurrence/ Death
Up to 1 mm	237	0.4%	0/0
1.1 to 3 mm	375	1.3%	0.5%/0
3.1 to 5 mm	132	6.8%	2.3%/1.5%

Adapted from Fu and Reagen (108).

microinvasive carcinoma, and *microcarcinoma* have been proposed, and controversy continues over whether depth of invasion or volumetric measurements should be used to define the lesion (80,115,131,135,158). Because of the lack of agreement over the criteria for the diagnosis, it is difficult to compare the results of studies aimed at determining the optimal treatment. Which lesions can be safely treated by simple hysterectomy or even cone biopsy and which require radical hysterectomy and pelvic lymphadenectomy still needs to be determined.

The studies of Burghardt (90) and Burghardt and Holtzer (92) have demonstrated that the volume of tumor is a useful parameter of metastatic potential. Several studies have shown, however, that measuring the depth of invasion and determining the presence of vascular/lymphatic invasion accurately predicts the likelihood of lymph node metastasis (Table 4) (83,131,149,152,158). The likelihood of vascular invasion increases with the depth of invasion; therefore, it is not clear that vascular invasion is an independent risk factor. Nonetheless, although the 1985 FIGO staging states that the presence of vascular/lymphatic invasion does not exclude classification of a tumor as microinvasive, it also states that the presence of vascular/lymphatic invasion should be indicated in the report.

Estimates of the frequency of microinvasion relative to all invasive cervical squamous cancers average approximately 8 percent. The average has varied over the years because of changes in the definition of microinvasion and the increasing use of cytology screening, which has reduced the frequency of frankly invasive carcinoma by increasing the rate of detection and eradication of precursor lesions.

Gross Findings. The gross appearance of microinvasive carcinoma is similar to that of intraepithelial neoplasia, and is best appreciated on colposcopic examination. A variety of colposcopic patterns may be seen, but the presence of abnormal vessels is considered to be the most specific.

Microscopic Findings. Microinvasion is manifested by the presence of irregularly shaped tongues of epithelium projecting from the base of an intraepithelial neoplasm into the stroma (fig. 61). Usually, the intraepithelial lesion is CIN 3, but in rare instances, the overlying epithelium is more differentiated, and the lesion resembles CIN 1 or 2. In these instances, the abnormal cells in the overlying epithelium are confined to the basal and parabasal levels, whereas the superficial epithelium is mature (figs. 62, 63). Typically, differentiation of the neoplastic cells occurs at the point of invasion. The invasive cells contain more abundant eosinophilic cytoplasm than the cells of the adjacent intraepithelial tumor and may show keratinization (figs. 64, 65). An accompanying desmoplasia and inflammatory infiltrate may be evident. Involvement of vascular/lymphatic spaces has been reported in 39 percent of stage IA2 cases (91). Larger lesions tend to have more vascular/lymphatic space invasion than smaller lesions. Because of shrinkage during tissue processing, it may be difficult to differentiate vascular invasion from tissue retraction around tumor nests (figs. 66, 67). In these instances, immunoperoxidase reactions for factor VIII and *Ulex europaeus* facilitates the distinction (fig. 68).

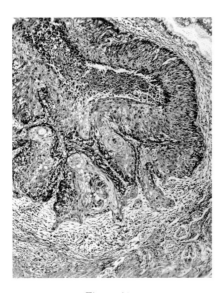

Figure 61

MICROINVASIVE SQUAMOUS CELL CARCINOMA

Multiple irregularly shaped tongues of squamous epithelium invade the underlying stroma from endocervical glands occupied by CIN 3. The loose reactive fibroblastic stroma beneath the epithelium also helps to identify invasion. (Fig. 4 from Leman MH, Benson WL, Kurman RJ, Park RC. Microinvasive carcinoma of the cervix. Obstet Gynecol 1976;48:571–8.)

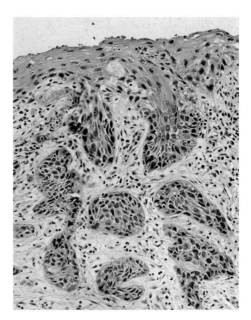

Figure 62

MICROINVASIVE SQUAMOUS CELL CARCINOMA

This lesion is characterized by irregularly shaped nests of epithelium infiltrating the stroma. The overlying squamous epithelium is differentiated, resembling CIN 1. (Figures 62 and 63 are from the same patient.)

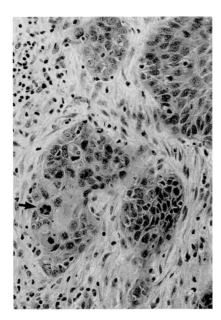

Figure 63

MICROINVASIVE
SQUAMOUS CELL CARCINOMA

A high magnification of figure 62 shows irregularly shaped nests of epithelium invading the stroma. Cytologic atypia is limited to the basal and parabasal cells. Note the presence of an abnormal mitotic figure (arrow).

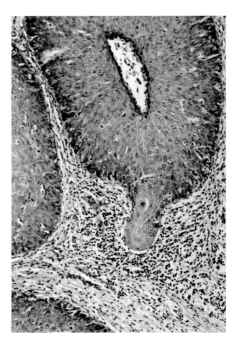

Figure 64

MICROINVASIVE SQUAMOUS CELL CARCINOMA

At the point of invasion, the cells contain more abundant eosinophilic cytoplasm than the overlying cells. This invasive bud measures less than 1 mm and the tumor therefore qualifies as stage IA1.

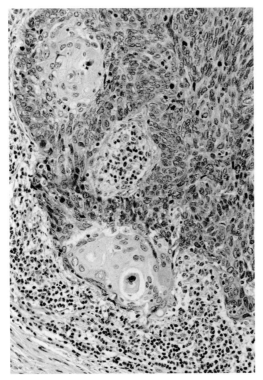

Figure 65
MICROINVASIVE SQUAMOUS CELL CARCINOMA
In this microinvasive carcinoma, there is squamous differentiation at the point of invasion.

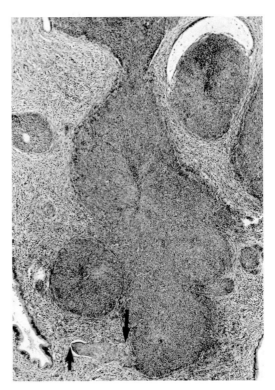

Figure 66
MICROINVASIVE SQUAMOUS CELL CARCINOMA
Microinvasion is present at the base of a gland that has been entirely replaced by CIN 3. The depth of invasion should be measured from the base of the gland at the point of invasion (large arrow) to the tip of the invasive bud (small arrow). In this instance, the invasive bud measures less than 1 mm and the tumor therefore qualifies as stage IA1. (Figures 66 and 67 are from the same patient.)

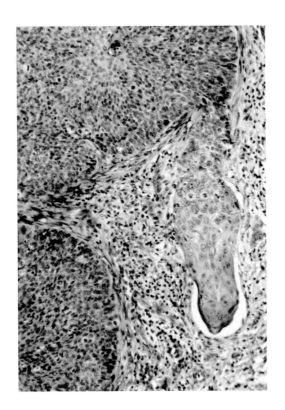

Figure 67
MICROINVASIVE
SQUAMOUS CELL CARCINOMA
This high magnification demonstrates the presence of invasive squamous epithelium within a space that is suggestive but not diagnostic of vascular invasion.

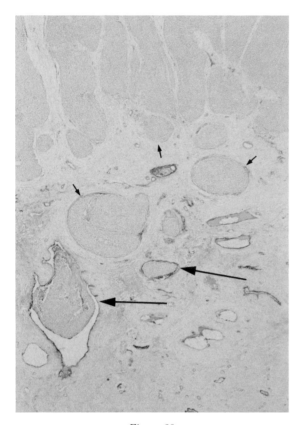

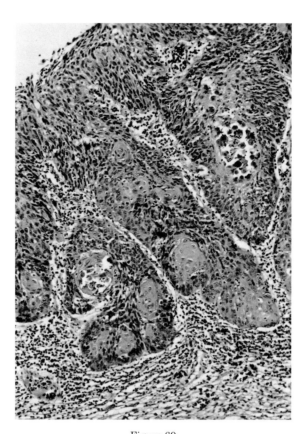

Figure 68

MICROINVASIVE SQUAMOUS CELL CARCINOMA

Immunoperoxidase reaction for factor VIII clearly delineates endothelial-lined spaces (large arrows) and helps in identifying vascular invasion. Note the absence of a positive reaction surrounding the nests of carcinoma at the top and center of the field (small arrows).

Figure 69

MICROINVASIVE SQUAMOUS CELL CARCINOMA

In this field, CIN 3 extensively involves endocervical glands. Multiple foci of squamous differentiation are present within the epithelium. This feature is often found in association with invasion and therefore should alert the pathologist to look for invasion nearby. (Figures 69 and 70 are from the same patient.)

Growth patterns of microinvasive carcinoma are usually described as finger-like or confluent, however, the distinction between these two patterns is too subjective to have any significance. Inflammation is present and admixed with the invading tumor in more than 50 percent of cases. In a study of 47 conization specimens, CIN extended to the margin of excision in nearly half the cases (130). In one case in which CIN was present at the margin of the cone biopsy, subsequent radical hysterectomy revealed residual carcinoma invading to 8 mm. Thus, involvement of the cone margin by invasive carcinoma or even by a high-grade CIN precludes a diagnosis of microinvasive carcinoma because deeper invasion may be present higher in the endocervix.

Differential Diagnosis. Microinvasion can be confused with CIN 3 with gland involvement

as a result of tangential cutting, sectioning, or crush artifacts. Prior biopsy with implantation of benign epithelium or CIN in the underlying regenerating stroma can also be confused with microinvasion. The most common problem, however, is overdiagnosis of CIN 3 as microinvasive carcinoma. The presence of necrosis or pearl formation within masses of squamous epithelium, interpreted as glandular involvement, are features useful in distinguishing high-grade CIN from microinvasive squamous carcinoma. Both of these features, if present in what appears to be CIN 3, suggest the presence of nearby microinvasion (figs. 69, 70). Although rarely present in intraepithelial processes, these features should prompt a careful search for the presence of microinvasion.

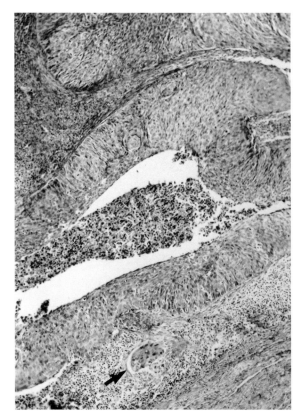

Figure 70
MICROINVASIVE SQUAMOUS CELL CARCINOMA
Central necrosis within an intraglandular CIN 3 lesion
should alert the pathologist to look for invasion (arrow).

Clinical Behavior and Treatment. The treatment for microinvasive carcinoma remains controversial. In the United States, treatment tends to be aggressive and most gynecologists follow the recommendations of the Society of Gynecologic Oncologists. Treatment is based on the depth of invasion and the presence of vascular invasion because the depth of invasion is easily measurable and is a reliable parameter of lymph node metastasis and survival. The method for measuring depth of invasion is shown in figure 71. A compilation of several series correlating depth of invasion with lymph node metastasis is shown in Table 4. Based on these findings, tumors invading less than 1 mm are treated by a simple hysterectomy, whereas those invading to 3 mm without vascular invasion are treated by a moderately extended so-called type II radical hysterectomy (103). In Europe however, tumors with inva-

sion less than 1 mm, i.e., stage IA1, are treated by cone biopsy because such lesions are almost never associated with lymph node metastasis (0.4 percent) (127). Treatment for tumors that qualify as stage IA2 is individualized and ranges from a cone biopsy to a simple hysterectomy (91, 127). As Burghardt emphasizes, however, the FIGO staging recommendations are not intended as guidelines for treatment but rather as a method that facilitates comparison of the results of treatment from different institutions (91).

Invasive Squamous Cell Carcinoma

General Features. The incidence and mortality of invasive squamous cell cervical carcinoma has decreased dramatically in the United States over the last three decades. The incidence in the United States was 34/100,000 in 1947, 15/100,000 in 1970, and 10 to 12/100,000 in 1986 (102). Although the incidence was decreasing in the United States before the implementation of mass screening programs, screening has had an additional major impact on both the incidence and mortality (94,107). Twenty-one years after the initiation of a mass screening program in Jefferson County, Kentucky, the incidence decreased by 60 percent, and the mortality in women between the ages of 30 and 59 years decreased by 70 percent. During the same period, there was a 60 percent increase in CIN 3 (94). The significance of cytologic screening in reducing the incidence of cervical cancer is further underscored by comparing the 4.5/100,000 incidence per year in a screened population to the 29/100,000 incidence in an unscreened population. Both cohorts exhibited similar epidemiologic characteristics (107).

Invasive squamous cell carcinoma is the most common cancer in women worldwide, with the exception of skin cancer. The highest rates have been reported in Latin America, where cervical cancer accounts for half of all female cancers. Based on a population-based cancer registry in Panama, the annual incidence of invasive cervical cancer in women between 30 and 50 years of age in high-risk areas is 1 in 1000 (145). In developing countries throughout the world, cervical cancer is a major public health problem and is one of the leading causes of death (159). Recent increases in incidence and mortality rates have

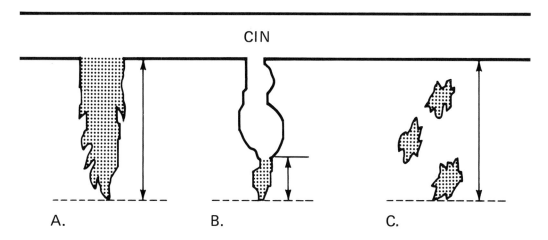

Figure 71
METHODS FOR MEASURING DEPTH OF STROMAL INVASION
These are the methods for measuring depth of stromal invasion for different patterns of stromal invasion. In (A) the invasion originates from the surface so depth of invasion is measured from the basal lamina of the surface epithelium to the deepest cell of the invasive focus. In (B) the invasion originates from a gland so depth of invasion is measured from the gland (not from the surface) to the deepest cell of the invasive focus. In (C) the origin of invasion is indeterminate so invasion is measured from the basal lamina of the surface to the deepest cell in the invasive focus. (Fig. 8.4 from Ferenczy A, Winkler B. Carcinoma and metastatic tumors of the cervix. In: Kurman RJ, ed. Blaustein's pathology of the female genital tract. 3rd ed. New York: Springer-Verlag, 1987.)

been observed in some Western countries including Canada, Great Britain, Sweden, and Norway (93,105,126,137). In the United States, the incidence among blacks and Hispanics is two times higher than among whites.

Socioeconomic, religious, sexual, obstetric, and dietary factors; immunosuppression; smoking, and oral contraceptive intake have been studied in relation to cervical cancer. Studies indicate that the risk of cervical cancer is increased by the number of sexual partners, the age at which sexual intercourse is initiated, and the promiscuity of the male partner. Husbands of women with cervical cancer have been found to have more sexual partners than husbands of controls (89). In a recent study, smokers had a twofold excess risk of cancer, with the risk linked to smoking intensity and duration (87). The effect was most striking among women who had smoked continuously up to the time of cancer diagnosis and women who began smoking late in life, suggesting that smoking played a promotional role in cervical cancer rather than an initiating role. Although studies evaluating the risk of cervical cancer and oral contraceptives are

difficult to evaluate because of potential confounding factors, the majority of recent case-control studies indicate that long-term users are at approximately a twofold increased risk (120). The role of venereally transmitted agents, particularly human papillomavirus, is discussed in the chapter Human Papillomaviruses and Cancer of the Lower Female Genital Tract. Finally, studies suggest that dietary carotenoids and vitamin C have a protective effect against cervical cancer (129,146). For a comprehensive review of the epidemiology of cervical cancer, the reader is directed to an excellent review by Brinton and colleagues (88).

Clinical Features. Invasive squamous cell carcinoma is uncommon before the age of 30 years. Half of the patients, however, are less than 50 years old (150), and most are between 45 and 55 years of age at the time of diagnosis. The majority of the patients present with intermittent painless vaginal bleeding, often first noted after sexual intercourse or douching. With advancing disease, bleeding may become continuous, and be accompanied by a malodorous discharge, and pain may supervene. Pain is frequently referred to the flank or leg as a result of tumor invasion of the pelvic wall or sciatic nerves. Involvement of the bladder and rectum during late stages in the evolution of the disease are associated with dysuria, hematuria, rectal bleeding, or obstipation. Involvement of lymphatics may result in edema of the lower extremities.

A cervical biopsy is mandatory for diagnosis. Although sampling problems and incorrect interpretation are partly responsible for false negative smears, necrosis and inflammation on the surface of the tumor may result in only an "atypical smear" that lacks obvious tumor cells. Consequently, the cervix that is abnormal by inspection or palpation is biopsied, even if the cytology smear is normal. In addition to biopsy of the ectocervix, an endocervical curettage is performed as an integral part of the evaluation because invasive carcinoma, particularly adenocarcinoma, frequently involves the endocervical canal and may not be visible on the ectocervix. Clinical tests utilized in the preoperative evaluation of patients with invasive cervical cancer relate to staging and are discussed further in the section on staging.

A number of tumor markers, including carcinoembryonic antigen, cancer antigen 125, and a subfraction of the TA-4 antigen called squamous cell carcinoma antigen, are elevated in patients with cervical cancer (124,157). The squamous cell carcinoma antigen appears to have the greatest utility as a serum tumor marker for squamous cell carcinoma because it is elevated in approximately 60 percent of cases and is rarely elevated in cases of adenocarcinoma (104). Carcinoembryonic antigen and cancer antigen 125 are much less commonly elevated. The frequency of elevated levels of carcinoembryonic antigen is directly related to the stage of disease and has no value in screening (157). Although serum levels of squamous cell carcinoma antigen are correlated with the response to treatment, changes in therapy are based on other diagnostic studies, including tissue biopsies, and not on tumor marker levels.

Gross Findings. Squamous carcinomas can occur either on the ectocervix or in the endocervical canal. They may be exophytic, infiltrative, or ulcerative. Exophytic tumors are polypoid or papillary (fig. 72). When the tumors are large and expand the endocervix, they produce a barrel-

shaped cervix (fig. 73). Infiltrative lesions invade the stroma extensively, resulting in very hard lesions with minimal surface change. Ulcerative lesions erode the cervix, causing an ulcer that involves a portion of the cervix and sometimes the upper vaginal vault (fig. 74).

Microscopic Findings. Invasive squamous cell carcinomas display considerable morphologic heterogeneity, resulting in great variation from one case to another. Most invasive squamous cell carcinomas are composed of compact masses and nests of neoplastic squamous epithelium that may show central keratinization or necrosis (fig. 75). Other tumors are composed of large masses of squamous cells with little intervening stroma. In still other cases, the neoplastic squamous epithelium invades as cords and individual cells (fig. 76), which may show considerable variation in size and shape and in the degree of keratinization. Generally, the cells are oval to polygonal, with eosinophilic cytoplasm. Cell borders are often sharp but may be indistinct, and intercellular bridges are usually not apparent. Nuclei may be relatively uniform or display considerable pleomorphism, and the chromatin tends to be coarse and granular. Mitotic figures are readily apparent, and abnormal mitotic figures are commonly encountered.

Subtypes. Squamous cell carcinomas have been subtyped according to both cell type and degree of differentiation. In the past, the most commonly employed system subdivided squamous cell carcinomas into three categories: large cell nonkeratinizing, large cell keratinizing, and small cell (144). The current classification places small cell carcinoma in a separate category and subdivides the remainder into keratinizing and nonkeratinizing squamous cell carcinomas. Nonkeratinizing carcinomas are characterized by rounded nests of neoplastic squamous cells often showing individual cell keratinization (fig. 77). These tumors are distinguished from keratinizing carcinomas by the absence of keratin pearls. The cells are relatively uniform, and the cell borders are indistinct. The nuclei are round to oval and contain coarse chromatin. Mitotic figures are numerous.

Keratinizing carcinomas are characterized by mature squamous cells arranged in irregularly shaped nests or cords that can vary considerably in size. The most striking feature is the presence

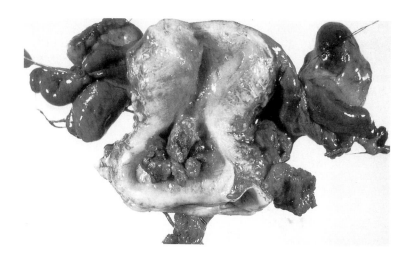

Figure 72
SQUAMOUS CELL CARCINOMA
This is a polypoid invasive squamous cell carcinoma of the cervix. (Courtesy of Dr. B.K. Chun, Washington, DC.)

Figure 73
SQUAMOUS CELL CARCINOMA
(BARREL-SHAPED CERVIX)
A bulky carcinoma expanding the endocervical portion of the endocervix creates a barrel-shaped cervix. Arrows delineate the margin of the tumor and the cervical stroma. (Courtesy of Dr. B.K. Chun, Washington, DC.)

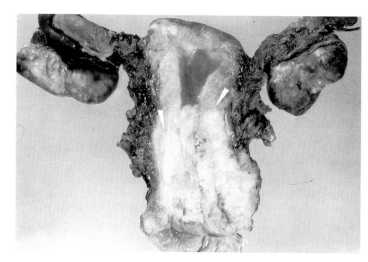

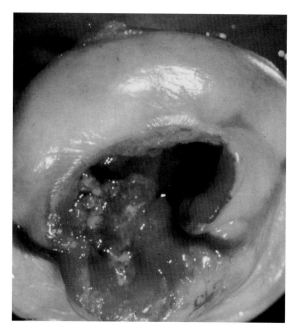

Figure 74
SQUAMOUS CELL CARCINOMA
This ulcerative invasive squamous cell carcinoma erodes the posterior lip of the cervix. (Courtesy of Dr. R.E. Scully, Boston, MA.)

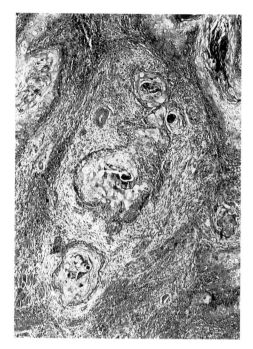

Figure 75
SQUAMOUS CELL CARCINOMA
Nests of this invasive squamous cell carcinoma show central keratinization.

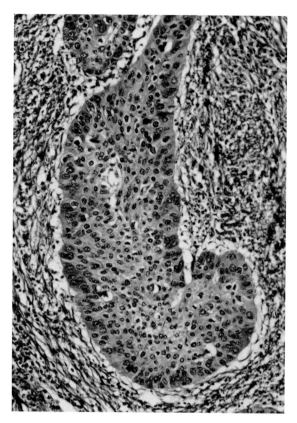

Figure 77
SQUAMOUS CELL CARCINOMA
This invasive squamous cell carcinoma is composed of nonkeratinized squamous epithelium.

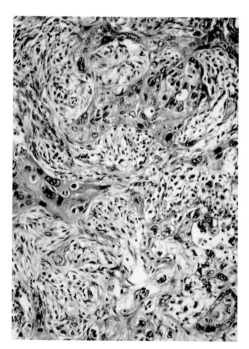

Figure 76
SQUAMOUS CELL CARCINOMA
This tumor is characterized by nests and individual squamous cells infiltrating the stroma. (Figures 76, 88, and 89 are from the same patient.)

of keratin pearls within the nests of neoplastic squamous epithelium (fig. 78). A keratin pearl is characterized by a rounded nest of squamous epithelium in which the cells are arranged in concentric circles surrounding a central focus of acellular keratin. The presence of one pearl is sufficient for a diagnosis of keratinizing squamous cell carcinoma (144). Individual squamous cells are large, with abundant eosinophilic cytoplasm, and many show individual cell keratinization. The cells are tightly adherent and often show prominent intercellular bridges. The nuclei may be enlarged or pyknotic. Mitotic activity is relatively low compared with the other tumor types.

Some squamous cell carcinomas are composed of small oval-shaped basaloid cells, with scant cytoplasm growing in masses and nests (fig. 79) (78). The nuclei are hyperchromatic and display abundant mitotic activity. Necrosis is frequently observed. Foci of more obvious squamous

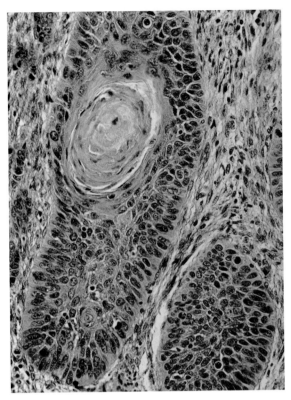

Figure 78
SQUAMOUS CELL CARCINOMA
This invasive squamous cell carcinoma is composed of irregularly shaped nests of keratinized squamous epithelium with a squamous pearl.

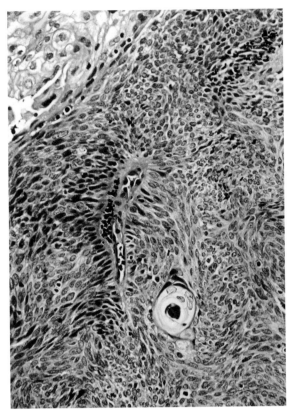

Figure 79
SQUAMOUS CELL CARCINOMA
This invasive squamous cell carcinoma is composed of small spindle-shaped squamous cells with scant cytoplasm. Squamous differentiation is present in the upper left and a squamous pearl is present in the lower right.

differentiation and keratinization are sometimes present, but keratin pearls are absent. These are similar to tumors occurring in the vagina and vulva which have been designated *basaloid carcinoma*. Squamous cell carcinomas composed of small cells should be distinguished from small cell undifferentiated or oat cell–like carcinomas. There is considerable potential for confusion when the term *small cell carcinoma* is used to describe a small cell nonkeratinizing squamous cell carcinoma in contrast to a small cell *undifferentiated* carcinoma similar to the oat cell carcinoma of the lung. It is therefore recommended that the term *small cell carcinoma* be reserved for tumors resembling small cell, i.e., neuroendocrine tumors in other anatomic sites such as the lung. Although the classification system by cell type has been found to have prognostic value by some investigators, particularly for patients treated by radiation (134,143), it has not been found useful by others (109,111).

Microscopic Grading. Most pathologists grade squamous cell carcinomas of the cervix with a modification of the Broder system. Well-differentiated tumors (grade 1) are composed predominantly of mature squamous cells, with abundant keratin and pearl formation and minimal mitotic activity (fig. 78). The nuclei are uniform and the cells occasionally display well-developed intercellular bridges.

Moderately differentiated carcinomas (grade 2) are composed of cells with less abundant cytoplasm. Cell borders are less distinct, and the nuclei have greater pleomorphism. Mitotic activity is higher than in well-differentiated tumors (fig. 76).

Poorly differentiated neoplasms (grade 3) are composed of masses and nests of small primitive-appearing oval cells with scant cytoplasm and hyperchromatic spindle-shaped nuclei with high mitotic activity. Keratinization is minimal or

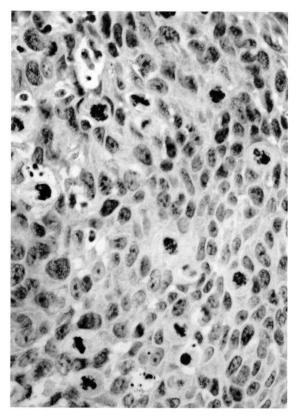

Figure 80
SQUAMOUS CELL CARCINOMA

This poorly differentiated invasive squamous carcinoma is composed of cells displaying minimal squamous differentiation and bizarre highly pleomorphic nuclei with abundant mitotic activity.

absent, and the neoplastic cells resemble those in high-grade CIN (fig. 79). Pleomorphic carcinomas that have minimal squamous differentiation, bizarre highly pleomorphic nuclei, and abundant mitotic activity (fig. 80) are also included in this category. There have been conflicting reports regarding the predictive value of this grading system (95,151), however recent studies have failed to show that this grading system correlates with outcome (96,97,161).

In an effort to improve the predictive value of histologic grading and to identify high-risk patients who might benefit from more aggressive therapy at the outset, a "malignancy grading system" has been described (79,154). This system evaluates eight different parameters: structure, cell type, nuclear atypia, mitotic activity, type of tumor margin, pattern of invasion, vascular invasion, and inflammatory reaction to assess the

tumor-host relationship more completely. Using this system and an abbreviated version, some investigators have reported that the malignancy grading system was superior to staging in predicting prognosis (84,153). Other groups have been unable to confirm these findings (96,97). Currently, the malignancy grading system is not used in clinical practice.

In summary, there has been no conclusive demonstration that a histologic grading system or the histologic typing system proposed by Reagan and associates (144) reliably predicts prognosis. Zaino and colleagues (161) found, however, that the presence of vascular invasion and depth of invasion were highly reliable predictors of behavior. Accordingly, in reporting squamous cell carcinomas, the depth of invasion (in millimeters or the proportion of the wall invaded), the presence or absence of vascular invasion, and the size of the tumor (greatest tumor dimension) should be reported. In contrast, histologic grading and classification into keratinizing and nonkeratinizing types are optional.

Immunohistochemical Findings. Immunoreactive cytokeratin and involucrin, a marker for squamous differentiation distinct from keratin, can be identified in invasive squamous cell carcinomas. In general, there is a correlation in the pattern of both of these proteins and the degree of cellular differentiation. Involucrin can be identified within the differentiated areas in the vast majority of squamous carcinomas (148). A variety of low- and high–molecular-weight cytokeratins, with differing patterns of distribution, can be found in poorly differentiated and nonkeratinizing carcinomas (99). High–molecular-weight keratins are present in well-differentiated keratinizing carcinomas (81).

Carcinoembryonic antigen and a cervical carcinoma tumor-associated antigen, TA-4, can be localized immunohistochemically in squamous cell carcinomas. Currently, tumor markers are not routinely used in clinical practice.

Finally, it has been shown that the *ras* oncogene product p21 can be localized at the cell membrane of invasive squamous cell carcinoma by immunohistochemical methods on formalin-fixed paraffin-embedded tissue. Overexpression of p21 in large cell keratinizing and nonkeratinizing squamous cell carcinomas has been associated with a poor prognosis (147).

Ultrastructural Findings. The malignant squamous cells of moderately and well-differentiated squamous carcinomas lose their well-developed intracytoplasmic tonofilaments, desmoplastic-tonofilament complexes, and intercellular microvilli with decreasing differentiation. There is also a decrease in gap-junction nexuses in squamous carcinomas compared with normal cervical squamous epithelium (106).

Morphometric Findings. Most squamous cell carcinomas are aneuploid, and approximately 20 to 40 percent are diploid. Unlike the results in other areas of the body, reports to date indicate that microscopic grading has not correlated well with ploidy levels possibly because of the morphologic heterogeneity of these tumors. Flow analyses show 25 percent disagreement in DNA values on the same tumor (121,155). There is a tendency for aneuploid tumors to be associated with vascular invasion, aggressive growth patterns, and advanced-stage disease, but the prognosis between aneuploid and diploid tumors is about the same (100,121,155), perhaps because the high proliferative activity of aneuploid tumors makes them more radiosensitive.

Differential Diagnosis. Invasive squamous cell carcinoma can be confused with benign lesions, including squamous metaplasia with extensive gland involvement and a marked decidual reaction. The features that distinguish these lesions from carcinoma are the absence of nuclear atypia and level of mitotic activity. Although immature squamous metaplasia may display a low level of mitotic activity, the cells are uniform in size and shape and lack significant nuclear atypia. Decidual cells lack mitotic activity and display no cytologic atypia. Immunoperoxidase reactions for cytokeratin are helpful in distinguishing decidua because decidual cells are negative, whereas carcinoma cells are strongly positive.

Placental-site nodules or plaques may also be confused with squamous cell carcinoma. These lesions represent incompletely resorbed hyalinized implantation sites and appear as well-circumscribed nodules or plaques containing intermediate trophoblastic cells (see figs. 175, 176) (160). Typically, the cells are arranged in nests surrounded by hyaline material and show no or minimal mitotic activity. Placental site nodules or plaques are focally positive immunocytochemically for placental lactogen. In contrast, squamous cell carcinomas are not well circumscribed, show at least some mitotic activity, and are rarely positive for placental lactogen.

There may be confusion with clear cell carcinoma when squamous cell carcinomas contain cells with abundant glycogen, resulting in masses of clear cells that resemble the solid areas of clear cell adenocarcinomas (fig. 81). In addition to the solid areas, clear cell adenocarcinomas usually have papillary or tubulocystic areas and hobnail as well as clear cells. Clear cell adenocarcinomas also lack squamous differentiation and, unlike squamous cell carcinoma, are often associated with in utero diethylstilbestrol exposure in young women.

Poorly differentiated squamous cell carcinomas that are composed predominantly of small cells merge with small cell (undifferentiated) carcinomas of neuroendocrine type (see Other Epithelial Tumors – Small Cell Carcinoma). Neurosecretory granules, evident by immunohistochemical staining or electron microscopy, are typically

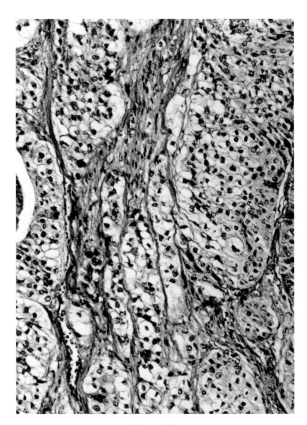

Figure 81
SQUAMOUS CELL CARCINOMA
In this invasive squamous cell carcinoma, the cytoplasm is clear due to the presence of abundant glycogen.

identified in small cell (undifferentiated) carcinoma. Occasionally, however, both of these methods are negative for dense-core granules. Conversely, some small cell carcinomas have squamous cell features on electron microscopy. In most cases, small cell carcinoma can be distinguished from a squamous cell carcinoma composed of small cells on the basis of conventional light-microscopic features. Small cell carcinomas have a distinctive growth pattern characterized by diffuse infiltration by small nests, sheets, and typically individual cells. Rosettes, trabeculae, and ribbons are also frequently present. Squamous cells are larger with larger nuclei and abundant cytoplasm. The nuclei lack prominent nucleoli and are intensely hyperchromatic, with smudged chromatin that obscures the nuclear detail. A characteristic crush artifact is another useful diagnostic clue. In contrast, squamous cell carcinomas composed of small cells have oval-shaped nuclei and granular chromatin arranged in cohesive nests. Squamous differentiation is occasionally seen in the centers of some nests. In addition, the cells in these nests tend to be perpendicular to the basement membrane (110). Occasionally, the distinction may be extremely difficult, in which case, immunohistochemistry and electron microscopy may be helpful.

Spread and Metastasis. Cervical carcinoma spreads primarily by local extension and lymphatic spread; hematogenous spread is unusual. Local extension may involve the adjacent vaginal mucosa, parametrial soft tissue and pelvic wall, lower uterine segment and corpus, and hypogastric, external iliac, and sacral lymph nodes and, secondarily, the common iliac, inguinal, and para-aortic nodes (figs. 82–84) (117). There is a close correlation between the stage and the frequency of lymph node metastasis. Lymph node involvement occurs in 15 to 20 percent of stage IB tumors, 25 to 40 percent of stage II tumors, and 50 percent of stage III and IV tumors. Approximately one third of patients with para-aortic node involvement have metastasis to the scalene nodes.

Staging. The current FIGO staging system is shown in Table 3 and illustrated in Plates I and II. Clinical staging is done primarily to permit comparison of the results of treatment and secondarily to provide guidelines for therapy. The stage approximates the extent of disease. Radiologic eval-

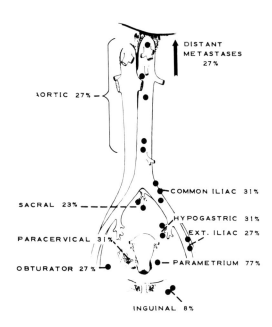

Figure 82
LYMPHATIC SPREAD OF CERVICAL CARCINOMA
This figure illustrates the frequency of lymph node involvement in 26 unrelated fatal cases of cervical carcinoma. (Fig. 2 from Henriksen E. The lymphatic spread of carcinoma of the cervix and of the body of the uterus. Am J Obstet Gynecol 1949;58:924–42.)

uation of the chest, intravenous pyelography, cystoscopy, proctosigmoidoscopy, and barium enema are performed routinely to determine the stage. Lymphangiography, ultrasound, and computerized tomography scanning are not used for clinical staging. Surgical staging is used to determine the presence of extrapelvic disease. Careful surgical staging reveals that the clinical stage is often inaccurate, with error rates ranging from 25 percent in stage I cases to 50 percent in stage III cases (150). These discrepancies explain why the clinical stage is a relatively insensitive predictor of prognosis.

Treatment. The treatment of frankly invasive squamous cell carcinoma is determined primarily from the clinical stage and consists of either radiation, a surgical operation, or both. Advanced-stage disease, i.e., beyond stage IIA, is treated primarily by radiotherapy, whereas the early-stage disease is treated by either radiation or a

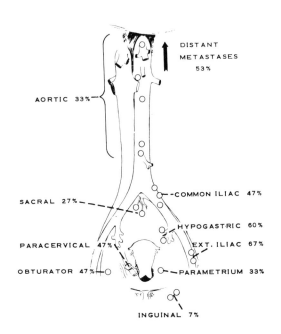

Figure 83
LYMPHATIC SPREAD OF CERVICAL CARCINOMA
This figure illustrates the frequency of lymph node involvement in 15 treated but fatal cases of cervical carcinoma. (Fig. 3 from Henriksen E. The lymphatic spread of carcinoma of the cervix and of the body of the uterus. Am J Obstet Gynecol 1949;58:924–42.)

radical surgical procedure. A combination of radiation and extrafascial hysterectomy is performed for large-volume and barrel-shaped stage IB lesions because the upper limits of the tumor often extend beyond the range of the field of radiation. The survival of stage IB patients is 80 to 85 percent, treated either by surgical therapy or radiation (101). A surgical procedure is preferred for younger patients because the ovaries can be conserved in view of the rarity of metastatic involvement. In addition, there is less likelihood of subsequent sexual dysfunction because the vagina is not altered, as it is after radiation. Radical hysterectomy is not performed for large stage IB tumors if the surgical margins may be involved or if extrapelvic disease is discovered at the time of operation. The radical hysterectomy performed for patients with stage IB or IIA disease consists of a wide excision of parametrial and paravaginal tissue, which requires partial mobilization of the bladder from the cervix and extensive dissection of the ureters. Upper vaginectomy and pelvic lymphadenectomy are also performed.

Prognosis. The prognosis after surgical treatment for stage IB squamous cell carcinoma depends on a variety of interrelated factors, the most important of which are the tumor size (138,156), depth of stromal invasion (119), and lymph node status. For patients with tumors less

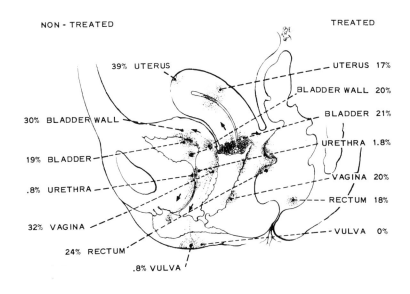

Figure 84
SPREAD OF CERVICAL CARCINOMA
This figure illustrates the frequency of involvement of adjacent tissues by cervical carcinoma from a series of 356 fatal cases. (Fig. 106 from Fascicle 33, Part 2, First Series.)

PLATE I

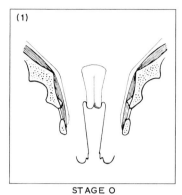

STAGE 0

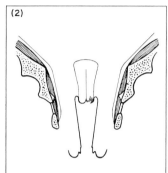

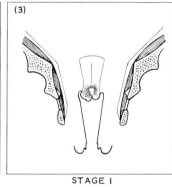

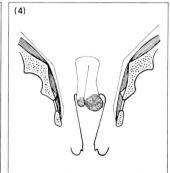

STAGE I

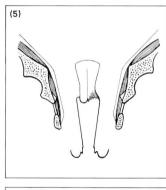

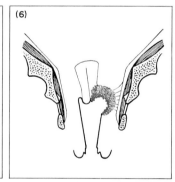

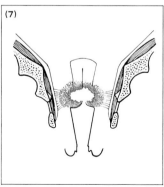

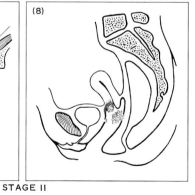

STAGE II

STAGES OF CERVICAL CARCINOMA

Cervical carcinoma stages 0, I, and II are represented by these drawings. (Pl. IV from Fascicle 33, Part 2, First Series. Adapted from Heyman J, ed. Atlas: inquiry into the results of radiotherapy in cancer of the uterus. Stockholm: League of Nations Health Organization, 1938.)

PLATE II

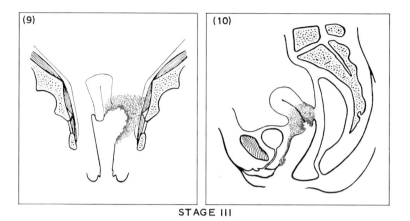

STAGE III

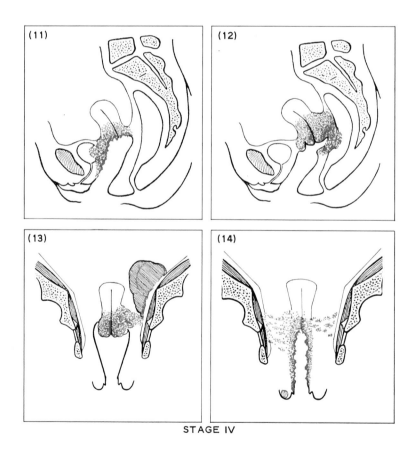

STAGE IV

STAGES OF CERVICAL CARCINOMA

Cervical carcinoma stages III and IV are represented by these drawings. (Pl. V from Fascicle 33, Part 2, First Series. Adapted from Heyman J, ed. Atlas: inquiry into the results of radiotherapy in cancer of the uterus. Stockholm: League of Nations Health Organization, 1938.)

than 2 cm in greatest dimension, the 5-year survival is approximately 90 percent, compared to 64 percent for patients with tumors 2 cm or greater (150). In one study, patients undergoing a radical hysterectomy for presumed stage I disease had a 95 percent 5-year survival with negative pelvic lymph nodes. Five-year survival fell to 62 percent with one positive node and to 17 percent with two or more positive nodes (150). Metastasis to para-aortic lymph nodes is a poor prognostic sign and is frequently associated with involvement of the scalene lymph nodes. Therefore, extended radiation treatment for patients with positive para-aortic nodes is of little value. The presence of vascular invasion and parametrial involvement also play a role in predicting prognosis (82,86). The grade of the tumor and the cell type, however, have not been reported to show a consistent effect on outcome. There is no consensus in the literature concerning the effect of age on survival.

Recurrence of squamous cell carcinoma develops in 10 to 20 percent of patients treated by radical hysterectomy and bilateral lymphadenectomy. Recurrence is more likely when lymph node metastasis is noted at the time of hysterectomy or if the tumor extends close to the parametrial margins. For patients with these findings, radiation treatment after radical hysterectomy does not appear to improve survival.

Most recurrences occur within 2 years of treatment, and 85 percent of patients who die of disease do so within 3 years (103). In view of the cellular changes induced by radiation, a diagnosis of carcinoma based on cytologic findings may be difficult. A diagnosis of recurrent disease should be based on histologic diagnosis, which permits evaluation of architectural and cytologic features. Nearly 75 percent of recurrences occur in the pelvis; of the remainder, approximately 6 percent involve the lungs (118). Ureteral obstruction with subsequent development of uremia is a complication of recurrent cervical carcinoma in 40 percent of patients (125). After recurrence, the 1-year survival is 10 to 15 percent. Recurrent disease that is confined to the upper vagina and parametrial area can be treated by pelvic exenteration, but with current sophisticated radiotherapy, isolated central pelvic recurrence rarely occurs. Consequently, recurrent disease is almost always treated palliatively.

Verrucous Carcinoma

Verrucous carcinoma is a distinctive type of very well-differentiated squamous cell carcinoma that characteristically tends to recur locally but does not metastasize (128). Because of the problems in diagnosis and the confusion in terminology, it is difficult to be certain how many authentic cases of verrucous carcinoma of the cervix have been reported, but it is probably around 20 to 30 (98). Because verrucous carcinomas are more common on the vulva, they are described in detail in the chapter Tumors of the Vulva.

Papillomavirus type 6 (136) and an unusual variant designated 6b (141) have been identified within verrucous carcinomas of the vagina and vulva by use of molecular hybridization. Clinically, verrucous carcinoma is a slow-growing locally invasive neoplasm that occasionally pursues a relentless course manifested by uncontrolled local recurrence that ultimately results in the death of the patient.

On gross examination, verrucous carcinomas have a warty, fungating appearance. Typically, the tumors are large and bulky and occasionally ulcerated. On cut section, the deep margin is characteristically sharply circumscribed.

Microscopically, verrucous carcinomas are exophytic, with an undulating hyperkeratinized surface composed of rounded or pointed papillary projections that lack central fibrovascular cores. The lack of fibrovascular cores is particularly useful in distinguishing a verrucous carcinoma from a condyloma acuminatum, which displays prominent fibrovascular cores (fig. 85). The deep margin of a verrucous carcinoma is composed of large bulbous masses that invade along a wide front in a "pushing" fashion (fig. 86). Laminated keratin whorls are present within the masses of epithelium. Typical features of the usual form of invasive squamous carcinoma, i.e., irregular prongs of squamous epithelium and small clusters of neoplastic squamous cells infiltrating the stroma, are absent unless a squamous cell carcinoma has supervened. The neoplastic squamous cells show almost no nuclear atypia (fig. 87). At best, the nuclei are slightly enlarged and may show some coarsening of the chromatin with some prominent nucleoli. Mitotic activity is usually low, and koilocytosis is usually not present.

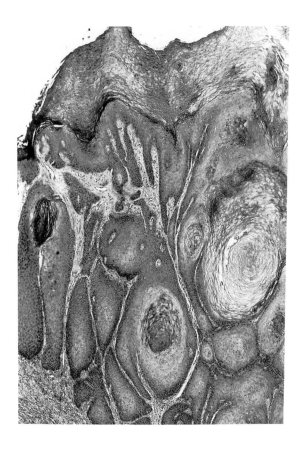

Figure 85
VERRUCOUS CARCINOMA
The tumor is composed of rounded masses of squamous cells with central keratinization lacking fibromuscular cores.

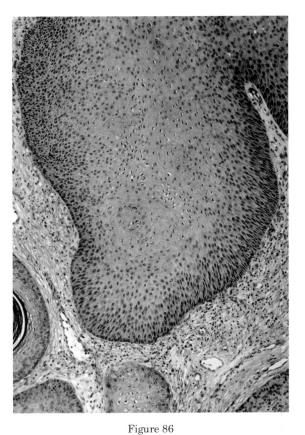

Figure 86
VERRUCOUS CARCINOMA
The tumor is characterized by large bulbous masses of squamous epithelium invading in a "pushing" fashion.

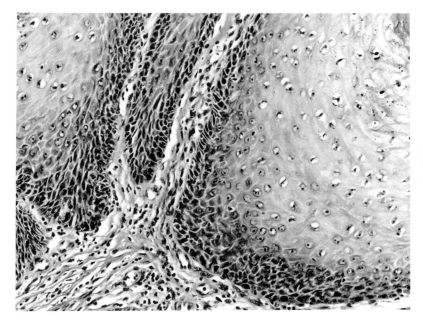

Figure 87
VERRUCOUS CARCINOMA
This high magnification of verrucous carcinoma shows that the neoplastic squamous cells have almost no nuclear atypia.

A benign condyloma may enlarge dramatically, particularly during pregnancy, and regress spontaneously. Such a neoplasm should be classified as a *condyloma acuminatum*, without the adjective *giant* to avoid confusion with verrucous carcinoma. Squamous cell carcinoma may arise in a condyloma, but this tumor is also not synonymous with verrucous carcinoma. Such a lesion should be classified as a *well-differentiated invasive squamous carcinoma arising in a condyloma acuminatum*. Squamous cell carcinoma may also arise immediately adjacent to a verrucous carcinoma and merge with it. Such a tumor should be termed a *mixed verrucous and invasive squamous cell carcinoma*.

Warty (Condylomatous) Carcinoma

Warty (condylomatous) carcinoma is a squamous cell carcinoma that has a striking condylomatous or warty appearance on microscopic examination. In the vulva, this tumor has been designated *warty carcinoma* (142). These tumors may also occur in the cervix and vagina. Like verrucous carcinoma, warty carcinoma appears to have a less aggressive behavior than typical well-differentiated squamous carcinoma, although the experience with this tumor is extremely limited. Microscopically, warty carcinoma, unlike verrucous carcinoma, has the features of a squamous cell carcinoma at the deep margin. Many of the malignant cells display koilocytotic atypia (see Tumors of the Vagina and Tumors of the Vulva).

Papillary Squamous (Transitional) Cell Carcinoma

Papillary squamous cell carcinoma is a rare variant of invasive squamous cell carcinoma (140) and has a superficial resemblance to transitional cell carcinoma of the urinary bladder. The clinical behavior of papillary squamous cell carcinoma resembles typical invasive squamous carcinoma of the cervix, except that, in the small series reported by Randall and colleagues (140), three recurrences developed after 7 years. This is unusual for squamous carcinoma of the cervix.

Microscopically, papillary squamous cell carcinoma is characterized by a papillary architecture with papillae that are covered by several layers of atypical basaloid cells displaying abundant mitoses and little or no evidence of matura-

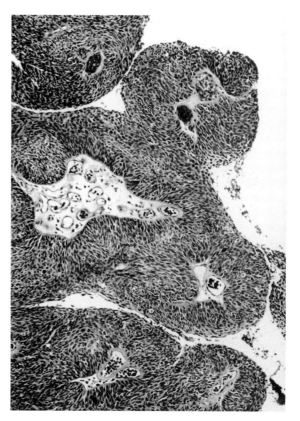

Figure 88
PAPILLARY SQUAMOUS CELL CARCINOMA
This tumor is characterized by papillary processes in which the papillae are covered by several layers of atypical basaloid cells. Invasion of the cervical stroma was present elsewhere (see fig. 76). (Figures 88, 89, and 76 are from the same patient.)

tion (figs. 88, 89). Occasionally, focal squamous differentiation is present (fig. 90). The cells have the appearance of a high-grade squamous intraepithelial lesion with hyperchromatic nuclei and scant cytoplasm and closely resemble transitional cell carcinoma of the urinary bladder. If there is no invasion of the underlying cervical stroma, the tumor qualifies as a *papillary squamous cell carcinoma in situ*. The in situ form of this tumor was erroneously reported in the past as a squamous papilloma (139). In tumors with broad papillae, invasion may also be detected within the fibrovascular core of the papillae. Invasive squamous carcinoma is usually evident at the base of the tumor. Sometimes invasion is manifested by well-circumscribed nests of epithelium in continuity with papillae extending deep

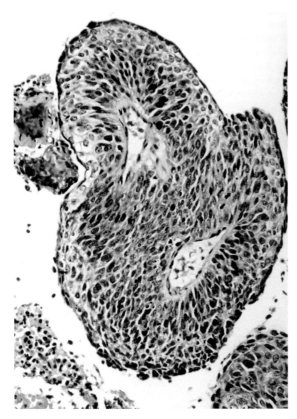

Figure 89
PAPILLARY SQUAMOUS CELL CARCINOMA
This high magnification of papillary squamous car-
cinoma shows basaloid cells with hyperchromatic nuclei.
Slight surface maturation is present.

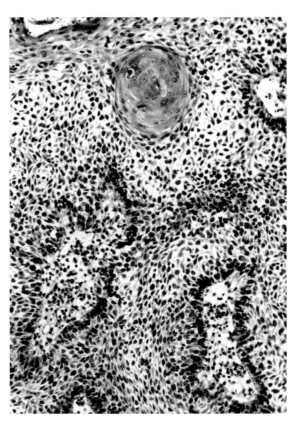

Figure 90
PAPILLARY SQUAMOUS CELL CARCINOMA
Focal squamous differentiation is present.

into the stroma. In other areas, the invasive
tumor resembles a typical (nonpapillary) squamous cell carcinoma (see fig. 76). It should be
emphasized that a superficial biopsy revealing a
papillary squamous cell carcinoma must be considered an invasive neoplasm until proved otherwise. At minimum this requires a cone biopsy.

It is important to recognize this entity because
it is aggressive and capable of metastasis. It
should therefore not be confused with a condyloma acuminatum with atypia, a squamous papilloma with atypia, or a verrucous carcinoma.
Unlike verrucous carcinoma, the projections of
papillary squamous cell carcinoma are covered by
basaloid-type cells with hyperchromatic atypical
nuclei rather than relatively bland epithelium. Similarly, a condyloma with atypia or a squamous papilloma with atypia shows evidence of maturation,
and the condyloma also displays koilocytosis.

Lymphoepithelioma-Like Carcinoma

Lymphoepithelioma-like carcinoma tends to
be well circumscribed and is composed of undifferentiated cells surrounded by a marked inflammatory infiltrate in the stroma (116). Histologically similar neoplasms occur in the
nasopharynx, salivary glands, breast, and thy-
mus, and the terms *lymphoepithelioma* and
medullary carcinoma have been applied to them
(112–114,133). We prefer the designation
lymphoepithelioma-like carcinoma. In the nasopharynx, these tumors have been shown to contain Epstein-Barr virus by in situ hybridization.
Epstein-Barr virus has not been identified in the
small number of cervical lymphoepithelioma-
like carcinomas examined. In one of the largest
studies from Japan, this neoplasm accounted for
5.5 percent of cervical carcinomas and was associated with a lower frequency of regional lymph
node metastasis and a significantly better prognosis when stratified according to stage (116).

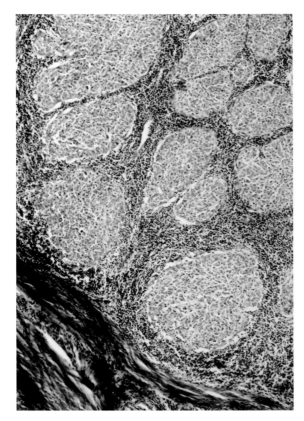

Figure 91
LYMPHOEPITHELIOMA-LIKE CARCINOMA
This tumor is characterized by nests of undifferentiated cells surrounded by a prominent lymphocytic infiltrate. The tumor margin is sharply circumscribed.

Microscopically, lymphoepithelioma-like carcinomas are characterized by a circumscribed margin and nests of undifferentiated cells with abundant cytoplasm and relatively uniform vesicular nuclei (fig. 91). The cell borders tend to be indistinct and form what has been described as a syncytium (133). The nests of neoplastic epithelium are surrounded by an intense inflammatory reaction consisting of lymphocytes, plasma cells, and eosinophils (fig. 91).

Some studies have analyzed the behavior of cervical tumors treated by surgical procedures and radiotherapy according to the extent of lymphoplasmacytic response (122,151) and stromal eosinophilia (85,123). Although the findings have been inconclusive due to the small number of cases, patients with tumors showing a marked lymphoplasmacytic response appear to have a higher survival rate than those in whom the response is minimal. A similar improvement in survival associated with a marked eosinophil infiltration has been suggested, but the results were not significant (123). These studies did not focus on lymphoepithelioma-like carcinoma specifically, although some tumors were probably included among the reported cases.

Lymphoepithelioma-like carcinoma should be distinguished from glassy cell carcinoma, which has a poorer prognosis. Glassy cell carcinoma is also characterized by nests of undifferentiated cells associated with a marked inflammatory response. However, unlike the cells of lymphoepithelioma-like carcinoma, the cells of glassy cell carcinoma have distinct cell borders, ground-glass cytoplasm, nuclei with prominent nucleoli, and a much higher mitotic activity. Lymphoepithelioma-like carcinoma is distinguished from the more commonly encountered nonkeratinizing squamous carcinoma, associated with marked inflammation by the less marked nuclear pleomorphism and hyperchromasia and by its lack of distinct cell borders. Confusion with a lymphoproliferative disorder can be avoided by immunohistochemical testing for cytokeratin, EMA, and leukocyte common antigen (LCA).

GLANDULAR LESIONS

Endocervical Polyp

Endocervical polyps are usually small but can sometimes attain a large size (207); typically, they are solitary, but may be multiple. Polyps often do not produce symptoms, but they may be associated with postcoital bleeding or discharge.

Microscopically, endocervical polyps are covered by varying amounts of squamous and columnar epithelium, depending on their location. Those that are high in the endocervical canal are covered by glandular epithelium, whereas those close to the transformation zone may also be covered by squamous epithelium. The stroma of polyps is composed of fibrous or fibromuscular tissue; thick-walled blood vessels are present at the base of the polyp. The stromal cells are typically bland but they are occasionally plump with prominent nucleoli, especially if inflammation is present. There is no increase in mitotic activity. On occasion, if CIN is present elsewhere in the cervix, it may also be found on the surface of a polyp and sometimes may involve underlying glands.

Müllerian Papilloma

This is a rare benign lesion of the cervix (194). It is identical to its counterpart in the vagina (see Tumors of the Vagina).

Glandular Atypia

Atypia involving endocervical glandular epithelium may occur in association with marked inflammation (fig. 92) or after radiation (figs. 93, 94). Characteristically, the epithelium lining the glands is not stratified. The nuclei are enlarged, pleomorphic, and hyperchromatic and may contain prominent nucleoli (fig. 92). Sometimes multinucleation is present, but mitotic figures are rarely observed. This lesion is distinguished from atypical endocervical hyperplasia and adenocarcinoma in situ by the lack of epithelial stratification, a lesser degree of nuclear atypia, and a paucity of mitotic activity. The smudged appearance of the chromatin and prominent nucleoli seen in glandular atypia also assist in distinguishing this lesion from atypical hyperplasia and adenocarcinoma in situ, which contain nuclei that have coarser chromatin.

Atypical Hyperplasia (Glandular Dysplasia)

Atypical hyperplasia closely resembles adenocarcinoma in situ but differs in that the nuclei are not cytologically malignant (figs. 95, 96) and mitotic figures are less numerous. Nuclear hyperchromatism and enlargement identify the involved glands and pseudostratification of cells is prominent. Cribriform and papillary formations are usually absent in atypical hyperplasia (191). If the cells are atypical but only one gland is involved, a diagnosis of atypical hyperplasia is recommended. By requiring involvement of

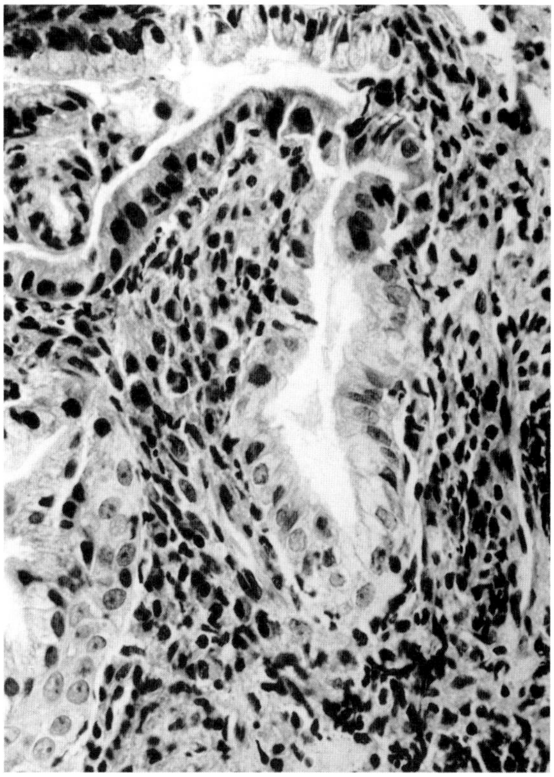

Figure 92
GLANDULAR ATYPIA
Glandular atypia characterized by glands lined by a single layer of epithelium with pleomorphic, hyperchromatic nuclei (upper center). Other cells have enlarged rounded nuclei with prominent nucleoli (lower left).

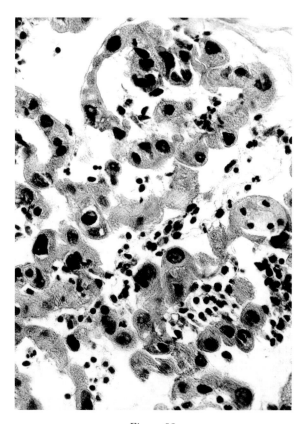

Figure 93
IRRADIATION EFFECT
This figure shows the irradiation effect on endocervical glandular epithelium characterized by nuclear enlargement, hyperchromatism, and granularity of the cytoplasm.

more than one gland for a diagnosis of adenocarcinoma in situ (AIS), there is less chance of confusion with reactive glandular epithelium. Reactive glandular atypia may have enlarged nuclei, macronucleoli and hyperchromatism, but it is associated with marked inflammation and is often near ulceration of the overlying surface.

Adenocarcinoma In Situ

Definition. Adenocarcinoma in situ (AIS) is characterized by the replacement of glandular epithelium by cytologically malignant epithelial cells.

General Features. Adenocarcinoma in situ represents 9 to 25 percent of adenocarcinomas of the cervix (170,215). Patients with AIS usually are a decade or two younger than those with invasive adenocarcinoma (168,169,192,220) but otherwise have the same epidemiologic profile. Most AIS is asymptomatic and found in patients with abnormal cervical smears. Many patients

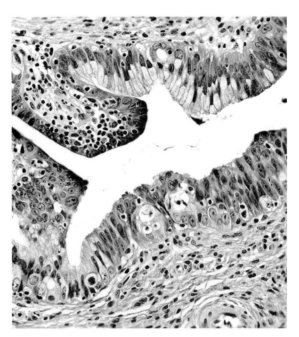

Figure 95
ATYPICAL ENDOCERVICAL HYPERPLASIA
This contrasts with adenocarcinoma in situ in that the cells display slight nuclear atypia but are not fully malignant. The cells retain polarity and have uniform size and shape.

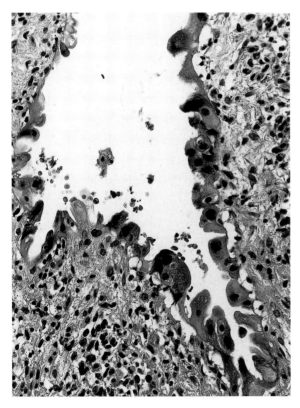

Figure 94
IRRADIATION EFFECT
These cells show marked nuclear pleomorphism but are not stratified and lack mitotic activity.

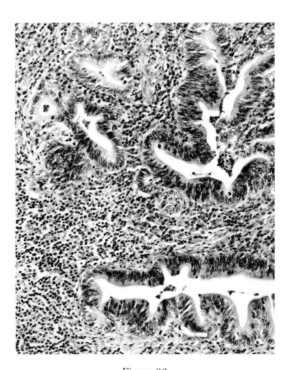

Figure 96
ATYPICAL ENDOCERVICAL HYPERPLASIA
The cells are hyperchromatic but not clearly cytologically malignant, and stratification is minimal.

with AIS present with symptoms from other gynecologic conditions. Thus, in patients with AIS, the most common symptom is vaginal bleeding, occurring in up to 60 percent of the patients (168), but discharge may be present as well (192).

Squamous intraepithelial lesions (cervical intraepithelial neoplasia [CIN]) (fig. 97) or invasive squamous cell carcinoma coexists with AIS in nearly two thirds of the cases (173). An association with CIN is less frequent in invasive adenocarcinoma, which tends to obliterate it. Coexisting high-grade CIN exfoliates atypical cells leading to clinical investigation, and thereby helps identify AIS and adenocarcinoma, which otherwise might be missed on visual examination and cytological smears. About 25 percent of the cases of AIS are accompanied by CIN 1 in the adjoining squamous epithelium (196). Approximately 90 percent of AIS contains HPV messenger RNA, mostly 16 and 18 (181).

Gross Findings. Adenocarcinoma in situ has no distinctive gross appearance (173). It often lies superior to the squamocolumnar junction, outside the transformation zone, and therefore is seldom visible colposcopically (215). When it is visible the epithelium appears only slightly thicker, with the crypts more irregular than normal. AIS is usually multifocal (163,167,175,215).

Microscopic Findings. Microscopically, AIS is characterized by glands lined by cytologically malignant cells. The glands of AIS do not extend below normal glands. AIS spreads along the surface of the endocervix without infiltrating the stroma and producing desmoplasia characteristic of invasive carcinoma (fig. 98).

Endocervical, intestinal, and endometrioid types of AIS have been reported (figs. 99, 100) (186,196). In addition, rare examples of adenosquamous carcinoma in situ (fig. 101) (227) and clear cell carcinoma in situ (189) have been described. The most common form of AIS is endocervical (mucinous) (figs. 99, 100), in which the cells resemble those of the endocervix with basal nuclei and pale granular cytoplasm containing mucin. There is striking nuclear enlargement, hyperchromasia and coarsening of the chromatin, prominent mitotic activity, and increased density of the cells lining the glands. Typically, there is a sharp demarcation of AIS from nearby uninvolved glands and from the uninvolved epithelium of the same gland. AIS of the intestinal type is character-

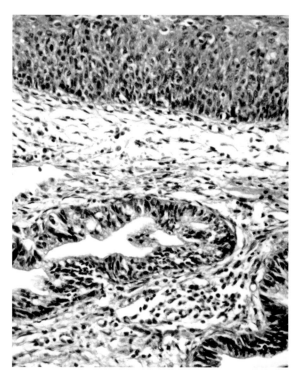

Figure 97
ADENOCARCINOMA IN SITU
UNDERLYING HIGH-GRADE CIN
Adenocarcinoma in situ is characterized by a disorderly stratification of cells and loss of polarity. The basement membrane is intact.

ized by the presence of goblet cells; argyrophilic cells may also be present (195). Endometrioid AIS is not well delineated from endocervical or intestinal AIS. In endometrioid AIS there are no goblet cells or cells with clear light-staining cytoplasm. The cytoplasm is scanty, shows no mucin production or goblet cells, and there is marked nuclear stratification. AIS can show significant morphologic variation. In some lesions there is a reduction in mucin, more marked cellular stratification, crowding, dispolarity, and formation of intraluminal bridges (167,169,182,185,196).

Carcinoembryonic antigen staining may be positive in AIS but is often absent and therefore not useful in the differential diagnosis. Ultrastructural and histochemical studies also do not contribute to the diagnosis (185,186).

Cytology. Adenocarcinoma in situ is often identified in smears as single columnar cells, clusters, or sheets of cells with the usual cytologic features of adenocarcinoma, without an

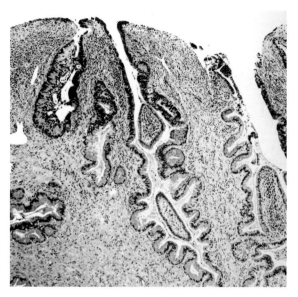

Figure 98
ADENOCARCINOMA IN SITU

The adenocarcinoma in situ (dark-staining epithelium near surface) is extending into endocervical glands. Multiple glands are involved.

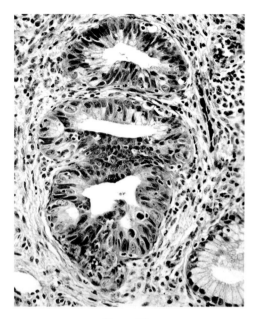

Figure 99
ADENOCARCINOMA IN SITU,
ENDOCERVICAL TYPE

This figure shows the mucinous type (top field), in which cells are enlarged and pseudostratified, and nuclei are hyperchromatic. Many of the cells contain mucin.

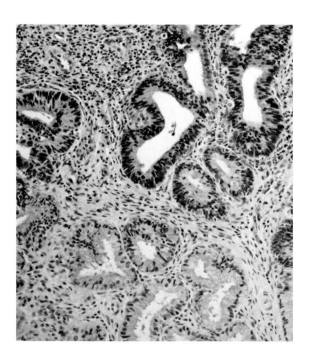

Figure 100
ADENOCARCINOMA IN SITU,
ENDOCERVICAL TYPE

Here the hyperchromatic enlarged nuclei (top field) contrast with those of relatively normal endocervical glands (bottom field).

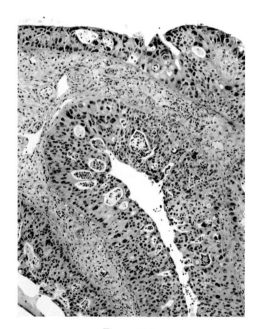

Figure 101
ADENOCARCINOMA IN SITU,
ADENOSQUAMOUS TYPE

Note the parallel orientation of the basal nuclei and lumens containing secretory material. Acute inflammatory cells are seen. The surface (top left) shows stratification of cells similar to a high-grade CIN.

81

accompanying tumor diathesis (173). Nuclear enlargement, pleomorphism, and hyperchromasia occur. The increased size of chromatin granules often obscures the enlarged nucleoli and the nuclear-cytoplasmic ratio is altered. In nearly 30 percent of the cases, abnormal cells are not evident (215).

Differential Diagnosis. Adenocarcinoma in situ must be distinguished from atypical hyperplasia, invasive adenocarcinoma, Arias-Stella reaction, glandular atypia due to inflammation or irradiation, microglandular hyperplasia, endometriosis, tubal metaplasia, and mesonephric remnants. Adenocarcinoma with early invasion is identified by the presence of irregularly infiltrating glands that lack the lobular architecture of endocervical glands with AIS. Glandular budding, papillarity and confluence, an inflammatory cell response, stromal desmoplasia, and extension of the glands beyond the normal glandular depth are additional features of invasion. In well-differentiated forms, however, an inflammatory or desmoplastic response may not be present. Early invasion may also occur in the form of small nests of cells in the stroma, or small buds of squamoid cells with eosinophilic cytoplasm projecting into the stroma.

Discrimination of AIS from the Arias-Stella reaction in glands of the endocervix may pose a problem because the latter is characterized by markedly enlarged cells with hyperchromatic nuclei. In contrast to AIS, the Arias-Stella reaction occurs in only sporadic areas in a gland or glands that are tortuous and hypersecretory. The nuclei of the cells characteristically protrude into the lumen with little accompanying cytoplasm, displaying a "hobnail" appearance; mitotic activity is rarely present, in contrast to AIS. Viral infections such as herpes and cytomegalovirus disease may result in nuclear enlargement (fig. 102). However, in contrast to the diffuse nature of the involvement by AIS, the affected cells are isolated and sporadic in cytomegalovirus infection and clustered in herpes. In AIS the cells are often stratified and form intraluminal bridges not evident in glands affected by viral changes. Inflammation and focal ulceration are also prominent in herpes infections.

Irradiation may produce marked glandular atypia. The lesion is characterized by a single layer of epithelial cells showing nuclear enlarge-

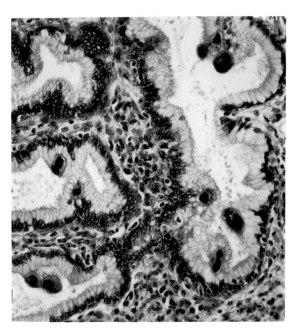

Figure 102
CYTOMEGALOVIRUS EFFECT
Only occasional cells contain large intranuclear inclusions.

ment, pleomorphism, hyperchromasia, and little or no polarity. The cytoplasm tends to be granular and vacuolated, and mitotic figures are absent (see figs. 93, 94).

Microglandular hyperplasia differs considerably from AIS because it is polypoid and characterized by a denser concentration of smaller, more uniform glands. The glands of microglandular hyperplasia are lined by vacuolated cells with uniform bland nuclei that lack mitotic activity. AIS, in contrast, is not polypoid, and has much more cytologic atypia and stratification, and the atypical cells occupy normally positioned glands. Unusual forms of microglandular hyperplasia may contain solid sheets of cells and include signet-ring cells, but they are typically accompanied by areas characteristic of microglandular hyperplasia (236).

Endometriosis is characterized by glands lined by endometrial-type cells with basally-oriented nuclei that lack atypia. There may be cellular stratification and some of the cells may have cilia, suggesting a benign diagnosis. Endometriotic glands are surrounded by endometrial-type stroma, which is often inconspicuous. Tubal metaplasia can be confused with AIS but it usually involves only a single gland or part of one, and the epithelium lacks significant nuclear atypia (see section on tubal metaplasia). Mesonephric remnants are usually deep in the stroma, although they occasionally impinge on normal endocervical glands near the mucosal surface. Mesonephric remnants also have bland unstratified nuclei unlike AIS. The intraluminal eosinophilic material and clustering arrangement of mesonephric remnants have little similarity to the features of AIS.

Clinical Behavior and Treatment. AIS is treated either by conization or hysterectomy. Relapse occurs more frequently after conization than hysterectomy, perhaps due to the multifocal distribution of AIS. Residual AIS is likely if the lesion involves the margins of the cone (191). If conservative treatment is chosen, follow-up is needed because residual AIS may be present in the hysterectomy specimen after conization (173). Progression to invasive carcinoma may occur over a variable period. One invasive carcinoma developed after an interval of 7 years (169).

Adenocarcinoma

General Features. Adenocarcinoma accounts for 8 to 26 percent of primary carcinomas of the cervix. The relative frequency has been increasing due to a decrease in the frequency of invasive squamous cell carcinoma, but there has also been an absolute increase in the incidence of adenocarcinoma (206,230,233). The overall increase in invasive adenocarcinoma has been 2 percent or more annually between 1972 and 1982 in several registries (217,223). An association with prior use of oral contraceptives, particularly those with a strong progestational component, has been described (172,177). The increase in adenocarcinoma of the cervix, unlike carcinoma of the cervix generally, has been greatest in young women in middle to upper income levels, who are likely to use oral contraceptives (217,223). Adenocarcinoma of the cervix shares a few of the epidemiologic factors associated with squamous cell carcinoma of the cervix and with endometrial carcinoma (202). For example, patients with cervical adenocarcinoma have a slight tendency toward obesity, hypertension, and nulligravidity, but the association is weaker than in women with endometrial carcinoma (172). Although cervical adenocarcinoma

does not have the socioeconomic or venereal associations of squamous cell carcinoma (193), closely related adenosquamous carcinoma is similar epidemiologically to squamous cell carcinoma in more respects than pure adenocarcinoma (172,216). Also, nearly 60 percent of cervical adenocarcinomas are associated with CIN or invasive squamous carcinoma (208,222), and about 89 percent of adenocarcinomas contain HPV nucleic acid sequences, the same proportion as in cases of squamous cell carcinoma (235). A subset of patients with clear cell adenocarcinoma have had in utero exposure to diethylstilbestrol. Patients with adenocarcinoma of the cervix, particularly those with minimum-deviation mucinous carcinoma, tend to have mucinous tumors of the ovary (200,237). Minimum-deviation mucinous adenocarcinomas are also associated with Peutz-Jeghers syndrome. The ovarian tumors that accompany adenocarcinoma of the cervix are usually independent primary neoplasms, but some are metastatic.

Clinical Features. The mean age of patients with adenocarcinoma of the cervix is between 47 and 53 years. Most reports suggest that women with adenocarcinoma are a few years older than those with squamous cell carcinoma. The symptoms of patients with adenocarcinoma of the cervix are similar to those having squamous cell carcinoma, i.e., typically a watery discharge or vaginal bleeding, but an equal proportion of patients are asymptomatic. Adenocarcinomas of different cell types are associated with similar symptoms. Adenocarcinoma is more difficult to detect in cytology smears than squamous cell carcinoma with the Ayre spatula technique. Use of improved methods to sample the endocervix enhances the detection of these lesions (170). At the time of discovery of the tumor, about 85 percent of women have disease limited to the cervix (stage I) or extending into the parametrium or upper vagina (stage II).

Gross Findings. About half of cervical adenocarcinomas are exophytic, polypoid, or papillary masses (fig. 103) (162). The others are nodular, with diffuse enlargement or ulceration of the cervix. Approximately 15 percent of patients have no visible lesion because the carcinoma is within the endocervical canal or infiltrative and small. Even in the absence of visible signs or symptoms, the lesion may infiltrate deeply into the wall (162).

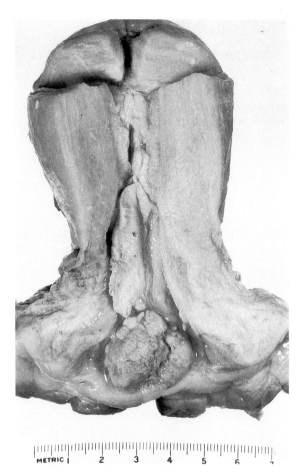

Figure 103
ADENOCARCINOMA OF THE CERVIX
Adenocarcinoma of the cervix is shown here with a polypoid configuration.

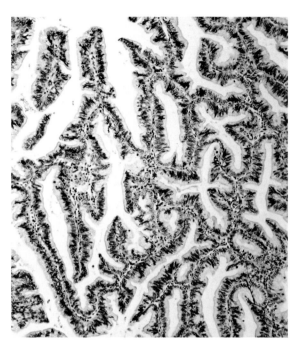

Figure 104
MUCINOUS ADENOCARCINOMA,
ENDOCERVICAL TYPE
This type of mucinous adenocarcinoma is composed of cells resembling those of the endocervix. Complex papillary processes reflect a well-differentiated adenocarcinoma.

Microscopic Findings. Adenocarcinomas exhibit a variety of patterns and are composed of diverse cell types, which often appear in combination. Because intermixtures are common, the designation of type is based on the predominant component. However, if a second type is 10 percent or more of the tumor, the tumor may be designated *mixed cell type* and the individual components listed in the diagnosis.

Mucinous Adenocarcinoma. This is the most common type of adenocarcinoma. It has three forms. One form is characterized by cells with pale granular cytoplasm and basal nuclei resembling the cells of the normal endocervix (so-called endocervical type) (figs. 104, 105). These tumors may be entirely papillary or papillary in part. In the second form, the cells resemble intestinal cells and line papillae or infiltrate as in carci-

noma of the colon (so-called intestinal type) (figs. 106–108). In the intestinal type, the epithelium tends to be pseudostratified, contains only small amounts of mucin, and may include goblet cells (fig. 108). In rare cases argentaffin cells are present. A third mucinous form is signet-ring cell carcinoma (fig. 109). This rarely occurs in a pure form because signet-ring cells are usually present as a minor component mixed with endocervical or intestinal patterns.

Endometrioid Adenocarcinoma. This tumor may at times be difficult to separate from an endocervical type adenocarcinoma that is not highly differentiated and contains little intracellular mucin (figs. 110–112). It is more easily recognized if it not only resembles a typical adenocarcinoma of the endometrium, but if it also shows squamous differentiation and lacks intracytoplasmic mucin. An in situ or invasive squamous cell carcinoma may coexist with an invasive adenocarcinoma (fig. 113). An adenocarcinoma with squamous differentiation is designated *adenosquamous carcinoma* if the cells of the squamous

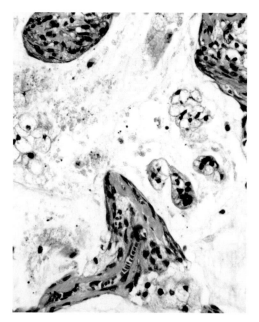

Figure 105
MUCINOUS ADENOCARCINOMA,
ENDOCERVICAL TYPE
This poorly differentiated mucinous adenocarcinoma has
clusters of malignant glandular cells floating in pools of mucin.

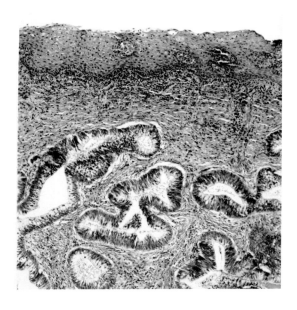

Figure 106
MUCINOUS ADENOCARCINOMA,
INTESTINAL TYPE
In this tumor, the spindle shape and stratification of the
nuclei and smaller amounts of intracytoplasmic mucin reflect
intestinal differentiation.

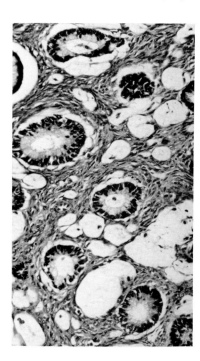

Figure 107
MUCINOUS ADENOCARCINOMA,
INTESTINAL TYPE
In this neoplasm the mucinous adenocarcinoma has
loculated pools of mucin in the stroma. Goblet cells are not
evident in this field.

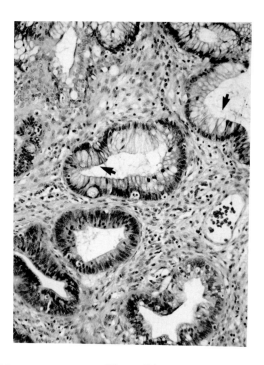

Figure 108
MUCINOUS ADENOCARCINOMA,
INTESTINAL TYPE
The arrows point to goblet cells.

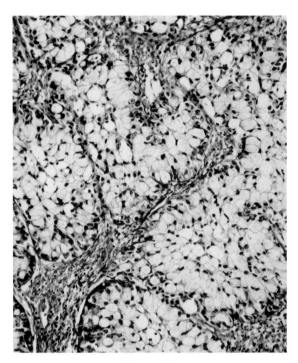

Figure 109
MUCINOUS ADENOCARCINOMA,
SIGNET-RING CELL TYPE
In this field nearly all of the cells are signet-ring cells.

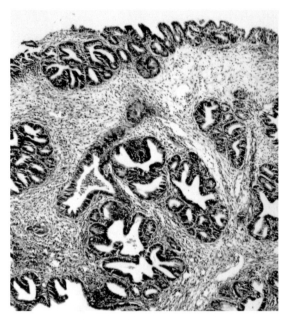

Figure 110
ADENOCARCINOMA, ENDOMETRIOID TYPE
The figure shows a small superficial portion of a larger, well-differentiated invasive carcinoma. The glands display papillary infoldings and branches. The cytoplasm lacks mucin, heightening the resemblance to an endometrial carcinoma.

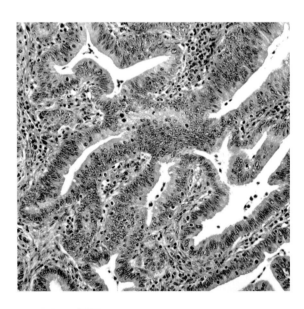

Figure 111
ADENOCARCINOMA, ENDOMETRIOID TYPE.
The glands resemble endometrial carcinoma in that the epithelium is stratified and cytoplasm is diminished and granular. Mucin is absent. Endometrioid differentiation is mainly reflected by relative loss of mucin production.

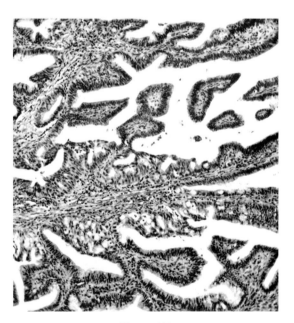

Figure 112
MUCINOUS ADENOCARCINOMA,
ENDOMETRIOID TYPE
This endometrioid or dedifferentiated mucinous adenocarcinoma has a focal papillary area. The cells are stratified, with oval nuclei having their long axis perpendicular to the basement membrane. Mucin is absent.

component are cytologically malignant. These tumors typically contain intracellular mucin, excluding a designation of *endometrioid carcinoma*. Because adenosquamous carcinoma may have special clinical and pathological characteristics, it is designated as a separate type of carcinoma. A *mucoepidermoid carcinoma* has been defined as a squamous carcinoma containing mucin (231).

Microscopic Grading. In the pathological evaluation of adenocarcinoma of the cervix, grading should be done either by nuclear or architectural grade. Architectural grade is based on the degree of gland formation. If less than 10 percent of the tumor is poorly differentiated, with areas not forming glands or tubules, it is well differentiated. If 10 to 50 percent of the tumor does not form glands or tubules, it is designated *moderately differentiated*. If the glands and tubules are not formed in more than half of the tumor, it is designated *poorly differentiated*.

By nuclear grading, cells with oval nuclei and evenly dispersed chromatin are considered grade 1. Cells with markedly enlarged nuclei displaying irregular coarse chromatin and prominent nucleoli are considered grade 3, and those displaying features between grades 1 and 3 are designated grade 2.

The depth of invasion should be expressed in percent of involvement of the wall. When invasion is superficial, a measurement of the depth in millimeters can be provided. Measurement of the depth of invasion of adenocarcinoma, however, is more subjective than in cases of microinvasive squamous cell carcinoma because of the difficulty in determining the point of origin. The presence or absence of vascular-space invasion should also be determined.

Immunohistochemical Findings. CEA positivity suggests a mucinous trend and is helpful in distinguishing adenocarcinoma of the cervix from benign lesions of the cervix and from carcinoma arising in the endometrium. About 75 percent of adenocarcinomas of the cervix contain CEA-positive areas; CEA is negative in normal endocervical mucosa and in most benign lesions of the cervix. Microglandular hyperplasia is an exception because it is uniformly CEA-positive. Only about 20 percent of carcinomas of the corpus contain CEA-positive areas, but when they show mucinous differentiation, the staining may be strongly positive (176). In an individual case, CEA is therefore not specific in distinguishing endometrial carcinoma from endocervical carcinoma, or in distinguishing a benign lesion from an adenocarcinoma, but it should be a consideration in difficult cases.

Differential Diagnosis. Major considerations in the differential diagnosis of adenocarcinoma of the cervix are microglandular hyperplasia and hyperplasia of mesonephric remnants among benign lesions and AIS, metastatic adenocarcinoma to the cervix, and extension of endometrial adenocarcinoma among malignant neoplasms.

Microglandular hyperplasia is polypoid and does not extend below the level of the normal endocervical glands. It tends to undergo squamous metaplasia and occurs mainly in young women who are usually pregnant or are taking oral contraceptives. Microglandular hyperplasia may occur in older women without a history of

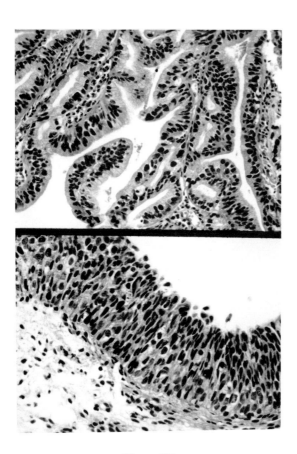

Figure 113
ADENOCARCINOMA,
ENDOCERVICAL TYPE WITH CIN
Here the adenocarcinoma (top) coexists with CIN 3 (bottom).

hormone intake, but it typically contains few mitotic figures. Mesonephric remnants generally occur in clusters and seldom extend to the surface. They usually contain prominent eosinophilic material within the tubular lumens, and the individual tubules typically have a well-demarcated peripheral basement membrane. Mitotic activity, cellular stratification, and nuclear atypia are minimal to absent in mesonephric remnants.

Adenocarcinoma in situ differs from invasive adenocarcinoma in that the glands of AIS do not extend below the deep margin of normal endocervical glands. Although irregularly positioned, the glands are still oriented perpendicular to the mucosal surface.

Nearly 90 percent of metastatic carcinomas to the cervix have evidence of widespread disease. In addition, there is usually extensive lymphatic permeation and absence of surface involvement.

Endometrial carcinoma may extend to the endocervix, but when it does, it usually has invaded the myometrium of the corpus and become sufficiently bulky to enlarge the uterus. Primary adenocarcinoma of the endocervix tends to expand the cervix, so if it, rather than the corpus, is enlarged, an endocervical primary site is clinically suggested. Mucinous differentiation suggests origin in the cervix, but may occur in endometrial carcinoma as well. Bland squamous differentiation within an adenocarcinoma favors an endometrial primary site because squamous differentiation in endocervical adenocarcinomas is usually poorly differentiated.

Clinical Behavior and Treatment. Adenocarcinoma of the cervix is treated the same as squamous cell carcinoma, stage for stage. Small, early-stage lesions can be treated equally well by irradiation or hysterectomy (219). Hysterectomy is advantageous for bulky lesions as it is more difficult to destroy those by irradiation alone (213,219). About 20 percent of lesions, stage II or higher, persist in the uterus after irradiation (165). Survival of patients with invasive adenocarcinoma is about the same or slightly worse than that of patients with squamous cell carcinoma when stage and type of therapy are controlled (165,166,178,203,206,213,224,233). Fewer patients with stage III and IV adenocarcinomas survive after 5 years compared to patients with squamous cell carcinomas of similar stages (171,192,213), although reports are inconsistent.

The stage, size, histologic grade, depth of invasion, and presence or absence of lymph node metastasis correlate with survival in most reports (206,219,230), although the evidence for a role for histologic grade is less convincing. Stage for stage, low-ploidy or diploid tumors have a better prognosis than high-ploidy or aneuploid tumors (183). High estrogen and progesterone receptor levels also correlate with improved survival in premenopausal women (218). Few, if any, tumors under 1 cm in diameter have metastasized to lymph nodes (219,224); lymphatic space involvement is an unfavorable finding (222).

Lymph node metastasis occurs in about 20 percent of patients with adenocarcinoma visibly confined to the cervix at operation (stage I), so radical hysterectomy and pelvic lymphadenectomy are appropriate for early stages (stages I–IIA). The examination of pelvic lymph nodes permits the identification of patients at high risk for recurrence and in need of adjuvant postoperative radiation. Autopsy study of fatal cases suggests a higher rate of metastasis to the adrenal gland and para-aortic lymph nodes than in fatal cases of squamous cell carcinoma (180). Outside of the pelvis, intraabdominal peritoneal spread, para-aortic lymph nodes, lung, and pleura are the most common sites of metastasis (192).

Clear Cell Carcinoma

General Features. Clear cell carcinoma accounts for about 4 percent of adenocarcinomas of the cervix (214). Almost two thirds of cases have occurred in women exposed in utero to diethylstilbestrol (DES) or a related substance. Those with a history of exposure have a median age of 19 years and a range of 7 to 31 years (221). The lesion has developed after doses as low as 1.5 mg/day and durations as short as 7 days, when given to the mother during the first trimester of pregnancy (190). Clear cell carcinoma of the cervix may also develop in the absence of in utero DES exposure, as demonstrated by its occurrence in women born before the use of DES during pregnancy (199). Of the cervical tumors related to DES exposure, about 50 percent are associated with vaginal adenosis and about 20 percent with gross structural cervicovaginal mesenchymal abnormalities such as hypoplasia, strictures, bands, fibroepithelial polyps, and malformations of the cervicovaginal interface (221). Chapter 6 discusses these tumors in more detail.

Gross Findings. Clear cell carcinomas vary from everting nodular reddish lesions (fig. 114) to small punctate ulcers (199,221).

Microscopic Findings. Papillary, microcystic, tubular, and solid patterns occur. The cells have clear (fig. 115) or eosinophilic granular cytoplasm, and often have a hobnail shape. Hobnail cells have prominent nuclei but scant cytoplasm so that the nucleus appears to protrude into the lumen of neoplastic tubules and cysts. The tubules are typically lined by a single layer of relatively bland cells (fig. 116). The microscopic features are the same as in clear cell carcinoma of the vagina. As in the vagina, most clear cell carcinomas of the cervix are closely associated with vaginal adenosis or with tuboendometrial glands in the exocervix (cervical ectropion).

Ultrastructural Findings. The ultrastructural findings in clear cell carcinoma are similar in all locations (cervix, vagina, ovary, endometrium), regardless of whether there is a history of DES exposure (179). Abundant glycogen and blunt microvilli are the main features of the clear cells. Large amounts of glycogen mainly account for the clear cytoplasmic appearance by light microscopy.

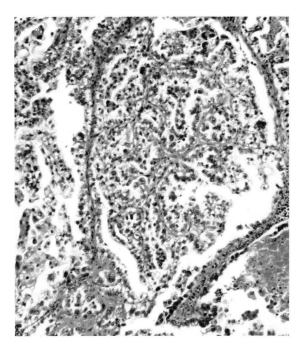

Figure 115
CLEAR CELL CARCINOMA
The papillary branching processes are lined by clear cells with dark nuclei. Cytoplasmic vacuolization, largely by glycogen, produces the clear cytoplasm.

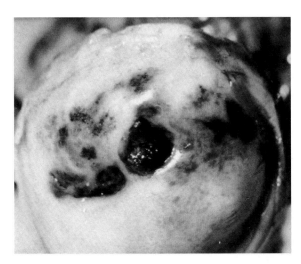

Figure 114
CLEAR CELL CARCINOMA
This tumor is protruding through the endocervical canal and involving portions of the exocervix. The small punctate dark areas represent benign endocervical glands in the exocervix. (Fig. 2 from Kaminski PF, Maier RC. Clear cell adenocarcinoma of the cervix unrelated to diethylstilbestrol exposure. Obstet Gynecol 1983;62:720–7.)

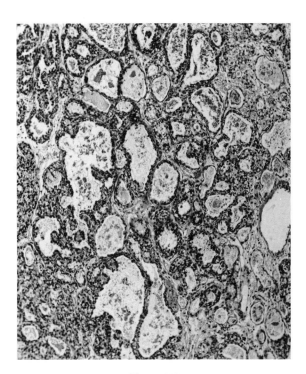

Figure 116
CLEAR CELL CARCINOMA
The tubulocystic pattern of clear cell carcinoma is shown.

Differential Diagnosis. Some squamous cell carcinomas are composed of cells that contain abundant glycogen, but glands and tubules are not formed (fig. 117). Of benign lesions, the differential diagnosis includes microglandular hyperplasia, Arias-Stella reaction, and mesonephric remnants. Microglandular hyperplasia is polypoid, with small glands that are markedly crowded, lined by a single layer of bland cuboidal cells, and usually accompanied by squamous metaplasia. If sheets of clear cells are formed in microglandular hyperplasia, the small bland nuclei and very low mitotic activity should distinguish it from clear cell carcinoma. Adenosis and ectropion, stigmata of DES exposure in utero, are usually absent with microglandular hyperplasia but common with clear cell carcinoma. Arias-Stella reaction occurs with intrauterine or ectopic pregnancy and gestational trophoblastic disease. In the Arias-Stella reaction, the nuclei are focally enlarged and have hyperchromatic smudged chromatin; mitotic figures are absent (see Arias-Stella reaction). The glands are secretory and the cytoplasm of affected cells is distended by clear secretory vacuoles with little of the granularity or eosinophilic cytoplasm seen in clear cell carcinoma. There may be an associated decidual change in the cervical stroma near the glands showing an Arias-Stella reaction.

Mesonephric remnants tend to be clustered relatively deep in the lateral wall of the cervix below the level of the endocervical glands and are often arranged around a central duct. They are not associated with adenosis, nor is there surface ulceration, or cervicovaginal mesenchymal abnormalities, as in clear cell carcinoma. Occasionally, clear carcinoma invades or impinges on mesonephric remnants (fig. 118).

Clinical Behavior and Treatment. More than 85 percent of clear cell carcinomas are stage I or II when detected (221). Treatment is either radical hysterectomy and vaginectomy or radiation. Metastasis occurs to pelvic nodes in about 18 percent of patients with stage I disease, but the frequency of metastasis reaches nearly 50 percent in stage II tumors (221).

Survival of patients with stage I disease is about 90 percent. Most recurrences occur within 3 years after primary therapy. Metastases are more often to distant sites than with squamous cell carcinoma, in that 36 percent of initial recurrences

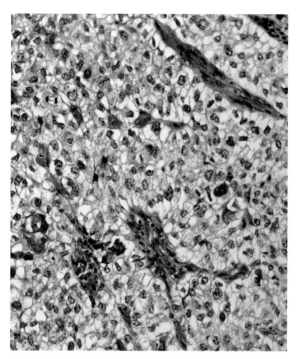

Figure 117
SQUAMOUS CARCINOMA SIMULATING
CLEAR CELL CARCINOMA
This squamous carcinoma has an unusual degree of vacuolization of the squamous cells. This pattern simulates clear cell adenocarcinoma, but gland lumens or tubules are not formed.

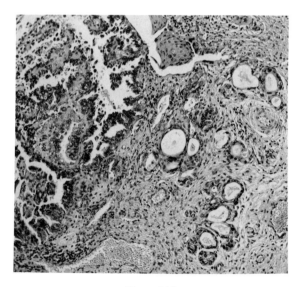

Figure 118
CLEAR CELL CARCINOMA
This clear cell carcinoma (left) is impinging on mesonephric remnants in the cervical stroma.

are to lung or supraclavicular nodes, in contrast to less than 10 percent in patients with squamous cell carcinoma. Features that are associated with a better prognosis include small size of the tumor, shallow depth of invasion (197), older age of the patient (≥19 years), a tubulocystic microscopic pattern (221), and lesser degrees of nuclear atypia (187).

Minimal Deviation Adenocarcinoma

Definition. Minimal deviation adenocarcinoma (MDA) is an unusually well-differentiated adenocarcinoma in which the cells lining the glands lack cytological features of malignancy. Originally termed *adenoma malignum* because of the resemblance of its glands to endocervical glands and its lack of malignant cellular features, the designation *minimal deviation adenocarcinoma* was proposed by Silverberg and Hurt in 1975 (225) as a more accurate reflection of the appearance of this form of adenocarcinoma. More recently, the definition of MDA has been expanded to include any cell type.

General Features. Minimal deviation adenocarcinoma is rare, representing about 1 to 3 percent of adenocarcinomas of the cervix and less than 18 percent of well-differentiated cervical adenocarcinomas (201). As in ordinary adenocarcinoma, a mucoid or watery vaginal discharge is common. Abnormal cervical glandular cells are evident in smears from most cases (198,229). More than any other type of cervical adenocarcinoma, MDA, particularly the mucinous form, is more likely to coexist with an ovarian neoplasm (201,239). The cervical tumor may occur synchronously or before the development of the ovarian tumor, which is usually a mucinous neoplasm or a rare ovarian sex cord stromal tumor (sex cord tumor with annular tubules) (209,239).

Gross Findings. Minimal deviation adenocarcinoma may be ulcerative or polypoid, but often it forms a suspicious-appearing irregularity or the cervix is stenotic without an evident mucosal lesion. With early lesions the cervix may appear normal (184,201).

Microscopic Findings. Identification of MDA is based on 1) cytologically bland glands that vary in size and shape (figs. 119–123), 2) increased mitotic activity, 3) a hyperplastic appearance of the glands at the surface, and 4) an increased number of glands positioned deeper than the lower level of normal endocervical glands. Normal glands seldom extend more than 5 mm below the endocervical surface. In nearly all instances, the diagnosis cannot be made reliably on biopsy material because deeply positioned glands are needed to confirm the presence of invasion, and a deep conization or hysterectomy specimen is needed (184).

Characteristically, the glands vary in size, ranging from small and round to large irregular and distorted forms with angular projections (figs. 119, 120, 122). Complex outlines and a minor component of desmoplasia are usually present. The glands are lined by a single layer of cells partially surrounded by a basement membrane. The cells are cytologically bland and near diploid DNA values are present (198).

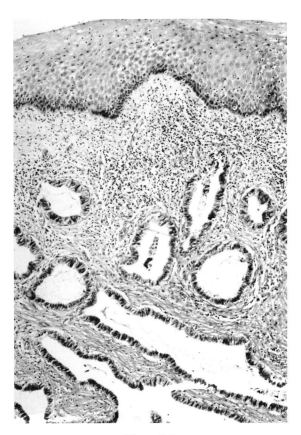

Figure 119
MINIMAL DEVIATION ADENOCARCINOMA, ENDOMETRIOID TYPE

In this tumor, the glands are relatively uniform, but the deeper ones are not oriented toward the surface. Identification of minimal deviation carcinoma requires evaluation of the deep margin for invasion.

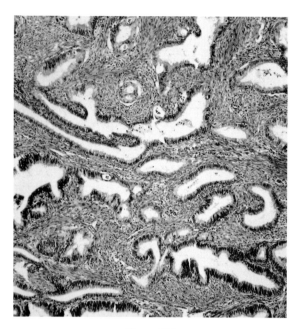

Figure 120
MINIMAL DEVIATION ADENOCARCINOMA,
ENDOMETRIOID TYPE
In this minimal deviation adenocarcinoma the glandular outlines are irregular and branched. The glands are infiltrating the stroma in a haphazard fashion.

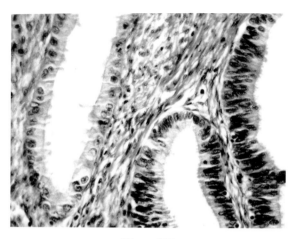

Figure 121
MINIMAL DEVIATION ADENOCARCINOMA,
NONSPECIFIC TYPE
This figure shows nonspecific epithelium (left) and endometrial-type epithelium (right).

Mucinous MDA is the most common form of MDA. In this carcinoma, the glands are lined by a single layer of columnar mucin-producing cells resembling the cells of endocervical glands that appear normal except for their shapes. Peculiar elongation or branching processes are common (fig. 122). The nuclei are basal with inconspicuous nucleoli.

MDA may also display an endometrioid (figs. 119–121), clear cell or nonspecific (figs. 121, 123) cellular type of differentiation. In endometrioid MDA, the tumor cells resemble those of proliferative endometrium or endometrial hyperplasia. In MDA with nonspecific cellular features, the glands are small and uniform, with gaping lumens often containing a homogeneous hyaline material. The cells lining the glands show little or no atypia, and the nuclei are bland and flattened (figs. 121, 123).

Immunohistochemical Findings. Minimal deviation adenocarcinoma is highly variable in its staining for CEA. It is usually positive in focal areas, whereas well-differentiated cervical adenocarcinoma is usually more diffusely positive. All benign lesions tested to date, except for microglandular hyperplasia, are negative for CEA (211,226). Immunostaining may therefore be helpful in some instances, but because of its variable pattern in MDA, the results must be interpreted cautiously.

Differential Diagnosis. Deeply positioned nabothian cysts, nodular clustering of endocervical glands (see section on tunnel clusters), microglandular hyperplasia, and mesonephric hyperplasia are the major considerations in the differential diagnosis. Endocervical glands are normally confined to within 5 mm of the surface, but may nearly extend to the serosal surface. These differ from MDA by having a single layer of flat to cuboidal inactive-appearing bland cells (174). MDA differs from nodular collections of endocervical glands, so-called tunnel clusters, by the greater variation in size, shape, and depth of its glands, and by the irregularity at its infiltrating margin. Microglandular hyperplasia differs from MDA in that it is more everting, polypoid, and superficial and does not extend below the level of endocervical glands. Microglandular hyperplasia also has greater crowding of glands, squamous metaplasia is usually present, and enlarged branching glands are absent. In contrast to mesonephric remnants and mesonephric hyperplasia, MDA lacks a lobular or clustered arrangement and the glands of MDA have more irregularly shaped outlines.

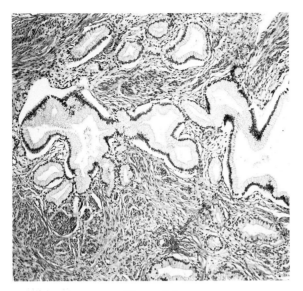

Figure 122
MINIMAL DEVIATION ADENOCARCINOMA,
ENDOCERVICAL TYPE
In this figure the mucinous glands are irregular in size
and shape.

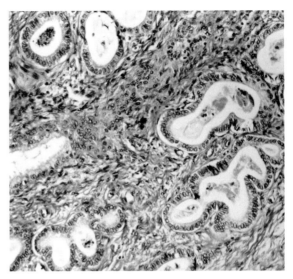

Figure 123
MINIMAL DEVIATION ADENOCARCINOMA
In this nonspecific cell type, the glands within this field
resemble hyperplasia of mesonephric remnants, but elsewhere they were more irregular in shape, and the deep
margin reflected invasion.

Other benign lesions that can be confused with MDA are intestinal metaplasia, atypical hyperplasia, and AIS. Intestinal metaplasia, often seen in atypical hyperplasia of endocervical glands and AIS, displays atypia and mitotic activity in excess of that found in MDA. Both intestinal metaplasia and atypical hyperplasia are limited and do not extend below the level of endocervical glands. A positive CEA stain favors a diagnosis of MDA over atypical hyperplasia.

Treatment and Prognosis. Ideally, the therapy for MDA should be the same as for ordinary adenocarcinoma of the same stage, but the lesion is seldom recognized before hysterectomy so that intracavitary radiation is seldom used.

The prognosis for MDA is unsettled. A majority of reports, particularly the early ones, found an unfavorable survival, but most neoplasms were discovered in late stages (210). Also, many MDAs fail to form a visibly evident lesion despite deep infiltration, leading to greater opportunity for vascular invasion and clinical understaging, resulting in undertreatment and a relatively poor prognosis. Some studies, however, report survival for MDA as good as for other forms of well-differentiated adenocarcinoma of the cervix at the same stage (201,225). A majority of reports find survival of patients with MDA an exception

to the rule that a well-differentiated carcinoma has a better prognosis than a poorly differentiated one (184). The distribution of metastases is similar to that of ordinary forms of cervical adenocarcinoma (184).

Well-Differentiated (Papillary) Villoglandular Adenocarcinoma

Definition. Well-differentiated villoglandular carcinoma is a newly described form of unusually well-differentiated papillary cervical adenocarcinoma found in young women and characterized by complex branching papillary processes.

General Features. Well-differentiated villoglandular adenocarcinoma is distinctive clinically because the patients are younger than most patients with adenocarcinoma, and none of the 37 reported cases have extended outside the uterus (196a,238). Despite the lack of proof of spread, villoglandular papillary adenocarcinoma may be deeply invasive and extend to the endometrium. Most patients are less than 40 years old and some are less than 30 years old. Patients have signs and symptoms similar to those of patients with stage I adenocarcinoma of the cervix.

Gross Findings. Well-differentiated villoglandular adenocarcinoma usually appears as a polypoid or broad-based papillary protuberance resembling a polyp. Some tumors are more subtle, however, appearing as eroded or friable nodular enlargements.

Microscopic Findings. Microscopically, the neoplasm exhibits a complex branching or arborescent pattern resembling an exaggeration of normal surface endocervical processes and crypts (figs. 124–126). The papillary fronds may be thin or thick with large branching papillae that give rise to smaller branching processes. Invasive portions are a continuation of the elongated branching glands separated by fibrous stroma. Papillary processes are usually lined by stratified columnar cells containing only sporadic mucinous cells. Pseudostratification of the cells in a single layer is common. Typically there is minimal cytologic atypia. The cells lining the fronds may be endocervical, endometrioid, or intestinal in type. The stroma may be desmoplastic or myxoid at the advancing margin. Serous and clear cell forms of villoglandular adenocarcinoma have not been described. AIS of the endocervix frequently occurs in association with this neoplasm.

Differential Diagnosis. Other papillary carcinomas (serous, mucinous, and clear cell types) differ in that their papillae are smaller, much thinner, and form a more complex lattice. Superficial neoplasms are difficult to distinguish from hyperplastic reactive glands, therefore a diagnosis of carcinoma should be reserved for those cases that show definite invasion. In areas where invasion is equivocally present, the cells lining the processes should be cytologically malignant.

Clinical Behavior and Treatment. In two series specifically devoted to villoglandular adenocarcinoma, the tumor was superficially invasive in the majority of cases (196a,238). In 3 women there was deep invasion. One of the deeply invasive lesions extended to the endometrium and invaded the myometrium apart from its origin in the endocervix, justifying the lesion as a form of carcinoma.

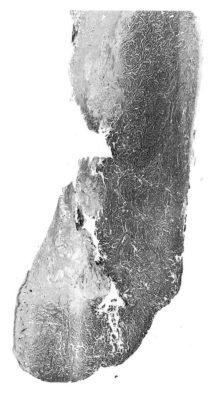

Figure 124
WELL-DIFFERENTIATED
VILLOGLANDULAR ADENOCARCINOMA

The lesion extends from the lower uterine segment to the exocervix and more than halfway through the cervix.

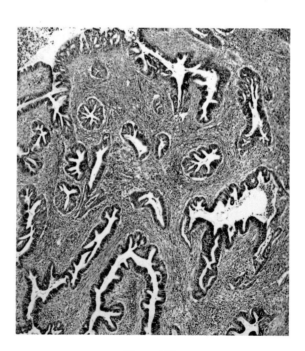

Figure 125
WELL-DIFFERENTIATED
VILLOGLANDULAR ADENOCARCINOMA

Here the broad papillae toward the surface are lined by stratified cells (top). Stroma is abundant.

Therapeutically, a conization is likely to be successful if 1) the margins of the cone are free of tumor, 2) invasion is no more than 3 mm, and 3) there is no vascular space invasion. Conservative therapy is advocated for superficially invasive lesions because none have metastasized and there has been no association with coexistent ovarian tumors (196a,238).

Serous Adenocarcinoma

This is a rare carcinoma identical to serous carcinoma of the ovary and endometrium. In the only series thus far reported none of the three tumors were deeply invasive, but in two of these pelvic nodal metastases were present (184a).

Mesonephric Adenocarcinoma

Carcinomas arising in mesonephric remnants of the cervix are rare (164,232). Older reports confused clear carcinomas with carcinomas arising in mesonephric remnants (188). Carcinomas arising from mesonephric remnants tend to be deeply positioned with the bulk of the tumor in the stroma forming tubular structures. The tu-

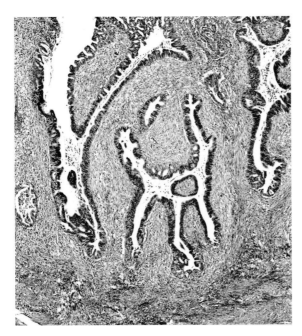

Figure 126
WELL-DIFFERENTIATED
VILLOGLANDULAR ADENOCARCINOMA
The broad villous processes are lined by multiple layers of cells.

bules are usually closely packed and diffusely infiltrate the stroma in a haphazard arrangement (figs. 127, 128) (205). The cells lining the tubules are cuboidal or columnar and form a single layer and most have darker, more granular cytoplasm than those in clear cell carcinoma. A prominent basement membrane about the periphery of tubules is often present (fig. 128), as in benign remnants. In contrast to benign mesonephric remnants, mesonephric carcinoma has an infiltrative pattern rather than maintaining a lobular architecture and the cells have malignant-appearing nuclei (see Mesonephric Remnants). A diagnosis of mesonephric carcinoma can be made if 1) the tumor is deeply situated in the lateral wall, 2) the endocervical mucosa is uninvolved, and 3) none of the stigmata of DES exposure are evident. Transition from mesonephric remnants is diagnostic but may be difficult to demonstrate.

OTHER EPITHELIAL TUMORS

Adenosquamous Carcinoma

Definition. Adenosquamous carcinoma is a form of carcinoma exhibiting both glandular and squamous differentiation. It is commonly classified as a *mixed carcinoma*, a designation for a cervical carcinoma showing glandular and squamous differentiation, rather than being listed within either adenocarcinoma or squamous cell categories. In this text adenosquamous carcinoma embraces any primary carcinoma containing malignant-appearing squamous and glandular elements. Thus, adenocarcinoma with bland squamous differentiation (adenoacanthoma) is not considered adenosquamous but endometrioid. Adenocarcinoma with bland squamous differentiation is rare as a primary carcinoma of the cervix because the squamous element is usually poorly differentiated and is the predominant element in adenosquamous carcinoma.

General Features. Adenosquamous carcinoma is 20 to 50 percent as common as adenocarcinoma of the cervix (271,276,282,284), depending on the microscopic criteria employed. Because of variability in the definition, the clinical features are unsettled. Adenosquamous carcinoma is found in both old and young women, and is often reported in association with pregnancy. Notable

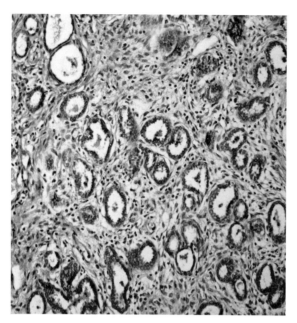

Figure 127
MESONEPHRIC ADENOCARCINOMA
The deep position of the tubules in the stroma and lack of surface involvement favor mesonephric duct origin. The cells are cuboidal, with dark nuclei and a high nuclear-cytoplasmic ratio.

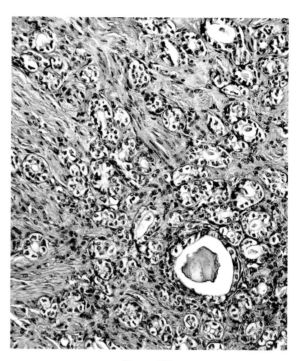

Figure 128
MESONEPHRIC ADENOCARCINOMA
The resemblance to mesonephric nests is apparent, but the extent of the proliferation and diffuse infiltration along with the variation in size and density of the tubules reflect a carcinoma.

differences in risk-factor profiles for adenosquamous carcinoma and other cervical adenocarcinomas have been reported (244), i.e., multiple sexual partners, low education level, and an association with smoking, which suggest that the risk factors are more like those of squamous cell carcinoma of the cervix than those of adenocarcinoma.

Gross Findings. Adenosquamous carcinoma does not differ grossly from adenocarcinoma of the endocervix, appearing as an ulceronodular or polypoid firm mass.

Microscopic Findings. The glandular component is usually poorly differentiated, showing some degree of mucinous differentiation in the form of minor cytoplasmic vacuolization and accumulation of mucin in gland lumens. The squamous component is poorly differentiated, showing little keratinization (figs. 129–131). The glandular component can be graded architecturally, as for adenocarcinoma, and by nuclear grade of the glandular and squamous components.

Differential Diagnosis. Extension of a poorly differentiated adenocarcinoma of the endometrium, with squamous differentiation to the en-

docervix, and adenocarcinoma coexisting with intraepithelial neoplasia or squamous cell carcinoma as collision tumors must be excluded. In cases of poorly differentiated adenocarcinoma with squamous differentiation of the endometrium extending to the cervix, the bulk of the tumor is in the endometrium because there is usually less clinical involvement of the cervix by a stage II endometrial carcinoma than by a stage I cervical carcinoma. The glandular component of the cervical tumor is much more often mucinous than endometrioid. In cases in which the neoplasm involves the corpus and cervix to an equal extent, it may be impossible to define the primary site even after hysterectomy. An adenocarcinoma coexisting with CIN lacks the intermingling of the two elements that is seen in cases of adenosquamous carcinoma.

Clinical Behavior and Treatment. The treatment for adenosquamous carcinoma is the same as that for other forms of carcinoma of the cervix. Reports of the survival of patients vary from no difference from that of patients with squamous

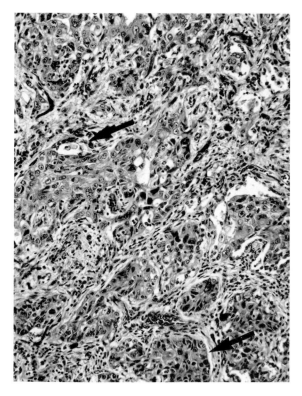

Figure 129
ADENOSQUAMOUS CARCINOMA
Poorly formed glands (upper arrow) and squamous differentiation (lower arrow) are present.

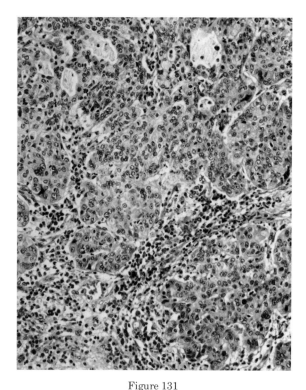

Figure 131
ADENOSQUAMOUS CARCINOMA
The glands in the upper field are formed by the same cells having solid differentiation in the lower field.

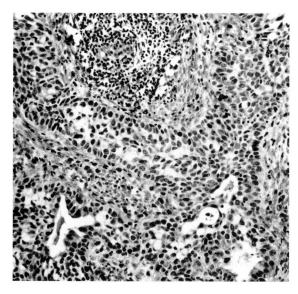

Figure 130
ADENOSQUAMOUS CARCINOMA
The epithelial cells in the upper field show squamous differentiation, but vague glands are formed in the lower field.

cell carcinoma or adenocarcinoma (256,271,276) to a much worse prognosis (249,250,272). In reports where the diagnosis is limited to neoplasms in which both glandular and squamous components appear malignant, a poor prognosis is found. Series are small and microscopic criteria vary, leading to inconsistent conclusions.

Glassy Cell Carcinoma

Definition. This is a poorly differentiated carcinoma characterized by sheets of cells having 1) a moderate amount of cytoplasm with a ground-glass or granular appearance, 2) a distinct cytoplasmic membrane, and 3) a large nucleus containing prominent single or multiple nucleoli.

General Features. Glassy cell carcinoma accounts for only 1 to 2 percent of all cervical carcinomas (252,258,261), but as much as 10 percent of adenocarcinomas (249,274). First recognized by Glucksmann and Cherry (252), who classified it within the group of mixed (adenosquamous) carcinomas, it occurs in patients with a younger mean age (31–41 years) than patients with squamous cell or ordinary adenocarcinoma of the cervix, and has been associated with pregnancy in an unexpected number of cases in early reports, but not in more recent series.

Gross Findings. Glassy cell carcinoma appears commonly as a bulky exophytic mass (fig. 132). Despite this presentation, there is characteristically less deep invasion than suspected from the size of the protuberant mass (281).

Microscopic Findings. The tumor is composed of invasive nests and sheets of cells, often separated by delicate fibrovascular septae (fig. 133). The neoplastic cells are relatively uniform, large, and polygonal, with a distinct cell border (fig. 134). The cells contain large oval nuclei, prominent nucleoli, and moderate amounts of finely granular, pale eosinophilic or amphophilic cytoplasm resembling ground glass. Mitotic figures are numerous. Minor degrees of keratinization (fig. 135), infrequent intercellular bridges, rare gland lumens, and intracellular mucin positivity may occur, but these are inconspicuous (261). A striking inflammatory infiltrate is present in the stroma, usually containing numerous eosinophils and plasma cells (258).

Cytology. Cervical smears reveal scattered clusters of cells and single cells with large nuclei, prominent single or multiple nucleoli, and a moderate amount of finely granular cytoplasm in a background of inflammatory cells and proteinaceous debris (267). Cytoplasmic membranes

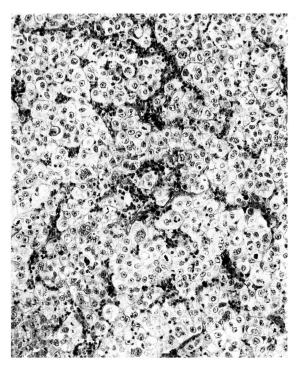

Figure 133
GLASSY CELL CARCINOMA
Sheets of cells with abundant lightly stained cytoplasm.

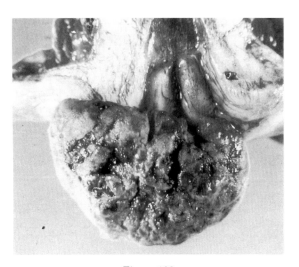

Figure 132
GLASSY CELL CARCINOMA
The tumor characteristically grows as a bulky exophytic mass.

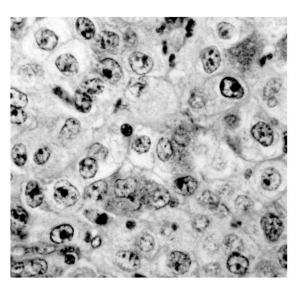

Figure 134
GLASSY CELL CARCINOMA
The well-defined cytoplasmic margin and nuclei with a prominent central nucleolus and absence of marked peripheral chromatin clumping distinguish this from nonkeratinizing squamous cell carcinoma.

are distinct, and mitotic figures are common. Distinction must be made from reactive atypia, which does not occur in isolated cells and non-keratinizing squamous cell carcinoma cells (268), which show more nuclear irregularity and an indefinite cytoplasmic margin.

Ultrastructural Findings. The cells are relatively uniform in size and outline, and nuclei have evenly dispersed chromatin and prominent nucleoli. The cytoplasm is distinctive in that numerous profiles of smooth endoplasmic reticulum dilated by an electron-dense secretory product are present. These features, along with the abundant tonofilaments, produce the ground-glass appearance seen by light microscopy (286, 292). Cell membranes are not convoluted, but a few have interdigitating microvillous processes. Occasional junctional complexes connect adjacent tumor cells. Glandular differentiation is confirmed by the presence of prominent Golgi apparatuses, abundant smooth endoplasmic reticula, secretory products, intracytoplasmic lumens, and microvillous surface projections (fig. 136). Squamous differentiation is evident in the form of focal concentrations of tonofilaments.

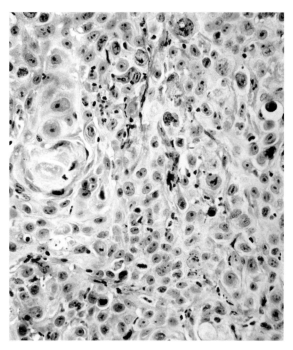

Figure 135
GLASSY CELL CARCINOMA
WITH SQUAMOUS DIFFERENTIATION
A suggestion of pearl formation is in the upper left. There is more variation in size of the cells and less uniformity of the cytoplasm than in the usual glassy cell carcinoma.

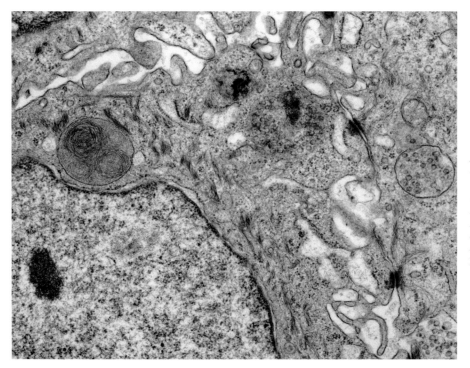

Figure 136
ELECTRON
MICROSCOPIC VIEW
OF GLASSY CELLS
Tonofilaments are located above the nucleus. Junctional complexes (right field) are common, and microvillous processes and secretory products are also present. (Fig. 6 from Zaino RJ, et al. Glassy cell carcinoma of the uterine cervix. Arch Pathol Lab Med 1982;106:250–4.)

Differential Diagnosis. The main differential diagnosis is with a poorly differentiated nonkeratinizing squamous cell carcinoma composed of cells similar in size to glassy cells but with more oval nuclei, syncytial growth of the cells, and fewer mitotic figures than glassy cell carcinoma. The chromatin of the cells of nonkeratinizing squamous cell carcinoma is coarser and distributed along the nuclear membrane. The cytoplasm is less finely granular, and the cytoplasmic membrane is less well defined than in glassy cell carcinoma (281). Poor fixation and pale staining of paraffin sections tends to obscure the features of nonkeratinizing squamous cell carcinoma to the degree that it may resemble glassy cell carcinoma. Not all investigators have found cytologically-distinctive features. It may be that glassy cell carcinoma is a form of poorly differentiated nonkeratinizing squamous cell carcinoma.

Clinical Behavior and Treatment. Therapy is the same as for invasive squamous cell carcinoma and adenocarcinoma of the same stage, but the prognosis is not as good. In a study of 29 stage IB glassy cell carcinomas, the survival was only 55 percent, about 20 percent lower than that of squamous cell carcinoma (268,281). The reputation of a poor prognosis, however, is based on only a few cases in each stage, so it can be questioned whether glassy cell carcinoma is worse than any other poorly differentiated carcinoma of the cervix (261). Part of the difficulty in assessing the results of therapy and relating it to prognosis is due to the variable microscopic criteria applied in the past and a degree of subjectivity in making the diagnosis.

Adenoid Cystic Carcinoma

General Features. Adenoid cystic carcinoma of the cervix is a rare tumor representing less than 1 percent of cervical adenocarcinomas (266). Most of the reported 120 examples are single-case reports or small series of cases (255). Early reports of adenoid cystic carcinoma contained examples of adenoid basal cell carcinoma because of overlapping pathological features. The two neoplasms, however, are distinct both clinically and pathologically and should be kept separate.

Patients with adenoid cystic carcinoma tend to be elderly, with few under 50 years of age (254,264). Reports from the United States contain a higher proportion of blacks than antici-

pated from the general population (247,266,288). Parity of patients with adenoid cystic carcinoma and the stage of tumor at its discovery are the same as for other patients with adenocarcinoma of the cervix. Ovarian epithelial tumors, particularly mucinous ones, are relatively common in women with adenoid cystic carcinoma.

Gross Findings. Adenoid cystic carcinomas usually form hard irregular polypoid friable masses, although some are endophytic and ulcerated.

Microscopic Findings. Microscopically, the cells form clusters, cords, and trabeculae with a circular or spiral pattern formed with lumens containing hyaline eosinophilic material (figs. 137, 138). The nuclei are small, dark, and relatively uniform and seldom show pleomorphism. Minor areas of squamous differentiation may be present. Mitotic figures and necrosis are common, and hyalinization of the stroma may be prominent. Overlapping patterns with ordinary adenocarcinoma and adenoid basal cell may be present (247,264,270). The mixture of patterns with ordinary forms of adenocarcinoma and the scarcity of myoepithelial differentiation indicates

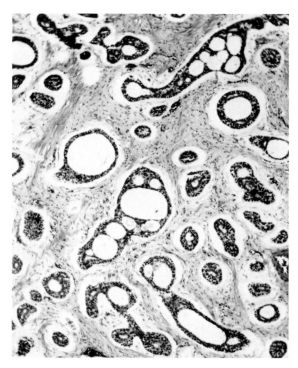

Figure 137
ADENOID CYSTIC CARCINOMA
This figure shows the characteristic cylindromatous pattern.

that most adenoid cystic carcinomas of the cervix are adenocarcinoma with adenoid cystic differentiation (247). Lymphatic invasion is usually evident (264).

Immunohistochemical and Ultrastructural Findings. Immunostains for cytokeratins are usually strongly positive, whereas CEA and EMA staining is focal. Ultrastructural analysis reveals less frequent myoepithelial differentiation than expected compared with adenoid cystic carcinoma of other sites, and actin and S-100 stains for myoepithelial cells are negative in most adenoid cystic carcinomas of the cervix, unlike adenoid cystic carcinomas in other locations (263).

Differential Diagnosis. The main differential diagnosis is with adenoid basal carcinoma.

Clinical Behavior and Treatment. Adenoid cystic carcinoma of the cervix is aggressive. In one study, 5 of 12 patients died of tumor or had local recurrence along with distant metastasis to lungs, liver, bone, or other sites (264). In other studies, the behavior is similar to, or worse than, adenocarcinoma and squamous cell carcinoma of the cervix (247,255,288).

Adenoid Basal Carcinoma

Definition. Adenoid basal carcinoma is a tumor characterized by nests and cords of small oval cells with a peripheral palisaded arrangement resembling that of basal cell and basosquamous cell carcinoma of the skin.

General Features. An uncommon neoplasm, adenoid basal carcinoma was first distinguished as an entity from adenoid cystic carcinoma in 1966 (242). Since then, only 20 cases have been reported (246,247,288). It justifies a separate designation because it tends to occur in elderly women and in all instances has been discovered while confined to the cervix. Metastasis has not been reported in patients whose tumors had the typical microscopic pattern. Despite this lack of aggressive behavior, it is regarded as a carcinoma because of its infiltrative pattern and its extension to the lower uterine segment in some instances.

Patients tend to be older than most with adenocarcinoma, having a median age of about 60 years. Nearly half of the patients are black. Patients with adenoid basal carcinoma differ markedly from those with ordinary adenocarcinoma of the cervix mainly in their early presentation (stage IA or IB) and lack of symptoms related to the lesion. The tumor is seen more often than expected in a cervical stump remaining after subtotal hysterectomy. Cytology smears are atypical or only suspicious in most cases and are related to an associated or overlying squamous intraepithelial lesion. In most cases, it is the associated CIN for which the uterus is removed.

Gross Findings. Grossly, the cervix appears normal or shows a mild nodular distortion.

Microscopic Findings. Microscopically, adenoid basal carcinoma resembles a basal cell carcinoma of the skin with squamous differentiation. The tumor is characterized by small nests and cords of uniform round or oval small cells with scant cytoplasm and small dark nuclei (fig. 139). Squamous differentiation occurs centrally, with the squamous cells surrounded or capped by smaller rounded basal cells (figs. 140, 141). A few of the cords or nests may contain small acini

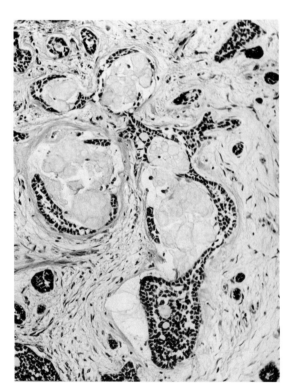

Figure 138
ADENOID CYSTIC CARCINOMA

Trabecular cords and nests of uniform cells are present. The hyaline stroma is a basement membrane material resembling amyloid (center).

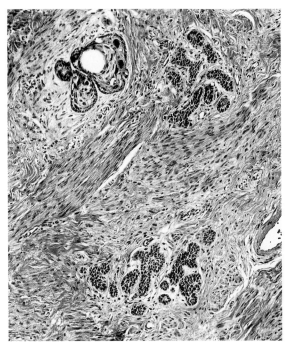

Figure 139
ADENOID BASAL CARCINOMA
Low power of groups of rounded nests of basaloid cells infiltrating the stroma. Squamous differentiation with microcyst formation (upper left) occurs along with nests of darker basaloid cells with scant cytoplasm.

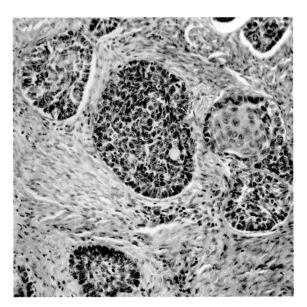

Figure 141
ADENOID BASAL CARCINOMA
Focal squamous differentiation is evident (right). There is no inflammation or desmoplasia accompanying tumor nests. Glands are not formed by the relatively uniform basaloid cells. Mitotic activity is also low.

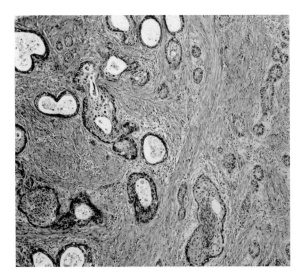

Figure 140
ADENOID BASAL CARCINOMA
Central squamous differentiation, microcyst formation, and dark peripherally-positioned small basaloid cells are characteristic features. Glands and the cylindromatous pattern of adenoid cystic carcinoma are not seen in adenoid basal carcinoma.

lined by a single layer of cuboidal to columnar cells; mitotic figures are infrequent. A desmoplastic stromal reaction is present in about half of the cases, but most nests produce no stromal reaction (fig. 140). Most are located at the lower level of endocervical glands or deeper because the overlying surface is usually minimally involved. There may be an intraepithelial squamous component with the tumor budding off the basal layer of the surface epithelium.

Differential Diagnosis. Adenoid basal carcinoma should be distinguished from pseudoepitheliomatous hyperplasia associated with inflammation. In pseudoepitheliomatous hyperplasia and acanthosis from healing erosions, nests of epithelium appear disconnected from the surface. Squamous metaplasia can fill superficial glands, producing bland nests resembling adenoid basal carcinoma. Adenoid basal carcinoma, however, forms nests and cords oriented haphazardly below the deepest level of endocervical glands. Furthermore, adenoid basal carcinoma involves the surface minimally or not at all, and is seldom associated with a significant degree of inflammation.

Adenoid basal carcinoma should be distinguished from adenoid cystic carcinoma and squamous cell carcinoma with basaloid features. Adenoid cystic carcinoma is more glandular, forming cystic spaces. Adenoid cystic carcinoma is also larger, involves the surface more extensively, is more widely infiltrative, and lacks squamous nests. Squamous cell carcinoma may contain a population of small squamous cells to the degree that it resembles adenoid basal carcinoma, but the squamous neoplasm is formed by frankly malignant cells and there is no gland formation. In contrast, nuclear abnormalities are minimal in adenoid basal carcinoma, and high mitotic activity is usually not a feature.

Clinical Behavior and Treatment. Treatment of adenoid basal carcinoma has been hysterectomy because of its deep location in most instances; sometimes it is an incidental finding in a hysterectomy specimen removed for other reasons. Conization may be appropriate under certain circumstances. Of the 20 reported cases, only one metastasized, and that one was unusual in that it had more glandular differentiation and a stromal morphea-like arrangement, unlike the usual adenoid basal carcinoma (247).

Carcinoid Tumor (Adenocarcinoma with Features of Carcinoid Tumor)

Definition. This designation applies to a carcinoma of the cervix with areas resembling a carcinoid and containing intracytoplasmic endocrine granules. It differs from typical carcinoids of the intestinal tract and elsewhere, and it is questionable whether a pure carcinoid of the cervix exists. Most reports of carcinoids in this location illustrate an adenocarcinoma with carcinoid features and prominent argyrophilic granules. This section summarizes the reports of so-called carcinoid of the cervix.

General Features. Initially described as a carcinoid tumor of the cervix because of a resemblance to an intestinal carcinoid and the presence of endocrine granules (240,241), it gradually became recognized that some cervical adenocarcinomas contain endocrine granules and have varying degrees of resemblance to a carcinoid (243,251, 253). It also became known that neuroendocrine granules were misnamed and are not specifically confined to cells derived from the neural crest.

Endocrine granules occur in 0.5 to 5 percent of cervical carcinomas (277). Most carcinomas with neuroendocrine granules are in the small cell carcinoma–atypical carcinoid spectrum, and many adenocarcinomas with carcinoid features have areas of small cell undifferentiated carcinoma and squamous differentiation (277). Even the original studies identified glandular, small cell, and mixed forms (240,241). Cases have been reported under the designation of *carcinoid, endocrine carcinoma, adenocarcinoma with endocrine granules, argyrophil cell carcinoma,* and *neuroendocrine carcinoma,* reflecting their diverse morphology and relationship to adenocarcinoma and small cell undifferentiated carcinoma.

The existence of a carcinoid tumor or adenocarcinoma with carcinoid features stems from the capacity of cells of the cervix to produce endocrine granules. Endocrine granules are identified by any of the following: 1) argyrophilia, 2) immunolocalization of polypeptides, or 3) electron microscopic evidence of secretory granules. Cells with argyrophilic granules are found in 20 to 40 percent of cervices, occurring more frequently in the squamous cells of the exocervix than in the glandular cells of the endocervix (248,273,283). Some of these cells are immunoreactive in the squamous portion of the cervix, whereas most argyrophilic cells of the cervix are Merkel type (248). In the glandular epithelium, the argyrophilic cells are chromogranin positive. The neoplasm reported as carcinoid in the cervix is derived either from these cells or from neometaplasia within a carcinoma (273).

The following polypeptides have been identified in cervical carcinoid tumors: somatostatin, calcitonin (285), vasoactive intestinal polypeptide, ADH, pancreatic polypeptide, β-melanocyte–stimulating hormone, ACTH, glucagon, insulin, gastrin (291), serotonin, and histamine (257,262,277). Some neoplasms produce as many as five immunoreactive substances (262).

Paraendocrine syndromes from cervical neoplasms are rare and include Cushing syndrome (259,262), carcinoid syndrome, and hypoglycemia. These are more likely to stem from small cell carcinoma than from a true carcinoid of the cervix.

Microscopic Findings. A wide morphological spectrum exists, ranging from adenocarcinoma dominated by a glandular pattern of carcinoid or islet cell tumor to a poorly differentiated small cell carcinoma similar to an oat cell carcinoma of the lung. Although carcinoid patterns have been illustrated, most if not all neoplasms are adenocarcinomas with carcinoid-like growth in cords and nests (fig. 142), ribbons (figs. 143, 144), solid sheets, and trabeculae, often with peripheral palisading of cells. All the patterns ascribed to neuroendocrine cells are seen, including islet cell tumor, medullary carcinoma of thyroid, and oat call carcinoma. Squamous metaplasia, adenosquamous differentiation (243,251,277), small cell carcinoma, and amyloid in the stroma (240,241) have all been reported. The cells that compose this tumor vary from small with scant cytoplasm to larger rounded or polygonal cells; some are spindle shaped. A variety of patterns in the same tumor is common. An AIS component has been identified in several instances (245,265,278). A pattern of goblet cell carcinoid has not been reported.

Clinical Behavior and Treatment. Carcinoid tumor of the cervix (adenocarcinoma with carcinoid features) is resistant to the traditional modes of therapy (243,277,291).

Small Cell Carcinoma

Definition. Small cell carcinoma is composed of a uniform population of small cells with a high nucleus-cytoplasm ratio resembling small cell carcinoma (oat cell carcinoma) of the lung.

General Features. Small cell carcinoma represents 2 to 5 percent of all cervical carcinomas. Patients are the same age or younger than women with ordinary forms of invasive cervical carcinoma. Noted for its aggressive behavior (253,269,289,290), small cell carcinoma is occasionally associated with polypeptide hormone production. A few paraendocrine syndromes have been reported in association with small cell carcinomas of the cervix, including Cushing syndrome (259), carcinoid syndrome, and Eaton-Lambert myasthenic syndrome (280). Ectopic secretion of ADH, insulin, and calcitonin also have been described, but it is not possible to determine whether the carcinomas responsible were small cell carcinomas, squamous cell carcinomas composed of small

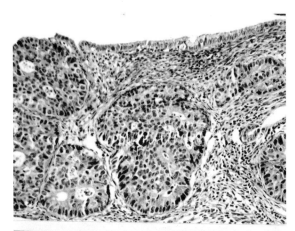

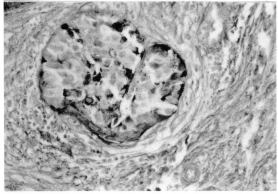

Figure 142

ADENOCARCINOMA WITH CARCINOID FEATURES

The upper field shows a glandular arrangement. The lower field shows argyrophilia in a solid nest (Cherukian-Schenk stain).

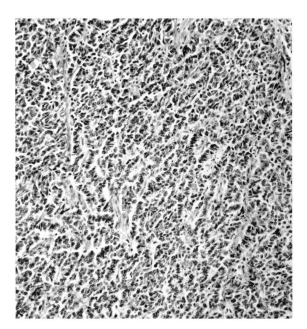

Figure 143

CARCINOID TUMOR

A ribbon-like arrangement is evident. This pattern usually merges with small cell undifferentiated carcinoma.

cells, or poorly differentiated adenocarcinomas with carcinoid features. Although human papillomavirus type 18 has been found in most of the small cell carcinomas with endocrine granules, type 16 has also been reported (162a).

Gross Findings. Grossly, small cell carcinoma is more often ulcerative and infiltrative than squamous or adenocarcinoma of the cervix. A barrel-shaped cervix is often formed.

Microscopic Findings. Microscopically, small cell carcinoma is highly cellular, composed of sheets of densely packed small cells with scant cytoplasm, and is identical to its counterpart in the vagina (see figs. 215, 216). In some examples, minor areas of glandular or squamous differentiation occur, but these, by definition, are less than 5 percent of the tumor. Nuclei are round-to-oval or slightly spindle shaped and densely hyperchromatic to the degree that nucleoli are inconspicuous and the nuclei appear smudged, obscuring nuclear detail. Morphometrically, small cell carcinoma has a mean nuclear diameter of 14.5 μm ± 2.1 (SD), versus a diameter of 18.6 ± 2.4 μm for keratinizing squamous cell carcinoma (290). The cytoplasm is scant and

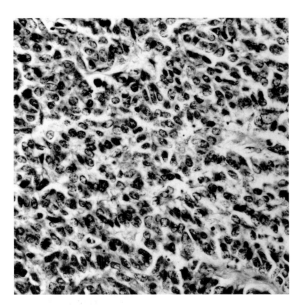

Figure 144
CARCINOID TUMOR
The small uniform cells are arranged in cords and gland-like units. This pattern merges with small cell undifferentiated carcinoma.

finely stippled. Cell outlines, like the nuclei, are spindle to oval. A few pleomorphic larger cells with more irregular nuclei and one or more nucleoli may be present. Mitotic activity is prominent, with three or more mitotic figures usually evident in each high-power field. Areas of necrosis are common. Capillary space invasion is observed in 60 to 90 percent of cases (289,290).

Immunohistochemical Findings. Nearly all neoplasms stain immunohistochemically for keratin. About one third to one half stain positively for one or more markers for endocrine granules such as chromogranin, serotonin, or somatostatin (287,290). The proportion that stains depends partly on the type of immunostain used. Neuron-specific enolase is too nonspecific to be a reliable marker for endocrine cells; nearly all small cell carcinomas stain for it. In one study of 10 small cell carcinomas of the cervix that were positive with neuron-specific enolase, argyrophilia was evident in only 3 of 10, chromogranin immunostaining was positive in half, and serotonin positivity was evident in only 2 of 10. Immunostains for neurofilaments were negative (287). Other investigators report an even higher degree of immunostaining for neuroendocrine granules (243,277).

Ultrastructural Findings. By electron microscopy, the cells are tightly packed with close apposition of cell membranes, leaving little intercellular space. The nuclei are round or oval, but some are irregular in outline. The chromatin is coarsely clumped and most dense adjacent to the nuclear membrane. The cytoplasm is scant but filled with mitochondria, Golgi, and profiles of smooth and rough endoplasmic reticulum. A few cells are dendritic with long tapering processes (251,260). These cells in particular tend to contain uniformly round or oval 120 to 250 nm dense core granules. The limiting membrane is separated from the core by a circumferential lucent space. Electron microscopy is less efficient in identifying endocrine granules than argyrophilic or immunohistochemical stains. Well-developed desmosomes with filamentous bundles resembling tonofilaments may be numerous in some tumors, reflecting squamous differentiation, but scant in others, and minor areas of the tumor may show intracytoplasmic lumens containing microvilli, a reflection of minor differentiation toward adenocarcinoma.

Differential Diagnosis. Distinguishing small cell carcinoma from other poorly differentiated neoplasms of the cervix is difficult because overlap exists with nonkeratinizing squamous cell carcinoma composed of small cells and poorly differentiated adenocarcinoma with carcinoid features (cervical carcinoid). This is particularly true in small biopsies. A diagnosis of small cell carcinoma should be limited to a small cell neoplasm in which squamous or glandular differentiation is minor or inconspicuous, i.e., less than 10 percent of the tumor. If 10 percent or more of the tumor has gland formation, a ribbon-like or trabecular pattern, or rosettes, the neoplasm should be regarded as a mixture with a component of adenocarcinoma or simply designated an adenocarcinoma with carcinoid features if trabecular areas are evident. Similarly, if 10 percent or more of the tumor has squamous differentiation, the tumor should be regarded as a mixture with a component of squamous cell carcinoma. These neoplasms all may contain endocrine granules.

Clinical Behavior and Treatment. The usual treatment is radical hysterectomy and bilateral pelvic and para-aortic lymphadenectomy. Pelvic radiation is given to patients with nodal metastasis. Metastasis occurs relatively early and frequently in the course of the disease, compared with ordinary cervical carcinoma. Lymph node metastasis is present in more than half of the patients with small cell carcinomas less than 2 cm in diameter and in a higher proportion of those with larger lesions (289,290). At least 40 percent of patients with stage I and II disease have recurrences, compared to about 30 percent of patients with other forms of cervical carcinoma of the same stages (290). In one study of 15 cases, there were only 3 patients free of tumor, and yet only one survivor had been followed more than 1 year (251). In another study, 12 of 14 women died of tumor even though most of the tumors were stage I or II (275). Distant metastasis to organs such as lung, liver, brain, and bone is common. Combination chemotherapy is added to the treatment for patients with stage II and higher stages, but metastases are seldom treated successfully.

Undifferentiated Carcinoma

All carcinomas that lack specific differentiation are placed in this category.

MESENCHYMAL TUMORS

Leiomyoma

Leiomyomas occur in the cervix in about 8 percent of uteri containing leiomyomas. Most cervical leiomyomas are asymptomatic, but some produce vaginal bleeding or discharge. Large cervical leiomyomas protrude below the os, fill the vagina, and may cause inversion of the uterus. Rare examples of squamous cell carcinoma arising on the irritated surface of a prolapsed leiomyoma have been reported.

Grossly, leiomyomas are typically discrete and firm and have a whorled appearance on sectioning. Microscopically, they differ little from those of the myometrium. Superficial erosions, edema (fig. 145), and infarction are more common in cervical leiomyomas than in those of the corpus. Increased mitotic activity may occur in those that are prolapsed or ulcerated. In these, mitotic activity is highest in a narrow zone, beneath the ulcer, but even in this zone it seldom exceeds 4 mitotic figures per 10 high-power fields.

Other Benign Mesenchymal Tumors

Both capillary hemangiomas (figs. 146, 147) and cavernous hemangiomas, as well as arteriovenous malformations occur in the cervix (296, 307,309). The malformations are generally small and secondary to biopsy or conization but may be part of a larger pelvic vascular abnormality.

Primary benign schwannomas of the uterine cervix have been reported (301) including one with pigment (319). Lipomas and lipoleiomyomas occur in the cervix but, other than in presentation, are similar to those of the uterine corpus. Most lipomatous differentiation in the uterus occurs within leiomyomas. Paragangliomas also occur, identified by their nesting arrangement, mixed population of chief and sustentacular cells, and endocrine granules (320). Individual cases of ganglioneuroma and rhabdomyoma have also been described (301).

Leiomyosarcoma

Leiomyosarcoma is the most common primary sarcoma in the cervix (295), although only 20 cases have been reported (297). Most leiomyosarcomas of the cervix are buried within reports of

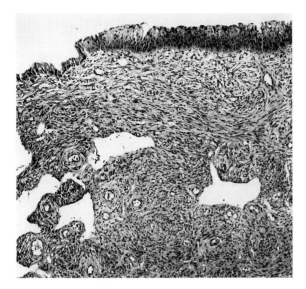

Figure 145
LEIOMYOMA
Spindle cells form a streaming pattern. Vascular channels are dilated in the leiomyoma.

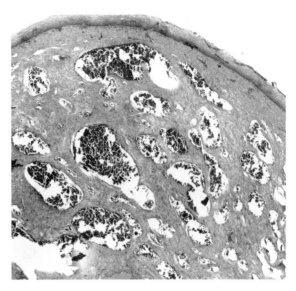

Figure 146
HEMANGIOMA OF THE CERVIX
The tumor is characterized by densely packed vascular channels of variable size lined by bland endothelial cells.

leiomyosarcoma of the uterine corpus. The youngest patient whose case has been reported was 36 years of age (316). Leiomyosarcoma of the cervix usually arises in perimenopausal women and presents with vaginal bleeding. Like other primary malignant tumors of the cervix, leiomyosarcoma may develop in a cervical stump after subtotal hysterectomy (316).

Grossly, leiomyosarcomas are polypoid but, in contrast to leiomyomas, are larger and softer, have a more irregular outline, and are more likely to contain areas of hemorrhage and necrosis.

Microscopically, leiomyosarcoma is composed of densely arranged interlacing bundles of smooth muscle cells with large, hyperchromatic, irregular nuclei. The microscopic criteria for leiomyosarcoma of the cervix are the same as for similar tumors of the uterine corpus. Nuclear atypia must be present, and mitotic figures in the most active areas must be 5 or more per 10 high-power fields, except for the rare myxoid leiomyosarcoma.

The treatment is the same as for leiomyosarcoma of the corpus. Survival is poor (295,316).

Endocervical Stromal Sarcoma

Twelve cases were reported by Abell and Ramirez (295). The patients ranged in age from 29 to 72 years, with an average of 54 years. All

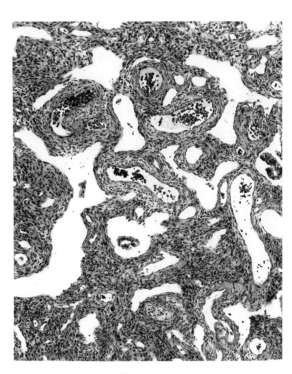

Figure 147
HEMANGIOMA OF THE CERVIX
The lesion extended from the level of the glands to deep in the endocervical stroma.

of them presented with vaginal bleeding, and some complained of pain. The tumors formed polypoid masses that protruded into the endocervical canal and infiltrated the wall of the cervix. Surface necrosis and hemorrhage were prominent. Microscopically, the tumors were composed of uniform small spindle cells with angular ill-defined outlines and tapered ends. The neoplasms resembled endometrial stromal sarcomas without the prominent background vascularity. Mitotic activity was high, usually exceeding 10 mitotic figures per 10 high-power fields. In the report of Abell and Ramirez, 6 of the 12 patients died of tumor. The illustrations are nonspecific, however, and there have been only three reports of endocervical stromal sarcoma since 1973, none of which described a specific entity (293,301,310).

Sarcoma Botryoides
(Embryonal Rhabdomyosarcoma)

Definition. This is a type of embryonal rhabdomyosarcoma characterized by grape-like clusters and an edematous myxoid background usually containing rhabdomyoblasts. A subepithelial cellular layer is characteristic.

General Features. Sarcoma botryoides usually arises in the vagina, but it may arise in the cervix (314). At times it is not possible to assign a primary site to a bulky tumor that involves both organs simultaneously. Older reports, summarized by Ober, obscure the fact that sarcoma botryoides of the cervix has a different clinical profile and prognosis from that of the vagina.

Clinical Features. Sarcoma botryoides of the cervix occurs in children and young women up to 26 years of age with a mean age of about 18 years. In contrast, sarcoma botryoides of the vagina is confined to infants and young children. Patients present with vaginal bleeding and a polypoid grape-like mass protruding from the cervix into the vagina. Some patients describe having passed tissue.

Gross Findings. Sarcoma botryoides forms multiple pedunculated or sessile soft grape-like clusters or single, multiple, and bilobed polyps covered by a glistening translucent surface. The sectioned surfaces vary from grayish white to light tan with punctate areas of hemorrhage. A stalk or pedicle is common.

Microscopic Findings. The surface is usually focally ulcerated. The stroma beneath the epithelium is overtly sarcomatous, showing a zone of increased cellularity (cambium layer) beneath the surface epithelium and around entrapped endocervical glands (fig. 148). The cells in the cambium layer are plump and spindle shaped with hyperchromatic nuclei and scant cytoplasm. Most sarcoma botryoides contain rhabdomyoblasts. These are large elongated cells with abundant eosinophilic cytoplasm, with and without cross striations. Immunohistochemical stains for desmin, muscle-specific actin and, less often, myoglobin are positive in rhabdomyoblasts. Deep to the cambium layer, the tumor is less cellular, with the cells loosely dispersed in an edematous or myxomatous stroma (fig. 149). Apart from the cambium layer, the stroma is usually vascular and edematous and is highly variable in its cellularity. The mitotic rate in the most cellular areas ranges from 2 to 12 mitotic figures per 10 high-power fields

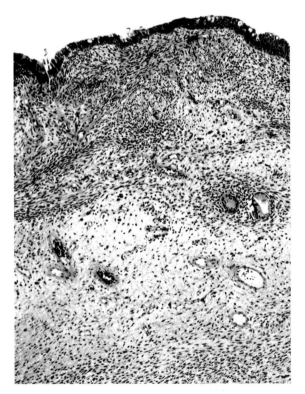

Figure 148
SARCOMA BOTRYOIDES
This figure shows sarcoma botryoides with a cellular cambium layer (top) and edematous stroma (lower center).

(304). Cartilaginous differentiation is a minor feature in about half of the cases (fig. 150). The grape-like areas evident clinically result from edema and myxoid change.

Differential Diagnosis. Sarcoma botryoides must be separated from adenosarcoma and an edematous mesodermal cervical polyp akin to those in the vagina (pseudosarcoma botryoides). Adenosarcoma may be found in young women and typically displays condensation of stromal cells beneath the surface epithelium and around glands that may resemble the cambium layer of sarcoma botryoides. Adenosarcoma, however, does not form grape-like clusters because the stroma is more fibrous and lacks the edematous aspect of sarcoma botryoides. Adenosarcoma also displays a prominent leaf-like pattern characterized by numerous epithelial-lined cysts and cleft-like invaginations of the surface resembling cystosarcoma of the breast. In contrast, if glands are present within a sarcoma botryoides, they are focal and the result of entrapment of surface epithelium.

Edematous cervical mesodermal polyps resemble sarcoma botryoides but differ in that polyps usually occur in adult women as solitary small, soft fleshy protuberances. They seldom exceed 1.5 cm in diameter. The edematous fibrous stroma of a polyp may resemble that of sarcoma botryoides, but a cambium layer or rhabdomyoblasts are not seen and there is more uniformity of the stroma within mesodermal polyps. Although polyps in pregnant women may contain atypical or multinucleate stromal cells, they are widely scattered and not part of a sarcomatous stroma (301,302,313).

Clinical Behavior and Treatment. Sarcoma botryoides of the cervix in young women is less aggressive than sarcoma botryoides of the vagina (304,314). Since 1950, the outlook for patients, particularly adults, has improved because of adjuvant chemotherapy. Of 29 patients in their second and third decades of life, all but four remained free of disease (303,304). In the series of 13 sarcoma botryoides reported by Daya and Scully (304), all patients were well 1 to 8 years postoperatively. The outlook for children with sarcoma botryoides of the cervix is less clear, although several have remained well after treatment (312,315). Therapy in recent years has tended toward less extensive operations than in the past, combined with multiagent chemotherapy (299,303,308). Radiation therapy had been unsuccessful when utilized before the

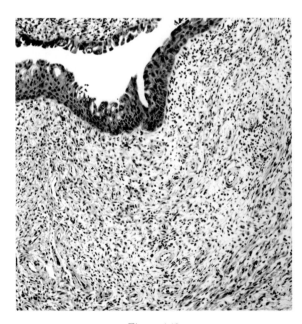

Figure 149
SARCOMA BOTRYOIDES
Edematous stroma produces a grape-like clinical appearance.

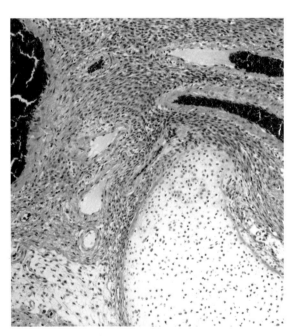

Figure 150
SARCOMA BOTRYOIDES
Cartilage occurs in nearly half of all cases. It is more immature in appearance than cytologically malignant.

use of modern adjuvant combination chemotherapy. Some patients with small stage I tumors have been well after conservative treatment such as polypectomy or cervicectomy. Daya and Scully (304) recommend adjuvant chemotherapy for large or deeply infiltrating stage I tumors and those in advanced stages.

Alveolar Soft-Part Sarcoma

General Features. More than 200 alveolar soft-part sarcomas (ASPSs) have been reported since its initial description in 1952, but only 6 have been located in the cervix (294,305,306,311,317). The patients have been between 30 and 40 years of age and have generally presented with bleeding. Five of the 6 had stage I disease. The origin of ASPS is uncertain; striated muscle, paraganglia, and nerve origins have all been suggested.

Gross Findings. Alveolar soft-part sarcoma forms a small, irregular, circumscribed, friable nodule on the cervix (294,317). The largest tumors reported were 4 cm in diameter (311).

Microscopic Findings. Microscopically, ASPS is relatively well demarcated, although infiltration of small groups of cells occurs at the periphery. The tumor is composed of cellular nests that are generally centrally cavitated, resembling alveoli, and separated by thin vascular septae. The cells are uniform and polyhedral, with abundant eosinophilic granular cytoplasm and small nuclei with prominent nucleoli. The cytoplasm is usually strongly PAS positive and diastase resistant. A characteristic and virtually diagnostic feature is the presence of PAS-positive, diastase-resistant rod-like crystals in the cytoplasm of about 80 percent of tumors.

Immunohistochemical and Ultrastructural Findings. Immunohistochemical examination shows myogenic characteristics in that muscle-specific actin and desmin are usually positive. In addition, a positive reaction with antibodies against neuron-specific enolase and S-100 have been described (294). Electron microscopy reveals basal lamina surrounding groups of tumor cells containing prominent mitochondria, abundant glycogen, lipid droplets, dense granules, and membrane-bound crystalline inclusions.

Differential Diagnosis. The main differential diagnosis includes metastatic renal cell carcinoma, clear cell carcinoma, and paraganglioma. Only two paragangliomas have been reported in the cervix (320). Paraganglioma is distinguished from ASPS by the presence of solid nests of chief and sustentacular cells and cells containing neuroendocrine granules. Metastasis to the cervix from renal cell carcinoma is rare. In addition, renal cell carcinoma lacks immunologic evidence of myogenic origin, it does not have the PAS-positive diastase-resistant crystals found in most ASPSs, and the ultrastructural features are entirely different. Clear cell carcinoma has a tendency to form papillary processes and small cysts. The cells are clearer than in ASPS, with relatively sparse PAS positivity in the cytoplasm. The PAS positivity in clear cell carcinoma also will dissolve with diastase digestion. Hobnail-appearing nuclear protrusions also occur in clear cell carcinoma but are rare or absent in ASPS.

Clinical Behavior and Treatment. Five patients underwent hysterectomy with bilateral salpingo-oophorectomy and were free of tumor at last contact. Only one of these patients received adjuvant chemotherapy.

Osteosarcoma

A pure osteosarcoma has been described in the cervix (298), akin to what has been described in the corpus (318). It occurred in a postmenopausal woman as a polypoid, fleshy, pinkish gray 3-cm neoplasm. Microscopically, malignant spindle cells were admixed with atypical cells within lacunae of osteoid.

Osteosarcoma should be distinguished from a malignant mesodermal mixed tumor and leiomyosarcoma with osteoclast-like giant cells. In a malignant mesodermal mixed tumor, malignant glands are intermingled with a sarcomatous stroma. Thorough sectioning may be necessary to identify an epithelial component in a sarcoma containing heterologous elements.

Osteoclast-like giant cells occur within some uterine leiomyosarcomas, but osteoid does not accompany them. Immunostains for actin and desmin should identify smooth muscle differentiation within a leiomyosarcoma. Desmin immunostains are negative in an osteosarcoma, but actin may be present if there is myofibroblastic differentiation within osteosarcoma.

Other Malignant Mesenchymal Tumors

These tumors include malignant schwannomas, liposarcomas, and malignant fibrous histiocytomas (301). A hemangiopericytoma involving the cervix has also been reported (300).

MIXED EPITHELIAL AND MESENCHYMAL TUMORS

Papillary Adenofibroma

General Features. Papillary adenofibromas are uncommon benign tumors. Originally described in 1971 (321), most occur in the endometrium (333). Those developing in the endocervix are less common but are similar to those of the endometrium. Of 10 adenofibromas of the uterus, only one arose from the cervix (334).

Gross Findings. Grossly, adenofibroma is papillary or sessile and protrudes into the endocervical canal. Some exceed 5 cm in diameter. Papillary adenofibroma is typically firm, rubbery, and tan-brown, with punctate areas of hemorrhage evident on the surface. The presence of small cysts on the sectioned surfaces imparts a spongy or mucoid appearance. Most are superficial and do not invade the underlying stroma.

Microscopic Findings. Microscopically, papillary adenofibroma has a nodular surface with a lobulated papillary configuration. Broad, fibrous, relatively acellular fronds are formed. The surface is covered by a flattened nonspecific cuboidal epithelium that is not significantly proliferative. Columnar mucinous cells and squamous differentiation occur focally in some tumors. The nuclei of the stromal cells are small, uniform, and bland; mitotic activity is low or absent; and there is no increased cellularity around entrapped glands.

Differential Diagnosis. The main differential diagnosis is adenosarcoma. Adenofibromas lack the stromal cellularity and invasiveness of adenosarcoma. In adenofibromas, the stromal cells have bland nuclei and little or no mitotic activity and there is much more intervening fibrous tissue.

Adenosarcoma

Only 2 of 24 adenosarcomas of the uterus arose in the cervix in the series of Zaloudek and Norris (334). Both occurred in 15-year-old patients. Nearly all of these tumors were confined to the uterus when discovered. Adenosarcomas in the cervix, as in the endometrium, are broad-based, sessile-polypoid growths that enlarge and distort the uterus.

Microscopically, papillary stromal fronds lined by epithelium form leaf-like processes that protrude into cysts and cleft-like spaces distributed within the stroma (figs. 151, 152). The epithelium is varied in adenosarcomas of the cervix, with a tendency to have more mucinous and squamous differentiation than in adenosarcomas of the endometrium. Adenosarcomas of the cervix, like those of the endometrium, are characterized by periglandular hypercellularity of the stromal component. The cellularity varies in different areas of the tumor. Differentiation to endometrial-type stroma occurs in focal areas of some tumors, but the stromal component is usually devoid of specific features. Atypia in the stromal cells varies throughout the tumor from mild to marked, and the frequency of mitotic figures also varies from sparse to 1 or 2 per

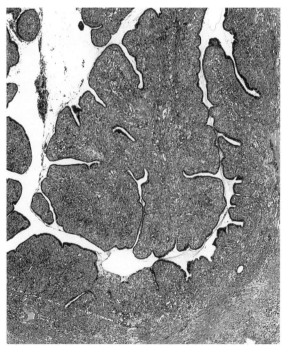

Figure 151
ADENOSARCOMA
The tumor is characterized by a leaf-like pattern resembling cystosarcoma phyllodes of the breast.

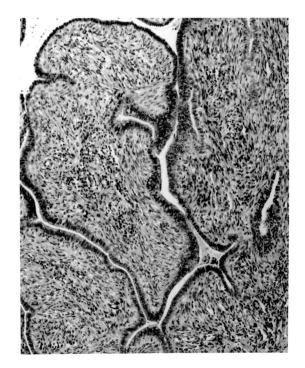

Figure 152
ADENOSARCOMA
The stromal component is uniformly cellular, fibrous and nonspecific in character. The cellularity is much greater than in an adenofibroma. The stromal cells are closely applied to the glandular epithelium.

high-power field in higher-grade areas. Most adenosarcomas have 4 or more mitotic figures per 10 high-power fields. About 25 percent contain heterologous elements in the form of rhabdomyoblasts, fat, cartilage, and osteoid, and smooth muscle differentiation is found in some.

The treatment of adenosarcoma is hysterectomy. Superficial adenosarcomas probably do not require radiation therapy, but those of the corpus invading more than halfway through the myometrium have a high likelihood of recurrence, so deeply invasive cervical adenosarcomas probably also require radiotherapy postoperatively. Because of the highly variable behavior and degree of atypia, individualized therapy is necessary. Two teenaged patients (334) and two adults (329) were well after having procedures less than hysterectomy for adenosarcoma of the cervix. Too few cases of adenosarcoma of the cervix have been documented, however, to

know whether the survival differs from that of adenosarcoma of the endometrium, recurrences of which develop in up to 25 percent of patients, mostly in the vaginal apex or pelvis. Death occurs in 10 to 25 percent of patients with adenosarcoma of the endometrium (324,327,334).

Malignant Mixed Mesodermal Tumor

General Features. Malignant mixed mesodermal tumors (MMMTs), both homologous (carcinosarcoma) and heterologous, develop as a primary sarcoma in the cervix less often than leiomyosarcoma. Most MMMTs involving the cervix represent extensions from the endometrium, because nearly 25 percent of endometrial MMMTs involve the cervix when initially seen. In the largest series of MMMTs of the uterus, only 1 of 202 was primary in the cervix (331). Most women with primary MMMT of the cervix are perimenopausal or menopausal.

Presenting symptoms of cervical MMMTs are the same as those of similar tumors arising in the corpus. Some patients were irradiated for squamous cell carcinoma of the cervix years earlier (322).

Gross Findings. Grossly, MMMT of the cervix forms a large polypoid partially necrotic mass that replaces the cervix.

Microscopic Findings. Microscopically, malignant glands are present along with sarcomatous differentiation. Much of the tumor is composed of undifferentiated small cells and malignant spindle cells. Fibroblastic and myofibroblastic differentiation is common (326). Squamous differentiation often occurs in small areas. About half of MMMTs contain a heterologous element, usually rhabdomyosarcoma. Chondrosarcoma occurs less frequently (331). Liposarcomatous differentiation and combinations of various heterologous components also occur. In one unusual MMMT of the cervix, ganglion cells and glial tissue were identified (325).

Clinical Behavior and Treatment. As in the corpus, MMMTs of the endocervix are highly malignant. Therapy usually consists of hysterectomy followed by combination chemotherapy or pelvic and abdominal irradiation, even if there is no evidence of metastasis, because of the high rate of relapse. The best outlook is for neoplasms that are small or pedunculated or are confined to polyps.

Wilms Tumor

Of the two reported cases of Wilms tumor of the uterus, one arose in the cervix (323). It occurred in a 13-year-old girl as a polypoid mass partially filling the vagina and producing vaginal bleeding. The lesion was 12 cm in diameter and attached to the endocervical canal by a short pedicle. Grossly, the neoplasm was gray, solid, and rubbery to gelatinous. Microscopically, it was focally ulcerated and composed of small cells with oval nuclei and scanty cytoplasm. A few admixed primitive tubules were present in a glomeruloid arrangement. A few areas of fetal-type skeletal muscle fibers with cross striations were present along with smooth muscle fibers and islands of mature cartilage. The patient was well at last contact, 9.6 years after operation. Wilms tumor is distinguished from MMMT by not containing areas of adenocarcinoma and by having glomeruloid differentiation and tubules.

MISCELLANEOUS TUMORS

Melanocytic Nevus

Nevi, similar microscopically to those arising in the skin, rarely occur in the cervix. These lesions are described in Tumors of the Vulva.

Blue Nevus

General Features. Blue nevus of the cervix was first described by Cid (341) in 1959, who subsequently found nine examples in 466 cervices, a frequency of 1.9 percent. The lesion varies considerably in frequency as revealed by Patel and Bhagavan (354), who found only 3 in 2500 hysterectomy specimens. At least 50 examples of this lesion have been described (343,354). Patients range from 22 to 73 years of age.

Gross Findings. Grossly, blue nevi are blue to black, flat, and usually only 2 or 3 mm in greatest dimension, but lesions as large as 1.5 and 2.0 cm have been described (354). About 20 percent are multiple. Typically, blue nevi appear as ill-defined lesions in the lower endocervix, usually posteriorly, but they have also been found in endocervical polyps. Most are incidental findings in biopsy, conization, or hysterectomy specimens (344).

Microscopic Findings. Microscopically, the lesion is similar to blue nevi in the skin, composed of collections of elongated, wavy dendritic cells arranged individually and in clusters just below and parallel to the endocervical epithelium (figs. 153, 154). Macrophages accompany the dendritic cells in the stroma. The cytoplasm of the nevus cells is filled with fine brown nonrefractile melanin pigment that stains green with Lillie's melanin stain and black with Grimelius and Fontana-Masson stains. The granules fail to react with Prussian blue and colloidal iron stains, excluding hemosiderosis. Immunostains for S-100 protein are usually positive. Ultrastructural examination confirms the dendritic nature of the elongated cytoplasmic processes and demonstrates electron-dense membrane-bound melanin granules and premelanosomes.

Differential Diagnosis. *Melanosis* is composed of benign, pigmented melanocytes in the basal layer of the epithelium and may be confused with blue nevus. At least five examples have been reported in the ectocervix (337). The lesion is flat and dark, and only 1–3 mm in diameter. Microscopically, the melanocytes are confined to the basal layer, but unlike melanosis in the skin, they are not accompanied by thickening of the epithelium. The melanocytes are usually densely pigmented and dendritic, but unlike blue nevus, they do not involve the stroma.

Malignant melanoma has junctional change and stromal infiltration by malignant cells. Hemosiderosis is similar microscopically, but the

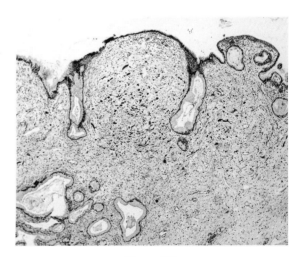

Figure 153
BLUE NEVUS
Low-power view showing dark, pigment-containing nevus cells in the cervical stroma.

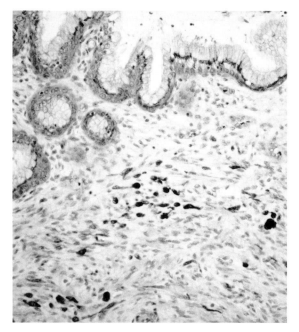

Figure 154
BLUE NEVUS
Dendritic melanocytes and melanophages are sparsely distributed in the stroma and are easily overlooked despite their dense cytoplasmic melanin.

hemosiderin granules are coarser, more refractile, and stain for iron. Furthermore, they do not stain positively with a Fontana-Masson stain and are found in macrophages rather than in dendritic spindle cells. Monsel's solution, a ferric subsulfate compound frequently used as a hemostatic agent after cervical biopsy, promotes the formation of hemosiderin deposition (342).

Malignant Melanoma

At least 24 primary melanomas have been reported in the cervix (335,340,348,353,355,359). It is one fifth as common as primary melanoma of the vagina and vulva. Melanoma of the cervix occurs in women ranging in age from 26 to 74 years who present with vaginal bleeding or discharge, often of short duration (345,351,352). About half of melanomas of the cervix involve the vagina (stage II) when discovered (351,352). Typically, melanomas appear as ulcerated grayish-blue or black protuberances or nodules. Microscopic examination reveals the tumor has a varied appearance similar to cutaneous melanomas and those arising in the vagina (see figs.

231–233). Small cell and spindle cell variants are relatively common. Even in the usual epithelioid cell type, areas of relatively small undifferentiated cells may occur. Junctional activity has been identified in less than half of the cases (352,355). Melanin pigment may be evident in hematoxylin and eosin stained slides. Melanoma-specific HMB-45 and S-100 immunostains are helpful in distinguishing melanoma from carcinoma, although a few poorly differentiated carcinomas are S-100 positive. Immunoreactions for keratin are negative in melanoma.

The differential diagnosis includes melanoma metastatic to the cervix. Most of these are primary in the vagina or vulvar skin. Metastatic melanoma, in contrast to primary melanoma, lacks junctional change.

Melanoma of the cervix has a poor prognosis. In summarizing melanomas of the cervix, Mordel et al. (351) found a 5-year survival of 40 percent for patients with stage I disease, but only 14 percent for higher stages. Most patients who die of tumor do so within 1 year of diagnosis. The most common and earliest site of spread from melanoma of the cervix is by direct extension and metastasis to the vagina. A successful treatment has not yet been found.

Lymphoma and Leukemia

General Features. Both lymphoma and rarely leukemia may become manifest initially in the cervix. More often, lymphoproliferative disorders involve the cervix secondarily in the course of systemic spread. More than 55 primary lymphomas of the cervix have been described (339,347,349,350). Less than 1 in 175 extranodal lymphomas present and possibly originate in the uterus or vagina. In reports, a distinction is seldom made between involvement of the cervix and involvement of the corpus. The cervix is more often affected as an initial manifestation of lymphoma than the uterine corpus or vagina (339,347). At necropsy, 2 to 9 percent of women with lymphoma have involvement of the uterus, about half of which is in the cervix (339).

Lymphomas of the cervix are staged by a modification of the Ann Arbor staging system for extranodal lymphomas (338) and by the International Federation of Gynecologists and Obstetricians (FIGO) system for staging of cervical carcinoma.

Clinical Features. The median age of women with lymphoma or leukemia is slightly over 40 years of age, with the age ranging from the third to ninth decade of life (339,347). More than 75 percent of patients present with a mass, 50 percent present with vaginal bleeding, and 33 percent have vaginal discharge. When the cervix is the initial site of disease, some patients also have anemia, splenomegaly, or other signs of lymphoma at the time of diagnosis. The duration of symptoms varies from 1 to 4 months. In about half the patients, the disease is stage II or more by FIGO criteria, being beyond the cervix with extension to the pelvic wall or lower third of the vagina. Most are stage IE by the modified Ann Arbor staging system for extranodal lymphomas; pelvic or para-aortic lymph node and ovarian involvement also occurs. Cervical cytology smears are usually negative (349,350).

Gross Findings. Lymphoma most commonly appears as a diffuse or multinodular enlargement of the cervix (fig. 155) without epithelial abnormality. The next most common presentation is as a polypoid endocervical mass protruding through the cervical os. Least commonly, the cervix has a granular, ragged or reddened surface as a result of ulceration of the tumor. Hodgkin disease, the rarest form of lymphoma of the cervix, tends to be more firm than that of the typical fish-flesh consistency of non-Hodgkin lymphoma (336). Granulocytic infiltrates may have a green color when freshly cut, giving rise to the term *chloroma*.

Microscopic Findings. Microscopically, lymphoma and leukemic infiltration produce two distinct patterns under low power, one infiltrating and one nodular. Follicular (nodular) lymphomas and diffuse large cell lymphomas are the most common subtypes. Granulocytic infiltrates in particular infiltrate the intrinsic structures of the cervix without destroying the landmarks (figs. 156, 157). Infiltration of vessel walls is characteristic. Extensive sclerosis also occurs in some infiltrates and crush artifact is common.

Immunohistochemical Findings. Immunostains recommended for a workup of lymphoma include LCA, investigation of monoclonality of immunoglobulin (light-chain restriction), and also L-26 for B cells, UCHL-1 for T cells, and Ki-1 for Hodgkin disease. Immunokeratin stains are negative in lymphoma and leukemia. A chloroacetate

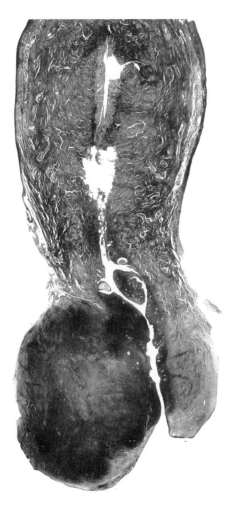

Figure 155
LYMPHOMA INVOLVING THE CERVIX
The tumor appears as a nodular enlargement of the cervix. (Fig. 1 from Chorlton I, Karnei RF, King FM, Norris HJ. Primary malignant reticuloendothelial disease involving the vagina, cervix and corpus uteri. Obstet Gynecol 1974;44:735–48.)

esterase stain as well as immunostains for myeloperoxidase for granulocytes helps to identify granulocytic infiltrates.

Differential Diagnosis. Lymphoma-like lesion (pseudolymphoma), small cell undifferentiated carcinoma, and metastatic carcinomas are the main considerations in the differential diagnosis. The cervix often is the site of an intense inflammatory response, but lymphoma-like lesions have a mixed cell infiltrate, indicative of a reactive process, and may form germinal centers.

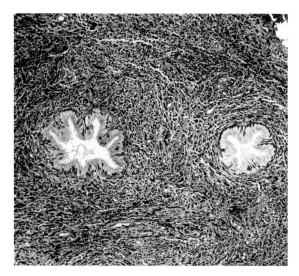

Figure 156
LYMPHOMA, LYMPHOCYTIC TYPE
The endocervical glands are preserved. (Fig. 2 from Chorlton I, Karnei RF, King FM, Norris HJ. Primary malignant reticuloendothelial disease involving the vagina, cervix and corpus uteri. Obstet Gynecol 1974;44:735–48.)

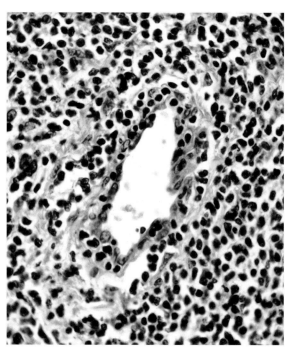

Figure 157
LYMPHOMA, LYMPHOCYTIC TYPE
High magnification of lesion illustrated in fig. 156, showing diffuse proliferation of small lymphocytes.

Lymphoma-like lesion is seldom, if ever, monomorphic. It is more superficial than lymphoma, is usually ulcerated, and almost always contains niduses of polymorphonuclear leukocytes and plasma cells. Lymphoma, in contrast, forms a larger lesion that deeply invades the stroma, often with associated sclerosis, deep perivascular infiltration, and a monomorphic cell population (358). A thin uninvolved subepithelial stromal layer is almost always present in cases of lymphoma. Immunostains may be needed to confirm the monoclonal nature of the infiltrate and thereby distinguish lymphoma from lymphoma-like lesions that are polyclonal.

A leukemic infiltrate may be difficult to distinguish from a poorly differentiated carcinoma. Leukemic cells do not have the cohesive quality resulting from cell membrane adherence that characterizes carcinoma. In addition, LCA positivity, when present, distinguishes a lymphoma or leukemia from primary or metastatic small cell carcinoma. A positive immunochemical stain for keratin identifies most carcinomas, but if the stain is negative, neuroendocrine markers may be positive in small cell carcinoma. Electron-microscopic examination was used to help differentiate lymphoma and leukemia from undifferentiated small cell carcinoma before the use of immunohistochemical stains. Imprint preparations and cytologic smears may be useful in distinguishing lymphoma and leukemic infiltrates from carcinoma in which the cells are adherent, clustered, and display epithelial characteristics, unlike the cells of lymphoma and leukemia.

Clinical Behavior and Treatment. The actuarial 5-year survival for stage IE lymphoma of the cervix alone is more than 75 percent (347,349,357). In one study, none of the 12 patients with stage IE lymphoma of the cervix or vagina who received definitive initial local treatment in the form of surgical excision or radiation therapy had relapse of their tumor (347). In another study, 4 of 6 patients with extranodal lymphoma had no evidence of disease after 1 year or more of follow-up (339). Granulocytic sarcoma presenting in the cervix may take 2

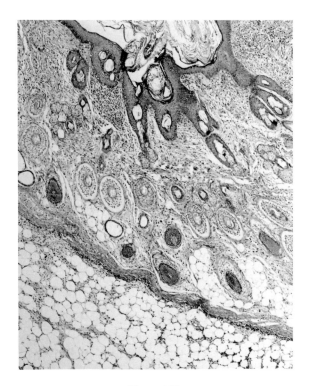

Figure 158
MATURE TERATOMA
This teratoma is composed of fat, mature squamous epithelium, and sebaceous glands.

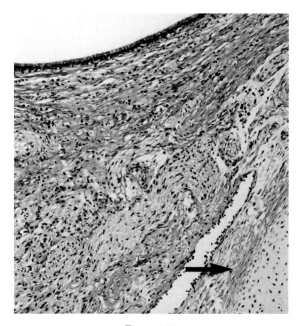

Figure 159
MATURE TERATOMA
This teratoma is composed of nerve tissue formed beneath a cystic endocervical gland. Cartilage is present in the lower right corner (arrow). This tumor is also illustrated in fig. 158.

years or more to become evident systemically (339,356). Radiation therapy is recommended for lymphoma, with combination chemotherapy advocated for patients with systemic disease (349).

Tumors of Germ Cell Type

Mature Teratoma. Teratomas of the uterus are uncommon in that only 10 examples have been reported, most of them primary polypoid lesions of the cervix, when the origin is known (346). Teratomas of the cervix are composed of mature elements including squamous epithelium organized as a skin surface with sebaceous glands and hair overlying fat (fig. 158). Bone, cartilage (fig. 159), mature lymphoid tissue, choroid plexus and ganglion cell differentiation also accompany the epidermal differentiation. Teratomas contain more than ectodermal derivatives, distinguishing them from epidermal metaplasia. All have been benign.

Yolk Sac Tumor (Endodermal Sinus Tumor). Yolk sac tumors occur as a primary tumor of the cervix, just as they do in the vagina. Although most yolk sac tumors arising in the vagina do not involve the cervix, some involve both areas at presentation. In many reports the primary site is not clearly defined, but approximately 10 to 15 percent of yolk sac tumors of the lower genital tract originate in the cervix and the majority arise in the vagina. The tumor develops in young children, usually from 14 to 27 months of age, and produces a blood-tinged vaginal discharge. Alpha-fetoprotein serum levels may be elevated. Grossly, yolk sac tumor is soft, friable, pedunculated or polypoid, and partially eroded. Microscopically, they are similar to those in the vagina (see figs. 234–236). Reticular, solid, and festoon patterns of yolk sac tumor are common, whereas the polyvesicular and hepatoid patterns have not been described. Schiller-Duval bodies are common in most neoplasms. Although early reports described a dismal outlook, modern combination chemotherapy and surgery offer a reasonable chance of cure.

117

SECONDARY TUMORS

About half of secondary tumors of the cervix stem from direct extension from an endometrial primary tumor (360). Poorly differentiated adeno-carcinoma of the endometrium is particularly likely to invade the cervix directly. Distinction from a primary carcinoma of the cervix extending to the endometrium may be difficult. A diagnosis of a primary endometrial carcinoma is made if the endometrial lesion is larger, if the cervical lesion is superficial, and if the microscopic pattern is consistent with an endometrial origin. The presence of coexistent endometrial hyperplasia supports an endometrial origin, whereas the presence of CIN or AIS of the cervix supports a primary cervical neoplasm. The clinical presentation usually provides clues as to the primary site, but at times, examination of the hysterectomy specimen is needed.

Of metastatic carcinomas to the cervix, ovarian carcinoma is the most common source (361, 362). Surface-implantation metastasis occurs from ovarian, tubal, and endometrial primary carcinomas.

Metastasis from extragenital tumors involves the ovary and vagina much more often than the cervix. Abrams et al. (360) reviewed the distribution of metastases from 1000 autopsies of patients dying with carcinoma and found metastases to the cervix in only 0.3 percent of cases. Of extragenital primary tumors that metastasize to the cervix, those of the breast, stomach, and colon are the most frequent, with scattered cases of metastasis from lung, pancreas, bladder, liver, kidney, and gallbladder also reported (360,362,365).

Carcinoma of the breast is the most common extragenital tumor to metastasize to the cervix (fig. 160). Yazigi and co-workers (366), in summarizing 24 cases of cervical metastasis from breast carcinoma, found that 80 percent occurred within 1 year after treatment of the breast tumor. Most of the other metastases were discovered at the time of diagnosis of the breast carcinoma, and in only one patient was the metastasis to the cervix the initial manifestation of the disease. The mean survival after identification of the metastatic tumor was only 1 year.

More than 30 cases of carcinoma of the stomach metastatic to the cervix have been reported (362,363), and about one third of them present in the cervix with suspicious or malignant cells in cervical smears (363). Of the carcinomas of the lung that have metastasized to the cervix, most have been of the small cell variety. More than 20 cases of carcinoma of the colon or rectum have metastasized to the cervix (365), but in only one case was the cervical involvement the initial presentation of the carcinoma.

Regardless of the primary site, nearly 90 percent of women with metastasis to the cervix have evidence of widespread disease (366). The most common symptom of metastasis to the cervix is vaginal bleeding, occurring in 75 percent of patients.

Grossly, the cervix usually appears normal, but it may reveal a minor eccentric thickening, small erosion, or slight irregularity of the mucosal surface. Microscopically, multiple nodular subepithelial infiltrates are evident. Most metastases are poorly differentiated, infiltrating around endocervical glands and involving lymphatic spaces. Features that suggest metastasis are the absence of an in situ component and relatively extensive lymphatic permeation in otherwise small superficial lesions. Immunostains for epithelial markers are often helpful in excluding a lymphoma or leukemic infiltrate.

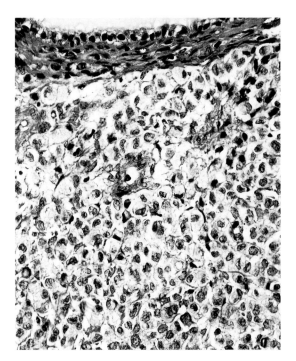

Figure 160
METASTATIC CARCINOMA

In this metastatic carcinoma from the breast, the dense aggregate of small round cells is located just beneath the surface. Signet-ring cells are also present.

TUMOR-LIKE LESIONS

Mesodermal Stromal Polyp (Pseudosarcoma Botryoides)

Mesodermal stromal polyps arise in the exocervix of women of reproductive age, particularly in pregnant women. They are much less common in the cervix than in the vagina, where they were initially described and designated vaginal polyps (382) (see Tumors of the Vagina). An exophytic lesion, mesodermal polyp is composed of edematous stroma covered by squamous epithelium. Scattered within the stroma are small spindle-shaped cells with scant cytoplasm and bland nuclei. The stroma may also contain occasional enlarged multinucleate hyperchromatic fibroblasts that may produce an alarming appearance, particularly in a patient at term (370). Unlike sarcoma botryoides, the lesion is not characterized by dense cellularity or a cambium layer, mitotic figures are rare, and rhabdomyoblasts are absent.

Microglandular Hyperplasia

General Features. Microglandular hyperplasia is a complex proliferation of endocervical glandular epithelium that was initially recognized in patients taking oral contraceptives (387,389). It may occur in pregnant women, but in pregnancy it is usually smaller than the lesion related to oral contraceptives (369,376). Postmenopausal women taking estrogen-progestogen replacement therapy may have microglandular hyperplasia. Women taking oral contraceptives are likely to have more extensive microglandular hyperplasia, squamous metaplasia, inflammation, and edema than those without a history of oral-contraceptive use. Oral contraceptive effects on endocervical glands include increased numbers of glands and hypersecretion with microglandular hyperplasia in about 3 percent of the cases (373).

Gross and Microscopic Findings. Microglandular hyperplasia is polypoid and may be single or multiple. Early lesions may appear sessile. Microscopically, densely crowded small glands are lined by a single layer of cuboidal cells containing varying amounts of mucin (figs. 161, 162). The cytoplasm is clear to finely granular, amphophilic to eosinophilic, and typically shows subnuclear vacuolization. Nuclei are uniformly small and round and have fine evenly dispersed chromatin. Nuclear enlargement and hyperchromatism are minimal or absent, unless an

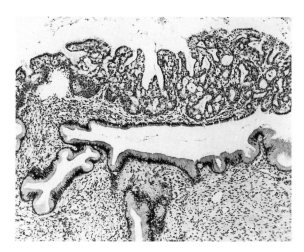

Figure 161
MICROGLANDULAR HYPERPLASIA
This figure shows the development from endocervical surface epithelium. (Fig. 5 from Taylor, HB, Irey NS, Norris HJ. Atypical endocervical hyperplasia in women taking oral contraceptives. JAMA 1967;202:637-9.)

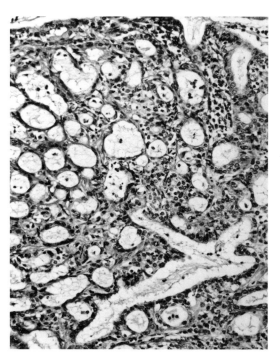

Figure 162
MICROGLANDULAR HYPERPLASIA
Glands are densely packed but not cytologically malignant.

Arias-Stella reaction has supervened. Mitotic figures are absent or sparse. The glandular cells stain weakly with mucicarmine, alcian blue, and PAS with diastase digestion, but the secretion within gland lumens is strongly positive. Neutrophils are typically present within gland lumens. Foci of squamous metaplasia may be present, and eosinophils and lymphocytes are scattered throughout. Stromal edema is common. A few stromal cells are present, compressed between glands.

Unusual forms of microglandular hyperplasia exist. These may be mucinous or solid or have areas of hyalinization (376,393). In the mucinous variant, islands and nests of detached cells float in pools of mucin. The solid pattern is characterized by sheets of clear cells with slightly vacuolated cytoplasm (fig. 163). The cells have small, centrally positioned, bland or slightly atypical nuclei. In both the mucinous and solid patterns, atypia is slight, and mitotic figures are largely absent. Abundant stromal hyalinization also occurs in some lesions. Fortunately, these unusual patterns are associated with areas of more typical microglandular hyperplasia.

Differential Diagnosis. Microglandular hyperplasia must be distinguished from clear cell carcinoma. The latter tends to form papillary processes and is composed of more open glands and tubules. In addition, clear cell carcinoma often contains hobnail cells with enlarged, hyperchromatic nuclei protruding into the lumens of glands and tubules. Clear cell carcinoma also has easily recognized mitotic figures. The absence of mitotic figures in densely packed glands of microglandular hyperplasia is a particularly helpful discriminating feature. The presence of a high glycogen content and absence of squamous metaplasia also help distinguish clear cell carcinoma from microglandular hyperplasia.

Adenocarcinoma may also arise in a cervix with microglandular hyperplasia, but the nuclear atypia, high mitotic activity, invasion into the cervical stroma, and histologic patterns consistent with adenocarcinoma of the cervix should help discriminate between the two.

Mesonephric Remnants

Mesonephric remnants occur in up to 22 percent of cervices (figs. 164–167). Their frequency varies with the type of specimen because they are seldom encountered in biopsy specimens, but are relatively common in conization and hysterectomy specimens in which deep portions of the

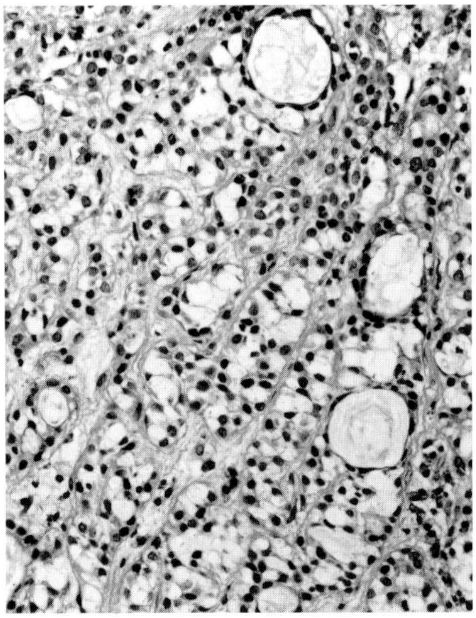

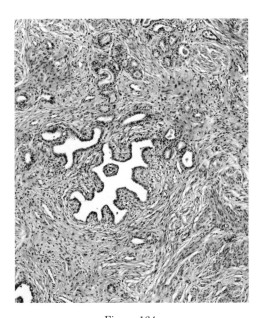

Figure 163
MICROGLANDULAR HYPERPLASIA
In this solid pattern, nests and sheets of vacuolated cells have formed between gland spaces.

Figure 164
MESONEPHRIC REMNANTS
A main branching duct is surrounded by clusters of mesonephric tubules.

cervix are routinely examined. Mesonephric remnants are asymptomatic incidental findings because they are too small to be seen visibly. Microscopically, they occur most commonly midway through the cervix in the lamina propria of the lateral wall beneath the junction of the exocervix with the endocervix. Mesonephric remnants often have a main branching duct with small tubular glands clustered in lobules around it. The main duct, when present, has an ampullary character (fig. 164). The tubules are distinctive and composed of a single layer of flat (fig. 165) to cuboidal cells (fig. 166) having cytoplasm that does not stain with PAS or mucicarmine. A prominent basement membrane surrounds the tubules, and a dense eosinophilic or hyaline secretion, also negative for mucicarmine, is usually present within lumens (figs. 165, 166).

Mesonephric tubules differ from endocervical glands by their small size, deep location, clustering about a main duct, absence of mucin production, presence of a basement membrane about tubules, and dense intraluminal eosinophilic secretion.

Cysts may develop from mesonephric remnants. These are solitary and lined by flattened or cuboidal epithelium. Squamous metaplasia rarely occurs in the cystic ampullary portion of mesonephric duct remnants (fig. 167).

Mesonephric Hyperplasia

Mesonephric remnants ordinarily occupy only a few millimeters of the deep cervical stroma. A diagnosis of hyperplasia is based on the presence of 1) a prominent increase in the number of tubules (figs. 168, 169), 2) an increase in lobule size (fig. 168), and 3) diffuse or extensive involvement of the cervix. The tubules may involve almost the full thickness of the cervix. In mesonephric hyperplasia the cells may show signs of activity and growth in the form of more variation in cell size and shape than usual (fig. 170). In addition, there is more variation in the staining intensity of the cytoplasm and nuclei and mitotic figures are observed at a rate of up to 2 per 10 high-power fields (367,378). Rare cases of mesonephric adenocarcinoma have been described.

Arias-Stella Reaction

The Arias-Stella reaction typically occurs in the endometrium in association with pregnancy, including ectopic gestations and gestational trophoblastic disease. Occasionally, it occurs in endocervical glands under these circumstances and

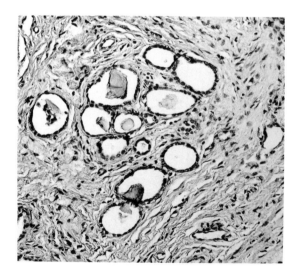

Figure 165
MESONEPHRIC REMNANTS
These mesonephric remnants are in a cluster. Tubules are lined by flat cells, and a dense hyaline secretion is present in some lumens.

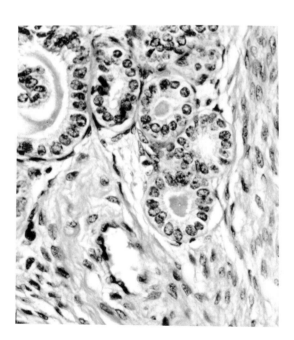

Figure 166
MESONEPHRIC REMNANTS
The cells are cuboidal and a basement membrane is evident around the tubules.

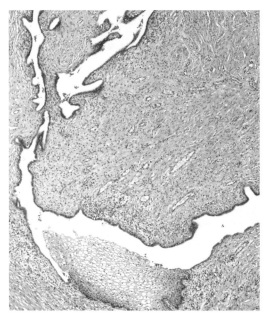

Figure 167
CYSTIC MESONEPHRIC DUCT REMNANT

This ampullary portion of a cystic mesonephric duct remnant has a small area of squamous metaplasia. The deep position, complex arrangement, flat to cuboidal lining cells, lack of surface connection, and absence of mucin production favor mesonephric origin.

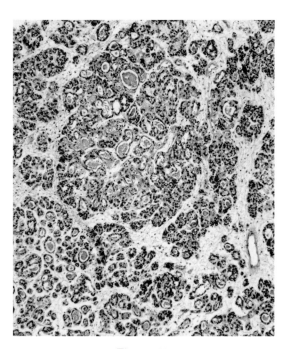

Figure 168
MESONEPHRIC HYPERPLASIA

Despite marked proliferation of tubules, there is retention of the lobular organization.

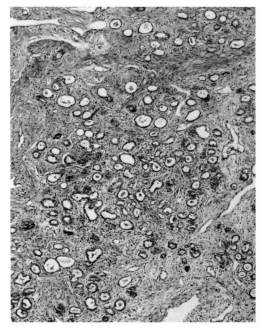

Figure 169
MESONEPHRIC HYPERPLASIA

These are characterized by a diffuse distribution of tubules, which extend throughout the inner two thirds of the cervix.

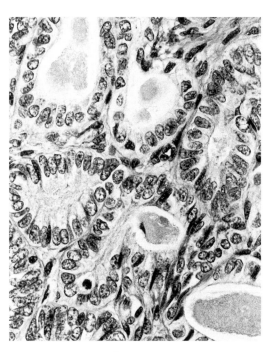

Figure 170
MESONEPHRIC HYPERPLASIA

The tubular cells are focally stratified, enlarged, and cuboidal to columnar, and there is variation in nuclear shape compared with mesonephric remnants.

is similar in appearance to the endometrial lesion. Microscopically, the Arias-Stella reaction is characterized by glands lined by vacuolated epithelial cells having a hypersecretory appearance (figs. 171, 172). The nuclei are pleomorphic, enlarged, hyperchromatic, and typically protrude into the glandular lumen with little accompanying cytoplasm, resulting in a hobnail appearance. The Arias-Stella reaction should not be confused with clear cell carcinoma. In contrast to clear cell carcinoma, the Arias-Stella reaction is associated with other morphologic alterations associated with pregnancy, such as hypersecretory glands and decidua. In addition, mitotic activity is rarely present in the Arias-Stella reaction compared with clear cell carcinoma.

Endometriosis

Usually located on the portio, the combination of endometrial glands and stroma, along with hemofuscin-laden or hemosiderin-laden macrophages, is diagnostic. If stroma is not present, the lesion cannot be identified with certainty. In this situation, the distinction from endometrial or tubal metaplasia or atypical hyperplasia of endocervical glands is based on the cell type and the position of the glands deep to the usual location of endocervi-

cal glands (fig. 173). In instances where only stroma is present (stromal endometriosis), the possibility of confusion with an endometrial stromal sarcoma exists, but stromal endometriosis is distinguished from endometrial and endocervical stromal sarcoma by its small size and failure to infiltrate widely at the periphery (372).

Cysts

Cysts of the cervix are usually the result of a dilated endocervical gland entrapped in the stroma. Some reach 1.5 cm in diameter. Most are multiple and contiguous with cystically dilated Nabothian cysts or normal-sized overlying endocervical glands. A cyst may extend through the endocervix to within 1 mm of the paracervical connective tissue (371). Most endocervical glandular cysts are lined by a single layer of endocervical-type cells that vary from columnar to flattened but are nonetheless mucinous in character. Mitotic figures and cell stratification are not observed. Mucin positivity of the luminal borders is usually present. Minimal deviation carcinoma

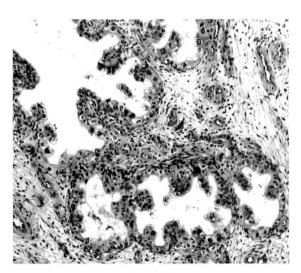

Figure 171
ARIAS-STELLA REACTION
The gland outlines are complex, resembling tortuous late secretory endometrial glands. The stroma is cervical not endometrial in character. The cytoplasm of glandular cells is vacuolated, and an occasional nucleus is enlarged, hyperchromatic, and protrudes into the lumen, i.e., so-called hobnail cells.

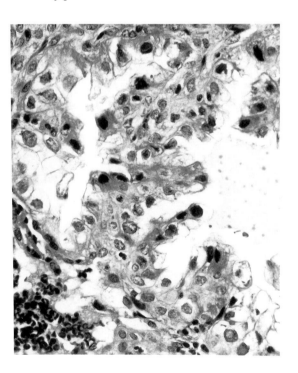

Figure 172
ARIAS-STELLA REACTION
This higher magnification of an Arias-Stella reaction shows nuclear enlargement and hyperchromasia similar to the Arias-Stella reaction in endometrial glands.

may form large mucinous cysts also, but in these the cells are large, the epithelium is hyperplastic in appearance, and the cysts are a component of a larger proliferation of glands of abnormal sizes and shapes. Less common types of benign cysts include a cystic gland within endometriosis or one showing tubal metaplasia. These are not grossly cystic and are superficial cystically dilated glands rather than true cysts. Cysts derived from the mesonephric duct are usually lined by flattened epithelium or cuboidal epithelium deep within the stroma unconnected to endocervical glands and do not contain mucin. Squamous metaplasia may rarely develop in some of these.

Decidual Nodule

Decidual nodules occur in the cervix during pregnancy just beneath the epithelium. They seldom exceed 3 or 4 mm in diameter. Decidual cells are uniform with abundant pale granular cytoplasm and a well-defined cell membrane (fig. 174). A decidual nodule may be confused with nonkeratinizing squamous cell carcinoma or a placental-site nodule (see below). The decidual cells, however, have no continuity with the surface epithelium and are not associated with an intraepithelial neoplasm. Decidual cells have uniform bland nuclei, differing from the more pleomorphic nuclei of the placental-site nodule and the nuclei of nonkeratinizing squamous cell carcinoma, which has coarsely clumped chromatin. Decidual cells also have no mitotic figures. An immunohistochemical stain for keratin is negative in decidual cells, whereas it is positive in squamous cell carcinoma and placental-site nodule.

Placental-Site Nodule

Early implantation sites are small and usually not visible grossly, and most are found incidentally in the endometrium of women of reproductive age (392). In the endometrium, they may be associated with menometrorrhagia. In the cervix, the placental-site nodule is located immediately beneath the epithelial surface and appears as a well-defined nodular hyalinized lesion composed of intermediate trophoblast showing

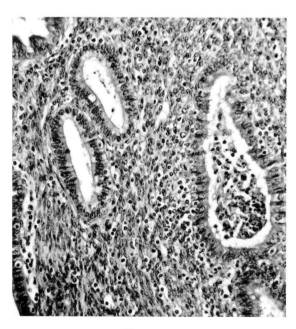

Figure 173
ENDOMETRIOSIS
The endometrial stromal cells are concentrated around the glands. The cells are round and more densely aggregated than cervical stromal cells.

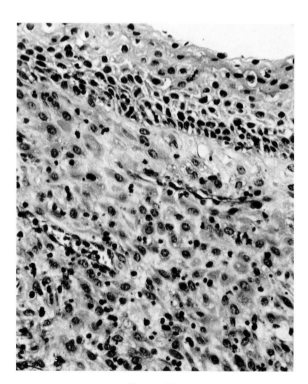

Figure 174
DECIDUALIZED STROMAL CELLS
These decidualized cells are in the stroma of the cervix in a pregnant woman. Decidual cells have abundant pink cytoplasm and may aggregate sufficiently to form a visible nodule.

cytoplasmic vacuolization and occasional inflammatory cells (figs. 175, 176). The intermediate trophoblastic cells are mainly mononucleate, but some are multinucleate. Confusion with early squamous cell carcinoma is possible. Placental-site nodules, however, lack significant atypia and only rarely contain mitotic figures. In addition, the cells are usually focally positive for human placental lactogen by immunostaining, in contrast to squamous cell carcinoma, which is negative. Because intermediate trophoblast reacts strongly with antibodies against keratin, a positive keratin immunostain should not lead to an erroneous diagnosis of carcinoma.

Amputation (Traumatic) Neuroma

A traumatic neuroma occurs in the cervix as a rare complication of conization (368). It forms an irregular firm gray area up to 2 mm in the region of the conization margin or scar. Microscopically, numerous haphazardly arranged tangles of nerves are evident within a scar composed of mature collagen and entrapped smooth muscle fibers. An immunohistochemical stain for S-100 confirms the presence of nerve fibers within the collagen.

Postoperative Spindle Cell Nodule

Postoperative spindle cell nodule may develop in the cervix after trauma, such as biopsy or curettage (377). The lesion develops more commonly in the vulva and vagina and only occasionally recurs after excision (383). A history of recent trauma or surgery is helpful in the diagnosis and should be present. The lesion resembles nodular fasciitis, being composed of loose actively proliferating spindle cells that may infiltrate at the periphery. The cells form bundles and fascicles, often separated by edema. A delicate network of capillaries is present within the lesion, and neutrophils and erythrocytes are often prominent, producing a resemblance to granulation tissue. The nuclei are oval to spindle shaped, but vary in size. Some are swollen or mildly hyperchromatic. Mitotic figures are common.

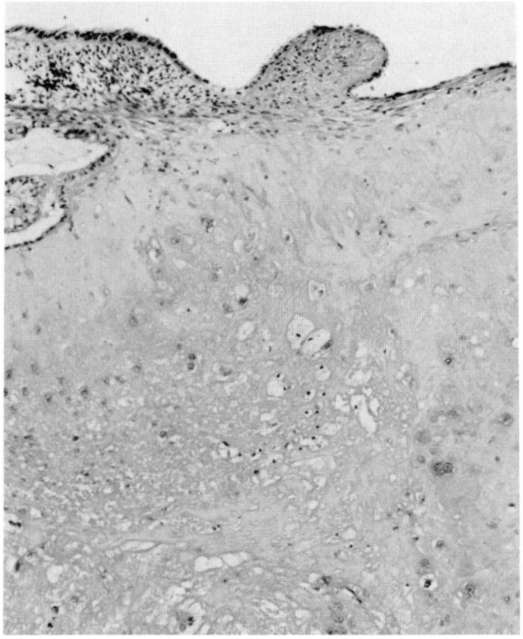

Figure 175
PLACENTAL-SITE NODULE
This nodule is located just below the surface. The lesion can be mistaken for keratinizing squamous cell carcinoma, but the sparsely cellular hyaline stroma helps to identify this lesion.

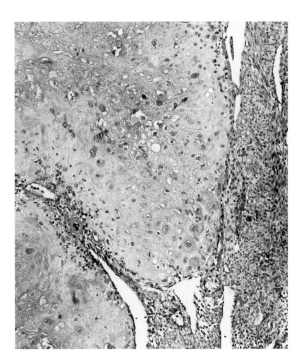

Figure 176
PLACENTAL-SITE NODULE
The higher magnification of intermediate trophoblast shows nuclear enlargement and cytoplasmic vacuolization.

Intestinal Metaplasia

Intestinal metaplasia may occur within atypical hyperplasia, AIS, and invasive adenocarcinoma of the endocervix. Goblet cells are present, and argentaffin and Paneth cells are occasionally seen (388). A lesion resembling a villous adenoma associated with nearby invasive adenocarcinoma has also been described (380).

Tubal Metaplasia

Tubal metaplasia is characterized by architecturally normal glands lined by cells resembling those of the fallopian tube mucosa. Ciliated or clear cells, nonciliated cells, and intercalary (peg) cells are often all present (fig. 177). Tubal metaplasia usually involves a single gland or a few glands near the squamocolumnar junction and is not associated with inflammation. The lesion is associated with minor foci of tubal metaplasia in the endometrium (386).

Epidermal Metaplasia

Epidermis, sebaceous glands, and hair follicles, alone or in combination, may occur in the cervix (fig. 178). Sebaceous glands alone have been described in eight cases (375). The origin of skin constituents in the cervix is controversial. Most investigators favor mesodermal metaplasia, but others favor a heterotopia. Epidermal differentiation in the form of sebaceous and eccrine glands and hair follicles has also been found within a squamous cell carcinoma of the cervix (375). This lesion should be distinguished from a mature teratoma, which also occurs in the cervix.

Glial Polyp

Glial tissue in the cervix is very rare; 33 cases have been reported (379,384,391). Glia containing bland astrocytes typically occurs as a discrete small polypoid lesion in the endocervix. In one instance, the endometrium and the endocervix were extensively infiltrated by soft white polypoid tissue 10 cm in extent (391). Most glial polyps are small and confined to the endocervix.

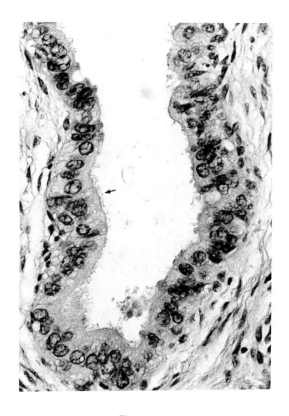

Figure 177
TUBAL METAPLASIA
This is characterized by pseudostratified epithelium with oval to round slightly enlarged nuclei. Some cells are ciliated (arrow).

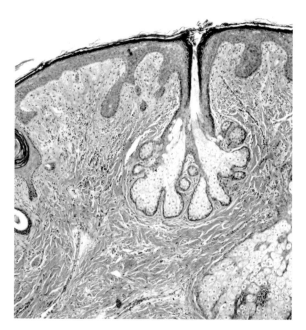

Figure 178
EPIDERMAL METAPLASIA
Here the epidermal metaplasia is in the form of sebaceous glands in the cervix. This phenomenon differs from teratoma in that only skin derivatives are present in epidermal metaplasia.

Microscopic examination shows glial tissue of low to moderate cellularity surrounding nearby endocervical glands and invading the stroma at the margin (fig. 179). Within the glia, astrocytes are relatively evenly spaced, multipolar with long radiating processes, and without atypia. Interwoven fine fibrillary processes that stain with phosphotungstic acid hematoxylin are present. Immunostains for glial acidic fibrillary protein may be positive in the cytoplasm of the astrocytic cells as well as in the glial stroma. All glial polyps have been benign, although several have recurred as late as 5 years after initial excision.

Three origins have been proposed for the presence of glia in the cervix. First, in some instances, fetal brain tissue implanted at the time of curettage or abortion and persisting as a graft probably occurs. Patients with a glial polyp, like those with heterotopic cartilage, are commonly of reproductive age and have a history of abortion or instrumentation, consistent with an origin of the glia or cartilage from retained fetal products (385). In some cases, the glia has been accompanied by choroid plexus, cartilage, bone, and even fatty tissue, further supporting the view that the lesion

is a result of fetal implantation (379). The finding of bulky glial differentiation within the endometrium in a young virgin implies a second origin from monophyletic overgrowth of a teratoma. The third origin suggested is mesodermal metaplasia. However, this is an unlikely possibility for the origin of glial polyps because there is no underlying neoplasm or other lesion to give rise to the glia via metaplastic transformation. Mesodermal metaplasia to glia has been identified in several malignant mesodermal mixed tumors (374).

Tunnel Clusters

This benign alteration of endocervical glands is composed of a nodular aggregate of dilated endocervical glands of the same size near the epithelial surface. The outline of the glandular aggregate is rounded, nodular, without infiltration at the periphery (fig. 180). The glands are uniformly round and dilated and contain a concentrated mucous fluid. They are lined by a single layer of flat to cuboidal mucinous cells with no mitotic activity, nuclear atypia, or stratification (fig. 181). The nodular aggregate of glands on low power may raise a question of hyperplasia or minimal deviation carcinoma, but the rounded noninvasive outline, superficial position, and lack of cytologic atypia confirm its benign nature (371). Tunnel clusters may result from involution of a cluster of formerly hyperplastic endocervical glands.

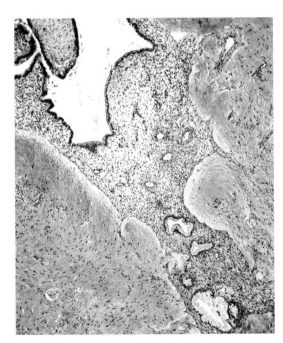

Figure 179
GLIAL POLYP
Polypoid masses of glia lie amid the endocervical glands below the epithelial surface.

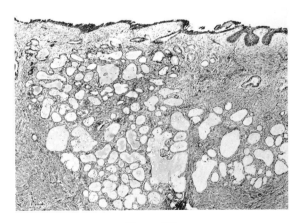

Figure 180
TUNNEL CLUSTERS
These are characterized by a nodular aggregate of uniform, round, open glands. The rounded outline of the aggregate is also characteristic.

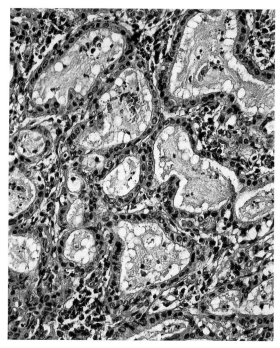

Figure 181
TUNNEL CLUSTERS
In this high magnification of the glands within a tunnel cluster the cells are uniform and cuboidal or flattened (not shown) and often contain dense secretion. There is no epithelial stratification, atypia, or mitotic activity.

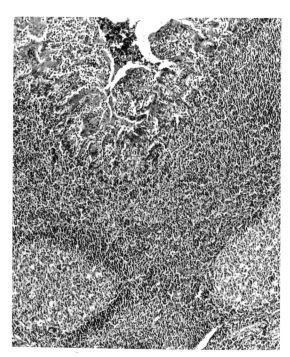

Figure 182
LYMPHOMA-LIKE LESION
A dense lymphocytic infiltrate involves the surface and glands. Lymphoid follicles are present.

Lymphoma-Like Lesion (Pseudolymphoma)

General Features. Inflammatory lesions in the cervix are seldom so extensive that they are confused with lymphoma. Rare lesions, however, have reached a size and uniformity of cell type that they can be confused with lymphoma. Designated lymphoma-like lesion or pseudolymphoma, 10 cases were reported in the cervix by Young et al. (390). The patients ranged from 19 to 65 years of age, with an average of 35 years. All but one were of reproductive age. Symptoms included vaginal bleeding, postcoital bleeding, discharge, and fever. One patient had infectious mononucleosis. Pelvic examination disclosed a normal-appearing cervix in some patients, but in most, it was abnormal and bled easily when touched.

Gross and Microscopic Findings. Lymphoma-like lesions are soft, nodular, superficial, and focally eroded. Microscopically, large clusters or diffuse sheets of large lymphoid cells admixed with mature lymphocytes, plasma cells, and neutrophils are seen. The infiltrate is band-like and superficial, usually only 3 mm in depth. The presence of macrophages and germinal centers supports a benign diagnosis (fig. 182). The infiltrate seldom extends below the level of the endocervical glands, a helpful point in distinguishing it from lymphoma. Immunoglobulin immunostains identify polyclonality, a useful feature in distinguishing lymphoma-like lesions from lymphoma. Rosai-Dorfman disease, a condition in which large histiocytes contain engulfed lymphocytes, has been described, as have histiocytosis and malakoplakia of the cervix. These seldom have the monomorphous appearance of lymphoma and the microscopic pattern is dominated by histiocytes rather than lymphocytes, as in lymphoma-like lesion (381).

REFERENCES

Benign Squamous Lesions

1. Bergeron C, Ferenczy A, Richart RM, Guralnick M. Micropapillomatosis labialis appears unrelated to human papillomavirus. Obstet Gynecol 1990;76:281–6.
2. Boxer RJ, Skinner DG. Condylomata acuminata and squamous cell carcinoma. Urology 1977;9:72–8.
3. Chuang TY, Perry HO, Kurland LT, Ilstrup DM. Condyloma acuminatum in Rochester, Minn., 1950–1978. I. Epidemiology and clinical features. Arch Dermatol 1984;120:469–75.
4. Crum CP, Egawa K, Fu YS, et al. Atypical immature metaplasia (AIM). A subset of human papilloma virus infection of the cervix. Cancer 1983;51:2214–9.
5. Davis GL, Hernandez E, Davis JL, Miyazawa K. Atypical squamous cells in Papanicolaou smears. Obstet Gynecol 1987;69:43–6.
6. Fetissof F, Serres G, Arbeille B, de Muret A, Sam-Giao M, Lansac J. Argyrophilic cells and ectocervical epithelium. Int J Gynecol Pathol 1991;10:177–90.
7. Gissmann L, deVilliers EM, zur Hausen H. Analysis of human genital warts (condylomata acuminata) and other genital tumors for human papillomavirus type 6 DNA. Int J Cancer 1982;29:143–6.
8. Goforth JL. Polyps and papillomas of the cervix uteri. Tex State J Med 1953;49:81–6.
9. Halpert R, Fruchter RG, Sedlis A, Butt K, Boyce JG, Sillman FH. Human papillomavirus and lower genital neoplasia in renal transplant patients. Obstet Gynecol 1986;68:251–8.
10. Kazal HL, Long JP. Squamous cell papillomas of the uterine cervix. A report of 20 cases. Cancer 1958;11:1049–59.
11. Lörincz AT, Temple GF, Patterson JA, Jenson AB, Kurman RJ, Lancaster WD. Correlation of cellular atypia and human papillomavirus deoxyribonucleic acid sequences in exfoliated cells of the uterine cervix. Obstet Gynecol 1986;68:508–12.
12. Marsh MR. Papilloma of the cervix. Am J Obstet Gynecol 1952;64:281–91.
13. Nuovo GJ, Nuovo MA, Cottral S, Gordon S, Silverstein SJ, Crum CP. Histological correlates of clinically occult human papillomavirus infection of the uterine cervix. Am J Surg Pathol 1988;12:198–204.
14. Nyirjesy I. Atypical or suspicious cervical smears. An aggressive diagnostic approach. JAMA 1972;222:691–3.
15. Potkul RK, Lancaster WD, Kurman RJ, Lewandowski G, Weck PK, Delgado G. Vulvar condylomas and squamous vestibular micropapilloma. Differences in appearance and response to treatment. J Reprod Med 1990;35:1019–22.
16. Reiter RC. Management of initial atypical cervical cytology: a randomized, prospective study. Obstet Gynecol 1986;68:237–40.
17. Sandmire HF, Austin SD, Bechtel RC. Experience with 40,000 Papanicolaou smears. Obstet Gynecol 1976;48:56–60.
18. Schafeek MA, Osman MI, Hussein MA. Carcinoma of vulva arising in condylomata acuminata. Obstet Gynecol 1979;54:120–3.
19. Schiffman MH, Kurman R, Barnes W, Lancaster W. HPV infection and early cervical cytological abnormalities in 3175 Washington, D.C. women. In: Howley PM, Broker TR, eds. Papillomaviruses. New York: Wiley-Liss, 1990:81–8. (Fox CF, ed. UCLA symposium on molecular and cellular biology; Vol 124.)

Squamous Intraepithelial Lesions

20. Bamford PN, Ormerod MG, Sloane JP, Warburton MJ. An immunohistochemical study of the distribution of epithelial antigens in the uterine cervix. Obstet Gynecol 1983;61:603–8.
21. Beral V. Cancer of the cervix: a sexually transmitted infection? Lancet 1974;1:1037–40.
21a. Burghardt E. Colposcopy - cervical pathology. Textbook and Atlas. New York: Thieme Medical Publishers, 1991:38–57.
22. Campion MJ, McCance DJ, Cuzick J, Singer A. Progressive potential of mild cervical atypia: prospective cytological, colposcopic, and virological study. Lancet 1986;2:237–40.
22a. Chapman WB, Lorinez AT, Willett GD, Wright VC, Kurman RJ. Evaluation of two commercially available in situ hybridization kits for detection of human papillomavirus in DNA of cervical biopsies: comparison of Southern blot hybridization. Mod Pathol (in press).
23. Christopherson WM. Concepts of genesis and development in early cervical neoplasia. Obstet Gynecol Surv 1969;24:842–50.
24. _____. Dysplasia, carcinoma in situ, and microinvasive carcinoma of the uterine cervix. Hum Pathol 1977;8:489–501.
25. _____, Lundin FE Jr, Mendez WM, Parker JE. Cervical cancer control: a study of morbidity and mortality trends over a twenty-one-year period. Cancer 1976;38:1357–66.
26. Crum CP, Egawa K, Fu YS, et al. Atypical immature metaplasia (AIM). A subset of human papilloma virus infection of the cervix. Cancer 1983;51:2214–9.
27. Evans AS, Monaghan JM. Spontaneous resolution of cervical warty atypia: the relevance of clinical and nuclear DNA features. Br J Obstet Gynaecol 1985;92:165–9.
28. Feldman MJ, Linzey EM, Srebnik E, Kent DR, Goldstein AI, Nelson M. Abnormal cervical cytology in the teenager: a continuing problem. Am J Obstet Gynecol 1976;126:418–21.
29. Ferenczy A, Braun L, Shah KV. Human papillomavirus (HPV) in condylomatous lesions of cervix. Am J Surg Pathol 1981;5:661–70.
30. _____, Richart RM. Female reproductive system: dynamics of scan and transmission electron microscopy. New York: John Wiley & Sons, 1974.
31. Fox CH. Biologic behavior of dysplasia and carcinoma in situ. Am J Obstet Gynecol 1967;99:960–74.
32. Fu YS, Reagan JW, Richart RM. Definition of precursors. Gynecol Oncol 1981;12:S220–31.

33. _____, Reagan JW, Richart RM, Townsend DE. Nuclear DNA and histologic studies of genital lesions in diethylstilbestrol-exposed progeny. I. Intraepithelial squamous abnormalities. Am J Clin Pathol 1979;72:503–14.

34. Hanselaar AG, Vooijs GP, Oud PS, Pahlplatz MM, Beck JL. DNA ploidy patterns in cervical intraepithelial neoplasia grade III, with and without synchronous invasive squamous cell carcinoma. Measurements in nuclei isolated from paraffin-embedded tissue. Cancer 1988;62:2537–45.

35. Heinzl S, Szalmay G, Jochum L, Roemer V. Observations on the development of dysplasia. Acta Cytol 1982; 26:453–6.

36. Ismail SM, Colclough AB, Dinnen JS, et al. Observer variation in histopathological diagnosis and grading of cervical intraepithelial neoplasia. Br Med J 1989;298: 707–10.

36a. Kiviat NB, Critchlow CW, Kurman RJ. Reassessment of the morphological continuum of cervical intraepithelial lesions: does it reflect different stages in the progression to cervical carcinoma? In: Muñoz N, Bosh F, Shah K, Mehens A, eds. The epidemiology of cervical cancer and human papillomavirus. Lyon: IARC, 1992:59–66.

37. Kolstad P, Klem V. Long-term followup of 1121 cases of carcinoma in situ. Obstet Gynecol 1976;48:125–9.

38. Koss LG. Carcinogenesis in the uterine cervix and human papillomavirus infection. In: Syrjänen K, Gissmann L, Koss LG, eds. Papillomaviruses and human disease. Berlin: Springer-Verlag, 1987:235–67.

39. _____. Diagnostic cytology and its histopathologic bases. 3rd ed. Philadelphia: JB Lippincott, 1979.

40. _____, Durfee GR. Unusual patterns of squamous epithelium of the uterine cervix: cytologic and pathologic study of koilocytotic atypia. Ann NY Acad Sci 1956; 63:1245–61.

41. Koutsky LA, Galloway DA, Holmes KK. Epidemiology of genital human papillomavirus infection. Epidemiol Rev 1988;10:122–63.

41a. Koutsky LA, Holmes KK, Critchlow CW, et al. Cohort study of risk of cervical intraepithelial neoplasia grade 2 or 3 associated with cervical papillomavirus infection. N Engl J Med 1992;327:1272–8.

42. Kurman RJ, Jenson AB, Lancaster WD. Papillomavirus infection of the cervix. II. Relationship to intraepithelial neoplasia based on the presence of specific viral structural proteins. Am J Surg Pathol 1983;7:39–52.

43. _____, Sanz LE, Jenson AB, Perry S, Lancaster WD. Papillomavirus infection of the cervix. I. Correlation of histology with viral structural antigens and DNA sequences. Int J Gynecol Pathol 1982;1:17–28.

44. Lindgren J, Wahlström T, Seppala M. Tissue CEA in premalignant epithelial lesions and epidermoid carcinoma of the uterine cervix: prognostic significance. Int J Cancer 1979;23:448–53.

45. Makin CA, Bobrow LG, Bodmer WF. Monoclonal antibody to cytokeratin for use in routine histopathology. J Clin Pathol 1984;37:975–83.

46. McIndoe WA, McLean MR, Jones RW, Mullins PR. The invasive potential of carcinoma in situ of the cervix. Obstet Gynecol 1984;64:451–8.

47. Meisels A, Fortin R, Roy M. Condylomatous lesions of the cervix. II. Cytologic, colposcopic and histopathologic study. Acta Cytol 1977;21:379–90.

48. _____, Roy M, Fortier M, et al. Human papillomavirus infection of the cervix: the atypical condyloma. Acta Cytol 1981;25:7–16.

49. Nash JD, Burke TW, Hoskins WJ. Biologic course of cervical human papillomavirus infection. Obstet Gynecol 1987;69:160–2.

50. Nasiell K, Nasiell M, Vaclavinkova V. Behavior of moderate cervical dysplasia during long-term follow-up. Obstet Gynecol 1983;61:609–14.

51. _____, Roger V, Nasiell M. Behavior of mild cervical dysplasia during long-term follow-up. Obstet Gynecol 1986;67:665–9.

52. National Cancer Institute Workshop. The 1988 Bethesda System for reporting cervical/vaginal cytological diagnoses. JAMA 1989;262:931–4.

53. Negrini BP, Schiffman MH, Kurman RJ, et al. Oral contraceptive use, human papillomavirus infection, and risk of early cytological abnormalities of the cervix. Cancer Res 1990;50:4670–5.

54. Nelson JH Jr, Hall JE. Detection, diagnostic evaluation, and treatment of dysplasia and early carcinoma of the cervix. Cancer 1970;20:150–63.

55. Patten SF Jr. Diagnostic cytopathology of the uterine cervix. 2nd rev ed. Basel: Karger, 1978. (Wied GL, ed. Monographs in clinical cytology; Vol 3.).

56. Peckham B, Greene RR. Follow-up on cervical epithelial abnormalities. Am J Obstet Gynecol 1957;74:804–15.

57. Purola E, Savia E. Cytology of gynecologic condyloma acuminatum. Acta Cytol 1977;21:26–31.

58. Randall ME, Andersen WA, Mills SE, Kim JA. Papillary squamous cell carcinoma of the uterine cervix: a clinicopathologic study of nine cases. Int J Gynecol Pathol 1986;5:1–10.

59. Reagan JW, Patten SF Jr. Dysplasia: a basic reaction to injury in the uterine cervix. Ann NY Acad Sci 1962; 97:662–82.

60. Richart RM. Natural history of cervical intraepithelial neoplasia. Clin Obstet Gynecol 1968;5:748.

61. _____, Barron BA. A follow-up study of patients with cervical dysplasia. Am J Obstet Gynecol 1969; 105:386–93.

62. Ringsted J, Amtrup F, Asklund C, et al. Reliability of histopathological diagnosis of squamous epithelial changes of the uterine cervix. Acta Pathol Microbiol Immunol Scand [A] 1978;86:273–8.

63. Robertson JH, Woodend BE, Crozier EH, Hutchinson J. Risk of cervical cancer associated with mild dyskaryosis. Br Med J 1988;297:18–21.

64. Rotkin ID. A comparison review of key epidemiological studies in cervical cancer related to current searches for transmissible agents. Cancer Res 1973;33:1353–67.

65. Sadeghi SB, Hsieh EW, Gunn SW. Prevalence of cervical intraepithelial neoplasia in sexually active teenagers and young adults. Results of data analysis of mass Papanicolaou screening of 796,337 women in the United States in 1981. Am J Obstet Gynecol 1984;148:726–9.

66. Saito K, Saito A, Fu YS, Cheng L, Hilborne LH. Immunoreactivity of involucrin in cervical condyloma and intraepithelial neoplasia. Int J Gynecol Pathol 1986; 5:308–18.

67. Sassoon AF, Said JW, Nash G, Shintaku IP, Banks-Schlegel S. Involucrin in intraepithelial and invasive squamous cell carcinomas of the cervix: an immunohistochemical study. Hum Pathol 1985;16:467–70.

67a. Schiffman MH, Bauer HM, Hoover RN, et al. Epidemiologic evidence that human papillomavirus causes most cervical intraepithelial neoplasia (in press).

68. Scott RB, Ballard LA. Problems of cervical biopsy. Ann NY Acad Sci 1962;97:767–81.

69. Soisson AP, Molina CY, Benson WL. Endocervical curettage in the evaluation of cervical disease in patients with adequate colposcopy. Obstet Gynecol 1988;71:109–11.

70. Spirtos NM, Schlaerth JB, d'Ablaing G III, Morrow CP. A critical evaluation of the endocervical curettage. Obstet Gynecol 1987;70:729–33.

71. Stegner HE, Kuhler C, Loning T. Tissue polypeptide antigen and keratins in cervical neoplasia. Int J Gynecol Pathol 1986;5:23–34.

72. Stern E. Epidemiology of dysplasia. Obstet Gynecol Surv 1969;24:711–23.

73. _____, Neely PM. Dysplasia of the uterine cervix. Incidence of regression, recurrence, and cancer. Cancer 1964;17:508–12.

74. Strang P. Cytogenetic and cytometric analyses in squamous cell carcinoma of the uterine cervix. Int J Gynecol Pathol 1989;8:54–63.

75. Syrjänen K, Vayrynen M, Saarikoski S, et al. Natural history of cervical human papillomavirus (HPV) infections based on prospective follow-up. Br J Obstet Gynaecol 1985;92:1086–92.

76. Twiggs LB, Clark BA, Okagaki T. Basal cell pseudopodia in cervical intraepithelial neoplasia; progressive reduction of number with severity: a morphometric quantification. Am J Obstet Gynecol 1981;139:640–4.

77. Warhol MJ, Antonioli DA, Pinkus GS, Burke L, Rice RH. Immunoperoxidase staining for involucrin: a potential diagnostic aid in cervicovaginal pathology. Hum Pathol 1982;13:1095–9.

Invasive Squamous Carcinoma

78. Abell MR. Invasive carcinoma of the uterine cervix. In: Norris HJ, Hertig AT, Abell MR, eds. The uterus. Baltimore: Williams & Wilkins, 1973:413–56 (Abell MR, ed. Monographs in pathology, no 14.).

79. Adelson MD, Johnson TS, Sneige N, Williamson KD, Freedman RS, Peters LJ. Cervical carcinoma DNA content, S-fraction, and malignancy grading. II. Comparison with clinical staging. Gynecol Oncol 1987;26:57–70.

80. Averette HE, Nelson JH Jr, Ng AB, Hoskins WJ, Boyce JG, Ford JH Jr. Diagnosis and management of microinvasive (stage IA) carcinoma of the uterine cervix. Cancer 1976;38(Suppl 1):414–25.

81. Bamford PN, Ormerod MG, Sloane JP, Warburton MJ. An immunohistochemical study of the distribution of epithelial antigens in the uterine cervix. Obstet Gynecol 1983;61:603–8.

82. Barber BR, Sommers SC, Rotterdam H, Kwon T. Vascular invasion as a prognostic factor in stage IB cancer of the cervix. Obstet Gynecol 1978;52:343–8.

83. Benson WL, Norris HJ. A critical review of the frequency of lymph node metastasis and death from microinvasive carcinoma of the cervix. Obstet Gynecol 1977;49:632–8.

84. Bichel P, Jakobsen A. Histopathologic grading and prognosis of uterine cervical carcinoma. Am J Clin Oncol 1985;8:247–54.

85. Bostrom SG, Hart WR. Carcinomas of the cervix with intense stromal eosinophilia. Cancer 1981;47:2887–93.

86. Boyce JG, Fruchter RG, Nicastri AD, et al. Vascular invasion in stage I carcinoma of the cervix. Cancer 1984;53:1175–80.

87. Brinton LA, Schairer C, Haenszel W, et al. Cigarette smoking and invasive cervical cancer. JAMA 1986;255:3265–9.

88. _____, Schiffman MH, Fraumeni JF. Uterine cervix. In: Schottenfeld D, Fraumeni JF Jr, eds. Cancer epidemiology and prevention. 2nd ed. New York: Oxford University Press, 1992; in press.

89. Buckley JD, Harris RW, Doll R, Vessey MP, Williams PT. Case-control study of the husbands of women with dysplasia or carcinoma of the cervix uteri. Lancet 1981;2:1010–5.

90. Burghardt E. Early histological diagnosis of cervical cancer. Philadelphia: WB Saunders, 1973. (Friedman EA, ed. Major problems in obstetrics and gynecology; Vol 6.).

91. _____, Girardi F, Lahousen M, Pickel H, Tamussino K. Microinvasive carcinoma of the uterine cervix (International Federation of Gynecology and Obstetrics Stage IA). Cancer 1991;67:1037–45.

92. _____, Holzer E. Diagnosis and treatment of microinvasive carcinoma of the cervix uteri. Obstet Gynecol 1977;49:641–53.

93. Carmichael JA, Clarke DH, Moher D, Ohlke ID, Karchmar EJ. Cervical carcinoma in women aged 34 and younger. Am J Obstet Gynecol 1986;154:264–9.

94. Christopherson WM, Lundin FE Jr, Mendez WM, Parker JE. Cervical cancer control: a study of morbidity and mortality trends over a twenty-one-year period. Cancer 1976;38:1357–66.

95. Chung CK, Stryker JA, Ward SP, Nahhas WA, Mortel R. Histologic grade and prognosis of carcinoma of the cervix. Obstet Gynecol 1981;57:636–42.

96. Crissman JD, Budhraja M, Aron BS, Cummings G. Histopathologic prognostic factors in stage II and III squamous cell carcinoma of the uterine cervix. An evaluation of 91 patients treated primarily with radiation therapy. Int J Gynecol Pathol 1987;6:97–103.

97. _____, Makuch R, Budhraja M. Histopathologic grading of squamous cell carcinoma of the uterine cervix. An evaluation of 70 stage Ib patients. Cancer 1985;55:1590–6.

98. Crowther ME, Lowe DG, Shepherd JH. Verrucous carcinoma of the female genital tract: a review. Obstet Gynecol Surv 1988;43:263–80.

99. Czernobilsky B, Moll R, Franke WW, Dallenbach-Hellweg G, Hohlweg-Majert P. Intermediate filaments of normal and neoplastic tissues of the female genital tract with emphasis on problems of differential tumor diagnosis. Pathol Res Pract 1984;179:31–7.

100. Davis JR, Aristizabal S, Way DL, Weiner SA, Hicks MJ, Hagaman RM. DNA ploidy, grade, and stage in prognosis of uterine cervical cancer. Gynecol Oncol 1989;32:4–7.

101. Delgado G. Stage IB squamous cancer of the cervix: the choice of treatment. Obstet Gynecol Surv 1978;33:174–83.

102. Devesa SS, Young JL Jr, Brinton LA, Fraumeni JF Jr. Recent trends in cervix uteri cancer. Cancer 1989;64:2184–90.

103. DiSaia PJ, Creasman WT. Clinical gynecologic oncology. 3rd ed. St Louis: CV Mosby, 1989.

104. Dodd JK, Henry RJ, Tyler JP, Houghton CR. Cervical carcinoma: a comparison of four potential biochemical tumor markers. Gynecol Oncol 1989;32:248–52.

105. Eide TJ. Cancer of the uterine cervix in Norway by histologic type, 1970–84. JNCI 1987;79:199–205.

106. Ferenczy A, Richart RM. Female reproductive system: dynamics of scan and transmission electron microscopy. New York: John Wiley & Sons, 1974.

107. Fidler HK, Boyes DA, Worth AJ. Cervical cancer detection in British Columbia. A progress report. J Obstet Gynaecol Br Commonw 1968;75:392–404.

108. Fu YS, Reagan JW. Pathology of the uterine cervix, vagina, and vulva. In: Bennington JL, ed. Major problems in pathology; Vol 21. Philadelphia: WB Saunders, 1989;71–82.

109. Goellner JR. Carcinoma of the cervix. Clinicopathologic correlation of 196 cases. Am J Clin Pathol 1976;66:775–85.

110. Groben P, Reddick R, Askin F. The pathologic spectrum of small cell carcinoma of the cervix. Int J Gynecol Pathol 1985;4:42–57.

111. Gunderson LL, Weems WS, Herbertson RM, Plenk HP. Correlation of histopathology with clinical results following radiation therapy for carcinoma of the cervix. Am J Roentgenol Radium Ther Nucl Med 1974;120:74–87.

112. Hafiz MA, Kragel P, Toker C. Carcinoma of the uterine cervix resembling lymphoepithelioma. Obstet Gynecol 1985;66:829–31.

113. Halpin TF, Hunter RE, Cohen MB. Lymphoepithelioma of the uterine cervix. Gynecol Oncol 1989;34:101–5.

114. Hamazaki M, Fujita H, Arata T, Takata S, Hamazaki M. Medullary carcinoma with marked lymphoid infiltration of the uterine cervix—pathological picture of a case of cervix cancer with a favorable prognosis. Jpn J Cancer Clin 1968;14:787–92.

115. Hasumi K, Sakamoto A, Sugano H. Microinvasive carcinoma of the uterine cervix. Cancer 1980;45:928–31.

116. _____, Sugano H, Sakamoto G, Masubuchi K, Kubo H. Circumscribed carcinoma of the uterine cervix, with marked lymphocytic infiltration. Cancer 1977;39:2503–7.

117. Henriksen E. The lymphatic spread of carcinoma of cervix and of the body of the uterus: a study of 420 necropsies. Am J Obstet Gynecol 1949;58:924–42.

118. Imachi M, Tsukamoto N, Matsuyama T, Nakano H. Pulmonary metastasis from carcinoma of the uterine cervix. Gynecol Oncol 1989;33:189–92.

119. Inoue T. Prognostic significance of the depth of invasion relating to nodal metastases, parametrial extension, and cell types. A study of 628 cases with stage IB, IIA, and IIB cervical carcinoma. Cancer 1984;54:3035–42.

120. Irwin KL, Rosero-Bixby L, Oberle MW, et al. Oral contraceptives and cervical cancer risk in Costa Rica. Detection bias or causal association? JAMA 1988;259:59–64.

121. Johnson TS, Adelson MD, Sneige N, Williamson KD, Lee AM, Katz R. Cervical carcinoma DNA content, S-fraction, and malignancy grading. I. Interrelationships. Gynecol Oncol 1987;26:41–56.

122. Kapp DS, Bibro MC, Lawrence R, Schwartz PE. Pretreatment histopathological virulence factors in radiation therapeutically managed carcinoma of the uterine cervix [Abstract]. Int J Radiat Oncol Biol Phys 1980;6:1427–8.

123. _____, LiVolsi VA. Intense eosinophilic stromal infiltration in carcinoma of the uterine cervix: a clinicopathologic study of 14 cases. Gynecol Oncol 1983;16:19–30.

124. Kato H, Tamai K, Morioka H, Nagai M, Nagaya T, Torigoe T. Tumor-antigen TA-4 in the detection of recurrence in cervical squamous cell carcinoma. Cancer 1984;54:1544–6.

125. Katz HJ, Davies JN. Death from cervix uteri carcinoma: the changing pattern. Gynecol Oncol 1980;9:86–9.

126. Kjellgren O. Mass screening in Sweden for cancer of the uterine cervix: effect on incidence and mortality. An overview. Gynecol Obstet Invest 1986;22:57–63.

127. Kolstad P. Follow-up study of 232 patients with stage Ia1 and 411 patients with stage Ia2 squamous cell carcinoma of the cervix (microinvasive carcinoma). Gynecol Oncol 1989;33:265–72.

128. Kraus FT, Perez-Mesa C. Verrucous carcinoma. Clinical and pathologic study of 105 cases involving oral cavity, larynx and genitalia. Cancer 1966;19:26–38.

129. La Vecchia C, Franceschi S, Decarli A, et al. Dietary vitamin A and the risk of invasive cervical cancer. Int J Cancer 1984;34:319–22.

130. Leman MH Jr, Benson WL, Kurman RJ, Park RC: Microinvasive carcinoma of the cervix. Obstet Gynecol 1976;48:571–8.

131. Maiman MA, Fruchter RG, DiMaio TM, Boyce JG. Superficially invasive squamous cell carcinoma of the cervix. Obstet Gynecol 1988;72:399–403.

132. Mestwerdt G. Die Frühdiagnose des Kollumkarzinoms. Zentralbl Gynäkol 1947;69:198–202.

133. Mills SE, Austin MB, Randall ME. Lymphoepithelioma-like carcinoma of the uterine cervix. A distinctive, undifferentiated carcinoma with inflammatory stroma. Am J Surg Pathol 1985;9:883–9.

134. Ng AB, Atkin NB. Histological cell type and DNA value in the prognosis of squamous cell cancer of uterine cervix. Br J Cancer 1973;28:322–31.

135. _____, Reagan JW. Microinvasive carcinoma of the uterine cervix. Am J Clin Pathol 1969;52:511–29.

136. Okagaki T, Clark BA, Zachow KR, et al. Presence of human papillomavirus in verrucous carcinoma (Ackerman) of the vagina. Immunocytochemical, ultrastructural, and DNA hybridization studies. Arch Pathol Lab Med 1984;108:567–70.

137. Parkin DM, Nguyen-Dinh X, Day NE. The impact of screening on the incidence of cervical cancer in England and Wales. Br J Obstet Gynaecol 1985;92:150–7.

138. Piver MS, Chung WS. Prognostic significance of cervical lesion size and pelvic node metastases in cervical carcinoma. Obstet Gynecol 1975;46:507–10.

139. Qizilbash AH. Papillary squamous tumors of the uterine cervix. A clinical and pathologic study of 21 cases. Am J Clin Pathol 1974;61:508–20.

140. Randall ME, Andersen WA, Mills SE, Kim JA. Papillary squamous cell carcinoma of the uterine cervix: a clinicopathologic study of nine cases. Int J Gynecol Pathol 1986;5:1–10.

141. Rando RF, Sedlacek TV, Hunt J, Jenson AB, Kurman RJ, Lancaster WD. Verrucous carcinoma of the vulva associated with an unusual type 6 human papillomavirus. Obstet Gynecol 1986;67 (Suppl 3):70–5S.

142. Rastkar G, Okagaki T, Twiggs LB, Clark BA. Early invasive and in situ warty carcinoma of the vulva: clinical, histologic, and electron microscopic study with particular reference to viral association. Am J Obstet Gynecol 1982;143:814–20.

143. Reagan JW, Fu YS. Histologic types and prognosis of cancers of the uterine cervix. Int J Radiat Oncol Biol Phys 1979;5:1015–20.

144. _____, Hamonic MJ, Wentz WB. Analytical study of cells in cervical squamous cell cancer. Lab Invest 1957;6:241–50.

145. Reeves WC, Brenes MM, De Britton RC, Valdes PF, Joplin CF. Cervical cancer in the Republic of Panama. Am J Epidemiol 1984;119:714–24.

146. Romney SL, Duttagupta C, Basu J, et al. Plasma vitamin C and uterine cervical dysplasia. Am J Obstet Gynecol 1985;151:976–80.

147. Sagae S, Kuzumaki N, Hisada T, Mugikura Y, Kudo R, Hashimoto M. Ras oncogene expression and prognosis of invasive squamous cell carcinomas of the uterine cervix. Cancer 1989;63:1577–82.

148. Sassoon AF, Said JW, Nash G, Shintaku IP, Banks-Schlegel S. Involucrin in intraepithelial and invasive squamous cell carcinomas of the cervix: an immunohistochemical study. Hum Pathol 1985;16:467–70.

149. Sedlis A, Sall S, Tsukada Y, et al. Microinvasive carcinoma of the uterine cervix: a clinical-pathologic study. Am J Obstet Gynecol 1979;133:64–74.

150. Shingleton HM, Orr JW. Cancer of the cervix: diagnosis and treatment. In: Monaghan J, Lind T, eds. Clinical obstetrics and gynecology. New York: Churchill Livingstone, 1987.

151. Sidhu GS, Koss LG, Barber RK. Relation of histologic factors to the response of stage I epidermoid carcinoma of the cervix to surgical treatment. Analysis of 115 patients. Obstet Gynecol 1970;35:329–38.

152. Simon NL, Gore H, Shingleton HM, Soong SJ, Orr JW Jr, Hatch KD. Study of superficially invasive carcinoma of the cervix. Obstet Gynecol 1986;68:19–24.

153. Stendahl U, Eklund G, Willen R. Prognosis of invasive squamous cell carcinoma of the uterine cervix: a comparative study of the predictive values of clinical staging IB–III and a histopathologic malignancy grading system. Int J Gynecol Pathol 1983;2:42–54.

154. _____, Eklund G, Willen H, Willen R. Invasive squamous cell carcinoma of the uterine cervix. III. A malignancy grading system for indication of prognosis after radiation therapy. Acta Radiol Oncol 1981;20:231–43.

155. Strang P. Cytogenetic and cytometric analyses in squamous cell carcinoma of the uterine cervix. Int J Gynecol Pathol 1989;8:54–63.

156. van Nagell JR Jr, Donaldson ES, Parker JC, van Dyke AH, Wood EG. The prognostic significance of pelvic lymph node morphology in carcinoma of the uterine cervix. Cancer 1977;39:2624–32.

157. _____, Donaldson ES, Wood EG, Goldenberg DM. The clinical significance of carcinoembryonic antigen in the plasma and tumors of patients with gynecologic malignancies. Cancer 1978;42 (Suppl 3):1527–32.

158. _____, Greenwell N, Powell DF, Donaldson ES, Hanson MB, Gay EC. Microinvasive carcinoma of the cervix. Am J Obstet Gynecol 1983;145:981–91.

159. Waterhouse J, Muir C, Stranmugaratnam K, Powell J, eds. Cancer incidence in five continent; Vol IV. IARC scientific publication series, no 42. Lyon: International Agency for Research on Cancer, 1982.

160. Young RH, Kurman RJ, Scully RE. Placental site nodules and plaques. A clinicopathologic analysis of 20 cases. Am J Surg Pathol 1990;14:1001–9.

161. Zaino R, Ward S, Frauenhoffer E. Histopathologic predictors of behavior of squamous carcinoma of the cervix [Abstract]. Lab Invest 1989;60:108A.

Glandular Lesions

162. Abell MR. Invasive carcinoma of the uterine cervix. In: Norris HJ, Hertig AT, Abell MR, eds. The uterus. Baltimore: Williams & Wilkins, 1973:413–56 (Monographs in pathology; no 14.).

162a Ambros RA, Park J-S, Shah KV, Kurman RJ. Evaluation of histologic, morphometric, and immunohistochemical criteria in the differential diagnosis of small cell carcinomas of the cervix with particular reference to human papillomavirus types 16 and 18. Mod Pathol 1991;4:586–93.

163. Andersen ES, Arffmann E. Adenocarcinoma in situ of the uterine cervix: a clinico-pathologic study of 36 cases. Gynecol Oncol 1989;35:1–7.

164. Barter RA. Carcinoma of the cervix arising from remnants of Gartner's duct. Aust N Z J Obstet Gynaecol 1961;1:64–72.

165. Berek JS, Castaldo TW, Hacker NF, Petrilli ES, Lagasse LD, Morre JG. Adenocarcinoma of the uterine cervix. Cancer 1981;48:2734–41.

166. _____, Hacker NF, Fu YS, Sokale JR, Leuchter RC, Lagasse LD. Adenocarcinoma of the uterine cervix: histologic variables associated with lymph node metastasis and survival. Obstet Gynecol 1985;65:46–52.

167. Bertrand M, Lickrish GM, Colgan TJ. The anatomic distribution of cervical adenocarcinoma in situ: implications for treatment. Am J Obstet Gynecol 1987;157:21–5.

168. Betsill WL Jr, Clark AH. Early endocervical glandular neoplasia. I. Histomorphology and cytomorphology. Acta Cytol 1986;30:115–26.

169. Boon ME, Baak JP, Kurver PJ, Overdiep SH, Verdonk GW. Adenocarcinoma in situ of the cervix: an underdiagnosed lesion. Cancer 1981;48:768–73.

170. _____, de Graaff Guilloud JC, Kok LP, Olthof PM, van Erp EJ. Efficacy of screening for cervical squamous and adenocarcinoma. The Dutch experience. Cancer 1987;59:862–6.

171. Brand E, Berek JS, Hacker NF. Controversies in the management of cervical adenocarcinoma. Obstet Gynecol 1988;71:261–9.

172. Brinton LA, Tashima K, Lehman HF, et al. Epidemiology of cervical cancer by cell type. Cancer Res 1987;47:1706–11.

173. Christopherson WM, Nealon N, Gray LA Sr. Noninvasive precursor lesions of adenocarcinoma and mixed adenosquamous carcinoma of the cervix uteri. Cancer 1979;44:975–83.

174. Clement PB, Young RH. Deep nabothian cysts of the uterine cervix. A possible source of confusion with minimal-deviation adenocarcinoma (adenoma malignum). Int J Gynecol Pathol 1989;8:340–8.

175. Colgan TJ, Lickrish GM. The topography and invasive potential of cervical adenocarcinoma in situ, with and without associated squamous dysplasia. Gynecol Oncol 1990;36:246–9.

176. Cooper P, Russell G, Wilson B. Adenocarcinoma of the endocervix—a histochemical study. Histopathology 1987;11:1321–30.

177. Dallenbach-Hellweg G. Occurrence and histological structure of adenocarcinoma of the endocervix after long-term use of oral contraceptives. Geburtshilfe Frauenheilkd 1982; 42:249–55.

178. Davidson SE, Symonds RP, Lamont D, Watson ER. Does adenocarcinoma of uterine cervix have a worse prognosis than squamous carcinoma when treated by radiotherapy? Gynecol Oncol 1989;33:23–6.

179. Dickersin GR, Welch WR, Erlandson R, Robboy SJ. Ultrastructure of 16 cases of clear cell adenocarcinoma of the vagina and cervix in young women. Cancer 1980;45:1615–24.

180. Drescher CW, Hopkins MP, Roberts JA. Comparison of the pattern of metastatic spread of squamous cell cancer and adenocarcinoma of the uterine cervix. Gynecol Oncol 1989;33:340–3.

181. Farnsworth A, Laverty C, Stoler MH. Human papillomavirus messenger RNA expression in adenocarcinoma in situ of the uterine cervix. Int J Gynecol Pathol 1989;8:321–30.

182. Fu YS, Berek JS, Hilborne LH. Diagnostic problems of in situ and invasive adenocarcinomas of the uterine cervix. Appl Pathol 1987;5:47–56.

183. _____, Reagan JW, Fu AS, Janiga KE. Adenocarcinoma and mixed carcinoma of the uterine cervix. II. Prognostic value of nuclear DNA analysis. Cancer 1982;49:2571–7.

184. Gilks CB, Young RH, Aguirre P, DeLellis RA, Scully RE. Adenoma malignum (minimal deviation adenocarcinoma) of the uterine cervix. A clinicopathological and immunohistochemical analysis of 26 cases. Am J Surg Pathol 1989;13:717–29.

184a._____, Clement PB. Papillary serous adenocarcinoma of the uterine cervix: a report of three cases. Mod Pathol 1992;5:426–31.

185. Gloor E, Hurlimann J. Cervical intraepithelial glandular neoplasia (adenocarcinoma in situ and glandular dysplasia). A correlative study of 23 cases with histologic grading, histochemical analysis of mucins, and immunohistochemical determination of the affinity for four lectins. Cancer 1986;58:1272–80.

186. _____, Ruzicka J. Morphology of adenocarcinoma in situ of the uterine cervix: a study of 14 cases. Cancer 1982;49:294–302.

187. Hanselaar AG, Van Leusen ND, De Wilde PC, Vooijs GP. Clear cell adenocarcinoma of the vagina and cervix. A report of the Central Netherlands Registry with emphasis on early detection and prognosis. Cancer 1991;67:1971–8.

188. Hart WR, Norris HJ. Mesonephric adenocarcinomas of the cervix. Cancer 1972;29:106–13.

189. Hasumi K, Erhmann RL. Clear cell carcinoma of the uterine endocervix with an in situ component. Cancer 1978;42:2435–8.

190. Herbst AL, Robboy SJ, Scully RE, Poskanzer DC. Clear-cell adenocarcinoma of the vagina and cervix in girls: analysis of 170 registry cases. Am J Obstet Gynecol 1974;119:713–24.

191. Hopkins MP, Roberts JA, Schmidt RW. Cervical adenocarcinoma in situ. Obstet Gynecol 1988;71:842–4.

192. _____, Schmidt RW, Roberts JA, Morley GW. Gland cell carcinoma (adenocarcinoma) of the cervix. Obstet Gynecol 1988;72:789–95.

193. Horowitz IR, Jacobson LP, Zucker PK, Currie JL, Rosenshein NB. Epidemiology of adenocarcinoma of the cervix. Gynecol Oncol 1988;31:25–31.

194. Janovski NA, Kasdon EJ. Benign mesonephric papillary and polypoid tumors of the cervix in childhood. J Pediatr 1963;63:211–6.

195. Jaworski RC. Endocervical glandular dysplasia, adenocarcinoma in situ, and early invasive (microinvasive) adenocarcinoma of the uterine cervix. Semin Diagn Pathol 1990;7:190–204.

196. _____, Pacey NF, Greenberg ML, Osborn RA. The histologic diagnosis of adenocarcinoma in situ and related lesions of the cervix uteri. Adenocarcinoma in situ. Cancer 1988;61:1171–81.

196a Jones MW, Silverberg SG, Kurman RJ. Well differentiated villoglandular adenocarcinoma of the uterine cervix. A clinicopathological study of 24 cases. Int J Gynecol Pathol (in press).

197. Jones WB, Koulos JP, Saigo PE, Lewis JL Jr. Clear-cell adenocarcinoma of the lower genital tract: Memorial Hospital 1974-1984. Obstet Gynecol 1987;70:573–7.

198. Kaku T, Enjoji M. Extremely well-differentiated adenocarcinoma ("adenoma malignum") of the cervix. Int J Gynecol Pathol 1983;2:28–41.

199. Kaminski PF, Maier RC. Clear cell adenocarcinoma of the cervix unrelated to diethylstilbestrol exposure. Obstet Gynecol 1983;62:720–7.

200. _____, Norris HJ. Coexistence of ovarian neoplasms and endocervical adenocarcinoma. Obstet Gynecol 1984;64:553–6.

201. _____, Norris HJ. Minimal deviation carcinoma (adenoma malignum) of the cervix. Int J Gynecol Pathol 1983;2:141–52.

202. Kessler II. Etiological concepts in cervical carcinogenesis. Appl Pathol 1987;5:57–75.

203. Kleine W, Rau K, Schwoeorer D, Pfleiderer A. Prognosis of the adenocarcinoma of the cervix uteri: a comparative study. Gynecol Oncol 1989;35:145–9.

204. Korhonen MO. Epidemiological differences between adenocarcinoma and squamous cell carcinoma of the uterine cervix. Gynecol Oncol 1980;10:312–7.

205. Lang G, Dallenbach-Hellweg G. The histogenetic origin of cervical mesonephric hyperplasia and mesonephric adenocarcinoma of the uterine cervix studied with immunohistochemical methods. Int J Gynecol Pathol 1990;9:145–57.

206. Leminen A, Paavonen J. Forss M. Walhström T, Vesterinen E. Adenocarcinoma of the uterine cervix. Cancer 1990;65:53–9.

207. Lippert LJ, Richart RM, Ferenczy A. Giant benign endocervical polyp: report of a case. Am J Obstet Gynecol 1974;118:1140–1.

208. Maier RC, Norris HJ. Coexistence of cervical intraepithelial neoplasia with primary adenocarcinoma of the endocervix. Obstet Gynecol 1980;56:361–4.

209. McGowan L, Young RH, Scully RE. Peutz-Jeghers syndrome with "adenoma malignum" of the cervix. A report of two cases. Gynecol Oncol 1980;10:125–33.

210. McKelvey JL, Goodlin RR. Adenoma malignum of the cervix. A cancer of deceptively innocent histological pattern. Cancer 1963;16:549–57.

211. Michael H, Grawe L, Kraus FT. Minimal deviation endocervical adenocarcinoma: clinical and histologic features, immunohistochemical staining for carcinoembryonic antigen, and differentiation from confusing benign lesions. Int J Gynecol Pathol 1984;3:261–76.

212. Milsom I, Friberg LG. Primary adenocarcinoma of the uterine cervix. A clinical study. Cancer 1983;52:942–7.

213. Moberg PJ, Einhorn N, Silfversward C, Soderberg G. Adenocarcinoma of the uterine cervix. Cancer 1986;57:407–10.

214. Noller KL, Decker DG, Dockerty MB, Lanier AP, Smith RA, Symmonds RE. Mesonephric (clear cell) carcinoma of the vagina and cervix. A retrospective analysis. Obstet Gynecol 1974;43:640–4.

215. Ostor AG, Pagano R, Davoren RA, Fortune DW, Chanen W, Rome R. Adenocarcinoma in situ of the cervix. Int J Gynecol Pathol 1984;3:179–90.

216. Parazzini F, La Vecchia C. Epidemiology of adenocarcinoma of the cervix. Gynecol Oncol 1990;39:40–6.

217. Peters RK, Chao A, Mack TM, Thomas D, Bernstein L, Henderson BE. Increased frequency of adenocarcinoma of the uterine cervix in young women in Los Angeles County. JNCI 1986;76:423–8.

218. Potish RA, Twiggs LB, Adcock LL, Prem KA, Savage JE, Leung BS. Prognostic importance of progesterone and estrogen receptors in cancer of the uterine cervix. Cancer 1986;58:1709–13.

219. Prempree T, Amornmarn R, Wizenbreg MJ. A therapeutic approach to primary adenocarcinoma of the cervix. Cancer 1985;56:1264–8.

220. Qizilbash AH. In-situ and microinvasive adenocarcinoma of the uterine cervix. A clinical, cytologic and histologic study of 14 cases. Am J Clin Pathol 1975;64:155–70.

221. Robboy SJ, Young RH, Herbst AL. Female genital tract changes related to prenatal diethylstilbestrol exposure. In: Blaustein A, ed. Pathology of the female genital tract. 2nd ed. New York: Springer-Verlag, 1982:99–118.

222. Saigo PE, Cain JM, Kim WS, Gaynor JJ, Johnson K, Lewis JL Jr. Prognostic factors in adenocarcinoma of the uterine cervix. Cancer 1986;57:1584–93.

223. Schwartz SM, Weiss NS. Increased incidence of adenocarcinoma of the cervix in young women in the United States. Am J Epidemiol 1986;124:1045–7.

224. Shingleton HM, Gore H, Bradley DH, Soong SJ. Adenocarcinoma of the cervix. I. Clinical evaluation and pathologic features. Am J Obstet Gynecol 1981;139:799–814.

225. Silverberg SG, Hurt WG. Minimal deviation adenocarcinoma ("adenoma malignum") of the cervix: a reappraisal. Am J Obstet Gynecol 1975;121:971–5.

226. Steeper TA, Wick MR. Minimal deviation adenocarcinoma of the uterine cervix ("adenoma malignum"). An immunohistochemical comparison with microglandular endocervical hyperplasia and conventional endocervical adenocarcinoma. Cancer 1986;58:1131–8.

227. Steiner G, Friedell GH. Adenosquamous carcinoma in situ of the cervix. Cancer 1965;18:807–10.

228. Suh KS, Silverberg SG. Tubal metaplasia of the uterine cervix. Int J Gynecol Pathol 1990;9:122–8.

229. Szyfelbein WM, Young RH, Scully RE. Adenoma malignum of the cervix. Cytologic findings. Acta Cytol 1984;28:691–8.

230. Tamimi HK, Figge DC. Adenocarcinoma of the uterine cervix. Gynecol Oncol 1982;13:335–44.

231. Thelmo WL, Nicastri AD, Fruchter R, Spring H, DiMaio T, Boyce J. Mucoepidermoid carcinoma of the uterine cervix stage IB. Long-term follow-up, histochemical and immunohistochemical study. Int J Gynecol Pathol 1990;9:316–24.

232. Valente PT, Susin M. Cervical adenocarcinoma arising in florid mesonephric hyperplasia: report of a case with immunocytochemical studies. Gynecol Oncol 1987;27:58–68.

233. Vesterinen E, Forss M, Nieminen U. Increase of cervical adenocarcinoma: a report of 520 cases of cervical carcinoma including 112 tumors with glandular elements. Gynecol Oncol 1989;33:49–53.

234. Weiss RJ, Lucas WE. Adenocarcinoma of the uterine cervix. Cancer 1986;57:1996–2001.

235. Wilczynski SP, Walker J, Liao SY, Bergen S, Berman M. Adenocarcinoma of the cervix associated with human papillomavirus. Cancer 1988;62:1331–6.

236. Young RH, Scully RE. Atypical forms of microglandular hyperplasia of the cervix simulating carcinoma. A report of five cases and review of the literature. Am J Surg Pathol 1989;13:50–6.

237. _____, Scully RE. Mucinous ovarian tumors associated with mucinous adenocarcinomas of the cervix. A clinicopathological analysis of 16 cases. Int J Gynecol Pathol 1988;7:99–111.

238. _____, Scully RE. Villoglandular papillary adenocarcinoma of the uterine cervix. A clinicopathologic analysis of 13 cases. Cancer 1989;63:1773–9.

239. _____, Welch WR, Dickersin GR, Scully RE. Ovarian sex cord tumor with annular tubules: review of 74 cases including 27 with Peutz-Jeghers syndrome and four with adenoma of the cervix. Cancer 1982;50:1384–402.

Other Epithelial Tumors

240. Albores-Saavedra J, Larraza-Hernandez O, Lopez SP, Rodriguez-Martinez H. Carcinoide primario del cuello uterine. Patologia 1975;13:67–89.

241. _____, Rodriguez-Martinez HA, Larraza-Hernandez O. Carcinoid tumors of the cervix. Pathol Ann 1979;14:273–91.

242. Baggish MS, Woodruff JD. Adenoid-basal carcinoma of the cervix. Obstet Gynecol 1966;28:213–8.

243. Barrett RJ II, Davos I, Leuchter RS, Lagasse LD. Neuroendocrine features in poorly differentiated and undifferentiated carcinomas of the cervix. Cancer 1987;60:2325–30.

244. Brinton LA, Tashima KT, Lehman HF, et al. Epidemiology of cervical cancer by cell type. Cancer Res 1987;47:1706–11.

245. Chan JK, Tsui WM, Tung SY, Ching RC. Endocrine cell hyperplasia of the uterine cervix. A precursor of neuroendocrine carcinoma of the cervix? Am J Clin Pathol 1989;92:825–30.

246. Daroca PJ Jr, Dhurandhar HN. Basaloid carcinoma of the uterine cervix. Am J Surg Pathol 1980;4:235–9.

247. Ferry JA, Scully RE. "Adenoid cystic" carcinoma and adenoid basal carcinoma of the uterine cervix. A study of 28 cases. Am J Surg Pathol 1988;12:134–44.

248. Fetissof F, Serres G, Arbeille B, de Muret A, Sam-Giao M, Lansac J. Argyrophilic cells and ectocervical epithelium. Int J Gynecol Pathol 1991;10:177–90.

249. Fu YS, Reagan JW, Hsiu JG, Storaasli JP, Wentz WB. Adenocarcinoma and mixed carcinoma of the uterine cervix. I. A clinicopathologic study. Cancer 1982; 49:2560–70.

250. Gallup DG, Harper RH, Stock RJ. Poor prognosis in patients with adenosquamous cell carcinoma of the cervix. Obstet Gynecol 1985;65:416–22.

251. Gersell DJ, Mazoujian G, Mutch DG, Rudloff MA. Small-cell undifferentiated carcinoma of the cervix. A clinicopathologic, ultrastructural, and immunocytochemical study of 15 cases. Am J Surg Pathol 1988;12:684–98.

252. Glucksmann A, Cherry CP. Incidence, histology, and response to radiation of mixed carcinomas (adenoacanthomas) of the uterine cervix. Cancer 1956; 9:971–9.

253. Groben P, Reddick R, Askin F. The pathologic spectrum of small cell carcinoma of the cervix. Int J Gynecol Pathol 1985;4:42–57.

254. Hoskins WJ, Averette HE, Ng AB, Yon JL. Adenoid cystic carcinoma of the cervix uteri: report of six cases and review of the literature. Gynecol Oncol 1979;7:371–84.

255. King LA, Talledo OE, Gallup DG, Melhus O, Otken LB. Adenoid cystic carcinoma of the cervix in women under age 40. Gynecol Oncol 1989;32:26–30.

256. Korhonen MO. Adenocarcinoma of the uterine cervix. Prognosis and prognostic significance of histology. Cancer 1984;53:1760–73.

257. Inoue T, Yamaguchi K, Suzuki H, Abe K, Chihara T. Production of immunoreactive-polypeptide hormones in cervical carcinoma. Cancer 1984;53:1509–14.

258. Littman P, Clement PB, Henriksen B, et al. Glassy cell carcinoma of the cervix. Cancer 1976;37:2238–46.

259. Lojek MA, Fer MF, Kasselberg AG, et al. Cushing's syndrome with small cell carcinoma of the uterine cervix. Am J Med 1980;69:140–4.

260. MacKay B, Osborne BM, Wharton JT. Small cell tumor of cervix with neuroepithelial features: ultrastructural observations in two cases. Cancer 1979;43:1138–45.

261. Maier RC, Norris HJ. Glassy cell carcinoma of the cervix. Obstet Gynecol 1982;60:219–24.

262. Matsuyama M, Inoue T, Ariyoshi Y, et al. Argyrophil cell carcinoma of the uterine cervix with ectopic production of ACTH, beta-MSH, serotonin, histamine, and amylase. Cancer 1979;44:1813–23.

263. Mazur MT, Battifora HA. Adenoid cystic carcinoma of the uterine cervix: ultrastructure, immunofluorescence, and criteria for diagnosis. Am J Clin Pathol 1982;77:494–500.

264. Miles PA, Norris HJ. Adenoid cystic carcinoma of the cervix. An analysis of 12 cases. Obstet Gynecol 1971;38:103–10.

265. Mullins JD, Hilliard GD. Cervical carcinoid ("argyrophil cell" carcinoma) associated with an endocervical adenocarcinoma: a light and ultrastructural study. Cancer 1981;47:785–90.

266. Musa AG, Hughes RR, Coleman SA. Adenoid cystic carcinoma of the cervix: a report of 17 cases. Gynecol Oncol 1985;22:167–73.

267. Nunez C, Abdul-Karim FW, Somrak TM. Glassy-cell carcinoma of the uterine cervix. Cytopathologic and histopathologic study of five cases. Acta Cytol 1985;29:303–9.

268. Pak HY, Yokota SB, Paladugu RR, Agliozzo CM. Glassy cell carcinoma of the cervix. Cytologic and clinicopathologic analysis. Cancer 1983;52:307–12.

269. Pazdur R, Bonomi P, Slayton R, et al. Neuroendocrine carcinoma of the cervix: implications for staging and therapy. Gynecol Oncol 1981;12:120–8.

270. Prempree T, Villasanta U, Tang CK. Management of adenoid cystic carcinoma of the uterine cervix (cylindroma): report of six cases and reappraisal of all cases reported in the medical literature. Cancer 1980;46:1631–5.

271. Randall ME, Constable WC, Hahn SS, Kim JA, Mills SE. Results of the radiotherapeutic management of carcinoma of the cervix with emphasis on the influence of histologic classification. Cancer 1988;62:48–53.

272. Saigo PE, Cain JM, Kim WS, Gaynor JJ, Johnson K, Lewis JL Jr. Prognostic factors in adenocarcinoma of the uterine cervix. Cancer 1986;57:1584–93.

273. Scully RE, Aguirre P, DeLellis RA. Argyrophilia, serotonin, and peptide hormones in the female genital tract and its tumors. Int J Gynecol Pathol 1984;3:51–70.

274. Seltzer V, Sall S, Castadot MJ, Muradian-Davidian M, Sedlis A. Glassy cell cervical carcinoma. Gynecol Oncol 1979;8:141–51.

275. Sheets EE, Berman ML, Hrountas CK, Liao SY, DiSaia PJ. Surgically treated, early-stage neuroendocrine small-cell cervical carcinoma. Obstet Gynecol 1988;71:10–4.

276. Shingleton HM, Gore H, Bradley DH, Soong SJ. Adenocarcinoma of the cervix. I. Clinical evaluation and pathologic features. Am J Obstet Gynecol 1981;139:799–814.

277. Silva EG, Kott MM, Ordonez NG. Endocrine carcinoma intermediate cell type of the uterine cervix. Cancer 1984; 54:1705–13.

278. Stassart J, Crum CP, Yordan EL, Fenoglio CM, Richart RM. Argyrophilic carcinoma of the cervix: a report of a case with coexisting cervical intraepithelial neoplasia. Gynecol Oncol 1982;13:247–51.

279. Stoler MH, Mills SE, Gersell DJ, Walker AN. Small-cell neuroendocrine carcinoma of the cervix. A human papillomavirus type 18–associated cancer. Am J Surg Pathol 1991;15:28–32.

280. Sutton GP, Siemers E, Stehman FB, Ehrlich CE. Eaton-Lambert syndrome as a harbinger of recurrent small-cell carcinoma of the cervix with improvement after combination chemotherapy. Obstet Gynecol 1988;72:516–8.

281. Tamimi HK, Ek M, Hesla J, Cain JM, Figge DC, Greer BE. Glassy cell carcinoma of the cervix redefined. Obstet Gynecol 1988;71:837–41.

282. _____, Figge DC. Adenocarcinoma of the uterine cervix. Gynecol Oncol 1982;13:335–44.

283. Tateishi R, Wada A, Hayakawa K, Hongo J, Ishii S. Argyrophil cell carcinomas (apudomas) of the uterine cervix. Light and electron microscopic observations of 5 cases. Virchows Arch [A] 1975;366; 257–74.

284. Tock EP, Shilkin KB. Pathological studies on adenocarcinoma of the uterine cervix in Singapore. Pathology 1974;6:275–86.

285. Tsukamoto N, Hirakawa T, Matsukuma K, et al. Carcinoma of the uterine cervix with variegated histological patterns and calcitonin production. Gynecol Oncol 1989; 33:395–9.

286. Ulbright TM, Gersell DJ. Glassy cell carcinoma of the uterine cervix. A light and electron microscopic study of five cases. Cancer 1983;51:2255–63.

287. Ulich TR, Liao SY, Layfield L, Romansky S, Cheng L, Lewin KJ. Endocrine and tumor differentiation markers in poorly differentiated small-cell carcinoids of the cervix and vagina. Arch Pathol Lab Med 1986;110:1054–7.

288. Van Dinh T, Woodruff JD. Adenoid cystic and adenoid basal carcinomas of the cervix. Obstet Gynecol 1985; 65:705–9.

289. Van Nagell JR Jr, Donaldson ES, Wood EG, Maruyama Y, Utley J. Small cell cancer of the uterine cervix. Cancer 1977;40:2243–9.

290. _____, Powell DE, Gallion HH, et al. Small cell carcinoma of the uterine cervix. Cancer 1988;62:1586–93.

291. Yamasaki M, Tateishi R, Hongo J, Ozaki Y, Inoue M, Ueda G. Argyrophil small cell carcinomas of the uterine cervix. Int J Gynecol Pathol 1984;3:146–52.

292. Zaino RJ, Nahhas WA, Mortel R. Glassy cell carcinoma of the uterine cervix. An ultrastructural study and review. Arch Pathol Lab Med 1982;106:250–4.

Mesenchymal Tumors

293. Abdul-Karim FW, Bazi TM, Sorensen K, Nasr MF. Sarcoma of the uterine cervix: clinicopathologic findings in three cases. Gynecol Oncol 1987;26:103–11.

294. Abeler V, Nesland JM. Alveolar soft-part sarcoma in the uterine cervix. Arch Pathol Lab Med 1989;113:1179–83.

295. Abell MR, Ramirez JA. Sarcomas and carcinosarcomas of the uterine cervix. Cancer 1973;31:1176–92.

296. Ahern JK, Allen NH. Cervical hemangioma: a case report and review of the literature. J Reprod Med 1978;21:228–31.

297. Ben David M, Dekel A, Gal R, Dicker D, Feldberg D, Goldman JA. Prolapsed cervical leiomyosarcoma. Obstet Gynecol Surv 1988;43:642–4.

298. Bloch T, Roth LM, Stehman FB, Hull MT, Schwenk GR Jr. Osteosarcoma of the uterine cervix associated with hyperplastic and atypical mesonephric nests. Cancer 1988;62:1594–600.

299. Brand E, Berek JS, Nieberg RK, Hacker NF. Rhabdomyosarcoma of the uterine cervix. Sarcoma botryoides. Cancer 1987;60:1552–60.

300. Buscema J, Rosenshein NB, Taqi F, Woodruff JD. Vaginal hemangiopericytoma: a histopathologic and ultrastructural evaluation. Obstet Gynecol 1985;66(Suppl 3):82–5S.

301. Clement PB. Miscellaneous primary tumors and metastatic tumors of the uterine cervix. Semin Diagn Pathol 1990;7:228–48.

302. _____. Multinucleated stromal giant cells of the uterine cervix. Arch Pathol Lab Med 1985;109:200–2.

303. Copeland LJ, Gershenson DM, Saul PB, Sneige N, Stringer CA, Edwards CL. Sarcoma botryoides of the female genital tract. Obstet Gynecol 1985;66:262–6.

304. Daya DA, Scully RE. Sarcoma botryoides of the uterine cervix in young women: a clinicopathological study of 13 cases. Gynecol Oncol 1988;29:290–304.

305. Flint A, Gikas PW, Roberts JA. Alveolar soft part sarcoma of the uterine cervix. Gynecol Oncol 1985;22:263–7.

306. Foschini MP, Eusebi V, Tison V. Alveolar soft part sarcoma of the cervix uteri. A case report. Pathol Res Pract 1989;184:354–60.

307. Ghosh TK. Arteriovenous malformation of the uterus and pelvis. Obstet Gynecol 1986;68(Suppl 3):40–3S.

308. Gordon AN, Montag TW. Sarcoma botryoides of the cervix: excision followed by adjuvant chemotherapy for preservation of reproductive function. Gynecol Oncol 1990;36:119–24.

309. Gusdon, JP. Hemangioma of the cervix. Am J Obstet Gynecol 1965;91:204–9.

310. Jaffe R, Altaras M, Bernheim J, Ben Aderet B. Endocervical stromal sarcoma—a case report. Gynecol Oncol 1985;22:105–8.

311. Kopolovic J, Weiss DB, Dolberg L, Brezinsky A, Ne'eman Z, Anteby SO. Alveolar soft-part sarcoma of the female genital tract. Arch Gynecol 1987;240:125–9.

312. Montag TW, d'Ablaing G, Schlaerth JB, Gaddis O Jr, Morrow CP. Embryonal rhabdomyosarcoma of the uterine corpus and cervix. Gynecol Oncol 1986;25:171–94.

313. Norris HJ, Taylor HB. Polyps of the vagina. A benign lesion resembling sarcoma botryoides. Cancer 1966;19: 227–32.

314. Ober WB. Sarcoma botryoides of the cervix uteri: a case report in a 75-year-old woman. Mt Sinai J Med 1971;38:363–74.

315. Ortner A, Weiser G, Haas H, Resch R, Dapunt O. Embryonal rhabdomyosarcoma (botryoid type) of the cervix: a case report and review. Gynecol Oncol 1982;13:115–9.

316. Rotmensch J, Rosenshein NB, Woodruff JD. Cervical sarcoma: a review. Obstet Gynecol Surv 1983;38:456–60.

317. Sahin AA, Silva EG, Ordonez NG. Alveolar soft part sarcoma of the uterine cervix. Mod Pathol 1989;2:676–80.

318. Scheffey LC, Levinson J, Herbut PA, et al. Osteosarcoma of the uterus: report of a case. Obstet Gynecol 1956;8:444–50.

319. Terzakis JA, Opher E, Melamed J, Santagada E, Sloan D. Pigmented melanocytic schwannoma of the uterine cervix. Ultrastruct Pathol 1990;14:357–66.

320. Young TW, Thrasher TV. Nonchromaffin paraganglioma of the uterus. A case report. Arch Pathol Lab Med 1982;106:608–9.

Mixed Epithelial and Mesenchymal Tumors

321. Abell MR. Papillary adenofibroma of the uterine cervix. Am J Obstet Gynecol 1971;110:990–3.

322. _____, Ramirez JA. Sarcomas and carcinosarcomas of the uterine cervix. Cancer 1973;31:1176–92.

323. Bell DA, Shimm DS, Gang DL. Wilms' tumor of the endocervix. Arch Pathol Lab Med 1985;109:371–3.

324. Clement PB. Müllerian adenosarcomas of the uterus with sarcomatous overgrowth. A clinicopathological analysis of 10 cases. Am J Surg Pathol 1989;13:28–38.

325. Gersell DJ, Duncan DA, Fulling KH. Malignant mixed müllerian tumor of the uterus with neuroectodermal differentiation. Int J Gynecol Pathol 1989;8:169–78.

326. Hall-Craggs M, Toker C, Nedwich A. Carcinosarcoma of the uterine cervix: a light and electron microscopic study. Cancer 1981;48:161–9.

327. Ostör AG, Fortune DW. Benign and low grade variants of mixed Müllerian tumour of the uterus. Histopathology 1980;4:369–82.

328. Roth E, Taylor HB. Heterotopic cartilage in the uterus. Obstet Gynecol 1966;27:838–44.

329. Rotmensch J, Rosenshein NB, Woodruff JD. Cervical sarcoma: a review. Obstet Gynecol Surv 1983;38:456–60.

330. Saier FL, Hovadhanakul P, Ostapowicz F. Giant cervical polyp. Obstet Gynecol 1973;41:94–6.

331. Silverberg SG, Major FJ, Blessing JA, et al. Carcinosarcoma (malignant mixed mesodermal tumor) of the uterus. A Gynecologic Oncology Group pathologic study of 203 cases. Int J Gynecol Pathol 1990;9:1–19.

332. Tang CK, Toker C, Harriman B. Müllerian adenosarcoma of the uterine cervix. Hum Pathol 1981;12:579–81.

333. Vellios F, Ng AB, Reagan JW. Papillary adenofibroma of the uterus: a benign mesodermal mixed tumor of Müllerian origin. Am J Clin Pathol 1973;60:543–51.

334. Zaloudek CJ, Norris HJ. Adenofibroma and adenosarcoma of the uterus: a clinicopathologic study of 35 cases. Cancer 1981;48:354–66.

Miscellaneous Tumors

335. Abell MR. Primary melanoblastoma of the uterine cervix. Am J Clin Pathol 1961;36:248–55.

336. Anderson GG. Hodgkin's disease of the uterine cervix. Report of a case. Obstet Gynecol 1967;29:170–2.

337. Barter JF, Mazur M, Holloway RW, Hatch KD. Melanosis of the cervix. Gynecol Oncol 1988;29:101–4.

338. Carbone PP, Kaplan HS, Musshoff K, Smithers DW, Tubiana M. Report of the Committee on Hodgkin's Disease Staging Classification. Cancer Res 1971;31:1860–1.

339. Chorlton I, Karnei RF Jr, King FM, Norris HJ. Primary malignant reticuloendothelial disease involving the vagina, cervix, and corpus uteri. Obstet Gynecol 1974;44:735–48.

340. Chua S, Viegas OA, Wee A, Ratnam SS. Malignant melanoma of the cervix. Gynecol Obstet Invest 1989;27:107–9.

341. Cid JM. La schwanosis uterina y el nevo azul del endocervix. An Cir 1964;29:8–18.

342. Davis JR, Steinbronn KK, Graham AR, Dawson BV. Effects of Monsel's solution in uterine cervix. Am J Clin Pathol 1984;82:332–5.

343. Diaz de Molnar AM, Guralnick M, Ferenczy A. Blue nevus of the endocervix: report of two cases and ultrastructure. Gynecol Oncol 1978;6:373–82.

344. Goldman RL, Friedman NB. Blue nevus of the uterine cervix. Cancer 1967;20:210–4.

345. Hall DJ, Schneider V, Goplerud DR. Primary malignant melanoma of the uterine cervix. Obstet Gynecol 1980;56:525–9.

346. Hanai J, Tsuji M. Uterine teratoma with lymphoid hyperplasia. Acta Pathol Jpn 1981;31:153–9.

347. Harris NL, Scully RE. Malignant lymphoma and granulocytic sarcoma of the uterus and vagina. A clinicopathologic analysis of 27 cases. Cancer 1984;53:2530–45.

348. Holmquist ND, Torres J. Malignant melanoma of the cervix. Report of a case. Acta Cytol 1988;32:252–6.

349. Komaki R, Cox JD, Hansen RM, Gunn WG, Greenberg M. Malignant lymphoma of the uterine cervix. Cancer 1984;54:1699–704.

350. Mann R, Roberts WS, Gunasakeran S, Tralins A. Primary lymphoma of the uterine cervix. Gynecol Oncol 1987;26:127–34.

351. Mordel N, Mor-Yosef S, Ben-Baruch N, Anteby SO. Malignant melanoma of the uterine cervix: case report and review of the literature. Gynecol Oncol 1989;32:375–80.

352. Morrow CP, DiSaia PJ. Malignant melanoma of the female genitalia: a clinical analysis. Obstet Gynecol Surv 1976;31:233–71.

353. Owens OJ, Pollard K, Khoury GG, Dyson JE, Jarvis GJ, Joslin CA. Primary malignant melanoma of the uterine cervix. Clin Radiol 1988;39:336–8.

354. Patel DS, Bhagavan BS. Blue nevus of the uterine cervix. Hum Pathol 1985;16:79–86.

355. Santoso JT, Kucera PR, Ray J. Primary malignant melanoma of the uterine cervix: two case reports and a century's review. Obstet Gynecol Surv 1990;45:733–40.

356. Seo IS, Hull MT, Pak HY. Granulocytic sarcoma of the cervix as a primary manifestation: case without overt leukemic features for 26 months. Cancer 1977;40:3030–7.

357. Stransky GC, Acosta AA, Kaplan AL, Friedman JA. Reticulum cell sarcoma of the cervix. Obstet Gynecol 1973;41:183–7.

358. Young RH, Harris NL, Scully RE. Lymphoma-like lesions of the lower female genital tract: a report of 16 cases. Int J Gynecol Pathol 1985;4:289–99.

359. Yu HC, Ketabchi M. Detection of malignant melanoma of the uterine cervix from papanicolaou smears. A case report. Acta Cytol 1987;31:73–6.

Secondary Tumors

360. Abrams HL, Spiro R, Goldstein N. Metastases in carcinoma: analysis of 1000 autopsied cases. Cancer 1950;3:74–85.

361. Kumar NB, Hart WR. Metastases to the uterine corpus from extragenital cancers. A clinicopathologic study of 63 cases. Cancer 1982;50:2163–9.

362. Lemoine NR, Hall PA. Epithelial tumors metastatic to the uterine cervix. A study of 33 cases and review of the literature. Cancer 1986;57:2002–5.

363. McGill F, Adachi A, Karimi N, et al. Abnormal cervical cytology leading to the diagnosis of gastric cancer. Gynecol Oncol 1990;36:101–5.

364. Singh P. Post menopausal bleeding secondary to metastatic disease in the endocervix from carcinoma of the breast [Letter]. Gynecol Oncol 1985;22:268–9.

365. Way S. Carcinoma metastatic in the cervix. Gynecol Oncol 1980;9:298–302.

366. Yazigi R, Sandstad J, Munoz AK. Breast cancer metastasizing to the uterine cervix. Cancer 1988;61:2558–60.

Tumor-Like Lesions

367. Ayroud Y, Gelfand MM, Ferenczy A. Florid mesonephric hyperplasia of the cervix: a report of a case with review of the literature. Int J Gynecol Pathol 1985;4:245–54.

368. Barua R. Post-cone biopsy traumatic neuroma of the uterine cervix. Arch Pathol Lab Med 1989;113:945–7.

369. Chumas JC, Nelson B, Mann WJ, Chalas E, Kaplan CG. Microglandular hyperplasia of the uterine cervix. Obstet Gynecol 1985;66:406–9.

370. Clement PB. Multinucleated stromal giant cells of the uterine cervix. Arch Pathol Lab Med 1985;109:200–2.

371. _____, Young RH. Deep nabothian cysts of the uterine cervix. A possible source of confusion with minimal-deviation adenocarcinoma (adenoma malignum). Int J Gynecol Pathol 1989;8:340–8.

372. _____, Young RH, Scully RE. Stromal endometriosis of the uterine cervix. A variant of endometriosis that may simulate a sarcoma. Am J Surg Pathol 1990;14:449–55.

373. Gall SA, Bourgeois CH, Maguire R. The morphologic effects of oral contraceptive agents on the cervix. JAMA 1969;207:2243–7.

374. Gersell DJ, Duncan DA, Fulling KH. Malignant mixed müllerian tumor of the uterus with neuroectodermal differentiation. Int J Gynecol Pathol 1989;8:169–78.

375. Grove A. Dermal adnexal differentiation in a squamous cell carcinoma of the uterine cervix. Histopathology 1988;13:109–14.

376. Jones MW, Silverberg SG. Cervical adenocarcinoma in young women: possible relationship to microglandular hyperplasia and use of oral contraceptives. Obstet Gynecol 1989;73:984–9.

377. Kay S, Schneider V. Reactive spindle cell nodule of the endocervix simulating uterine sarcoma. Int J Gynecol Pathol 1985;4:255–7.

378. Lang G, Dallenbach-Hellweg G. The histogenetic origin of cervical mesonephric hyperplasia and mesonephric adenocarcinoma of the uterine cervix studied with immunohistochemical methods. Int J Gynecol Pathol 1990;9:145–57.

379. Luevano-Flores E, Sotelo J, Tena-Suck M. Glial polyp (glioma) of the uterine cervix, report of a case with demonstration of glial fibrillary acidic protein. Gynecol Oncol 1985;21:385–90.

380. Michael H, Sutton G, Hull MT, Roth LM. Villous adenoma of the uterine cervix associated with invasive adenocarcinoma: a histologic, ultrastructural, and immunohistochemical study. Int J Gynecol Pathol 1986;5:163–9.

381. Murray J, Fox H. Rosai-Dorfman disease of the uterine cervix. Int J Gynecol Pathol 1991;10:209–13.

382. Norris HJ, Taylor HB. Polyps of the vagina. A benign lesion resembling sarcoma botryoides. Cancer 1966;19:227–32.

383. Proppe KH, Scully RE, Rosai J. Postoperative spindle cell nodules of genitourinary tract resembling sarcomas. A report of eight cases. Am J Surg Pathol 1984;8:101–8.

384. Roca AN, Guajardo M, Estrada WJ. Glial polyp of the cervix and endometrium. Report of a case and review of the literature. Am J Clin Pathol 1980;73:718–20.

385. Roth E, Taylor HB. Heterotopic cartilage in the uterus. Obstet Gynecol 1966;27:838–44.

386. Suh KS, Silverberg SG. Tubal metaplasia of the uterine cervix. Int J Gynecol Pathol 1990;9:122–8.

387. Taylor HB, Irey NS, Norris HJ. Atypical endocervical hyperplasia in women taking oral contraceptives. JAMA 1967;202:637–9.

388. Trowell JE. Intestinal metaplasia with argentaffin cells in the uterine cervix. Histopathology 1985;9:551–9.

389. Wilkinson E, Dufour DR. Pathogenesis of microglandular hyperplasia of the cervix uteri. Obstet Gynecol 1976;47:189–95.

390. Young RH, Harris NL, Scully RE. Lymphoma-like lesions of the lower female genital tract: a report of 16 cases. Int J Gynecol Pathol 1985;4:289–99.

391. _____, Kleinman GM, Scully RE. Glioma of the uterus. Report of a case with comments on histogenesis. Am J Surg Pathol 1981;5:695–99.

392. _____, Kurman RJ, Scully RE. Proliferations and tumors of intermediate trophoblast of the placental site. Semin Diagn Pathol 1988;5:223–37.

393. _____, Scully RE. Atypical forms of microglandular hyperplasia of the cervix simulating carcinoma. A report of five cases and review of the literature. Am J Surg Pathol 1989;13:50–6.

TUMORS OF THE VAGINA

SQUAMOUS LESIONS

Squamous Papilloma

Squamous papilloma is a benign papillary lesion similar in its gross and microscopic appearance to squamous papillomas involving the ectocervix and vulva. Accordingly, squamous papilloma is also described in the cervix and vulva chapters.

In the vagina, squamous papillomas are only a few millimeters in greatest diameter, may be single but more often are multiple, and typically occur in clusters. They occur anywhere in the vagina, but characteristically are located around the hymenal ring, often merging with similar lesions in the vulvar vestibule. Multiple lesions are referred to as *squamous papillomatosis*. As indicated in the previous chapter, squamous papillomas are not related to HPV infection. Although they resemble condylomas, they have distinctive features (fig. 183). In particular, they lack bona fide koilocytosis, and HPV DNA, by Southern blot hybridization, is only occasionally detected (13,18). Because HPV DNA sequences can be found by Southern blot hybridization in vaginal and vulvar scrapings in 10 to 20 percent of women without discernable lesions, the occasional presence of HPV DNA in squamous papillomas is probably coincidental.

Squamous papillomas are usually asymptomatic. When they are extensive, and particularly when they involve the vulvar vestibule, they may produce vulvar burning or dyspareunia characterized by an abrasive sensation localized to the introitus. Asymptomatic lesions require no treatment. Those associated with dyspareunia respond to ablative treatment with trichloroacetic acid or laser vaporization.

Condyloma Acuminatum

Vaginal condylomas are similar in their gross and microscopic appearance to condylomas arising on the ectocervix and vulva and are described in detail in the cervix and vulva chapters.

Transitional Metaplasia

This lesion is composed of basal and parabasal cells with ovoid nuclei resembling transitional epithelium. It is important to distinguish this lesion from high grade vaginal intraepithelial lesions (see Squamous Intraepithelial Lesions). In transitional metaplasia the cells are uniform, lack disorganization, and have bland-appearing nuclei. Usually there is little, if any, mitotic activity. A counterpart of this lesion occurs in the cervix.

Squamous Atypia

This lesion is similar to its counterpart in the cervix. It is characterized by a relatively uniform population of cells with nuclear enlargement and prominent nucleoli. The cells are not crowded and retain an orderly pattern of maturation (fig. 184).

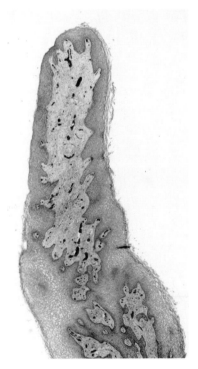

Figure 183
SQUAMOUS PAPILLOMA
The lesion is characterized by a thick fibrovascular core and covered by mature stratified squamous epithelium showing no cytologic atypia.

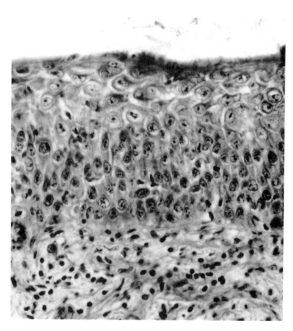

Figure 184
SQUAMOUS ATYPIA

There is slight nuclear enlargement and atypia. The most striking feature is the presence of prominent nucleoli. There is a normal maturation with no cellular disorganization. The retention of polarity, normal maturation, presence of prominent nucleoli, and absence of koilocytotic atypia in squamous atypia help to distinguish it from VAIN (figs. 185–187).

Typically there is marked acute and chronic inflammation in the stroma and leukocytes in the epithelium. This is helpful in distinguishing squamous atypia from VAIN because it is unusual to see leukocytes within the epithelium of VAIN, although there often is an inflammatory infiltrate in the stroma.

Squamous Intraepithelial Lesions

Definition. Proliferative intraepithelial squamous lesions with abnormal maturation, nuclear enlargement, and atypia. The latter is characterized by pleomorphism, coarse chromatin clumping, and irregular nuclear contours.

These lesions have been termed *dysplasia, carcinoma in situ* (CIS), and *vaginal intraepithelial neoplasia* (VAIN). In the Bethesda System, vaginal cytologic smears showing VAIN 1 are designated *low-grade squamous intraepithelial lesion* (SIL) and VAIN 2 and 3 are designated *high-grade SIL*. As discussed in the chapter on Classification of Tumors of the Lower Female

Genital Tract, to conform with the WHO histologic classification for tumors and tumor-like lesions of the vagina, the primary terminology in this text is VAIN.

General Features. Intraepithelial lesions of the vagina have been recognized relatively recently, probably because of a heightened awareness of their existence. The vast majority are not apparent on clinical examination but are diagnosed by cytologic smears. The average age-adjusted incidence rate in the United States is 0.20 per 100,000 for white and 0.31 for black women (5). The ratio of vaginal to cervical intraepithelial lesions is 1:23 (8). The mean age of women with VAIN 3 is 53 years, approximately 10 years older than women with CIN 3 (7). Although vaginal lesions are almost invariably diagnosed after treatment of cervical neoplasia, this may not reflect the natural history of the disease but may be an artifact of cytology screening; i.e., in women who have not had a hysterectomy, smears are generally obtained from the cervix. Only after a hysterectomy for malignant or benign disease are smears taken from the vagina, and therefore, preexisting VAIN may have been overlooked earlier.

VAIN 3 usually occurs in the upper third of the vagina and is multifocal or diffuse in nearly half the cases (2,9,23). One third of the patients have a history of prior CIN 3, sometimes as long as 22 years earlier. In addition, CIN coexists with VAIN in 10 to 20 percent of the cases (2,8,9,23). It has been suggested that the multicentric distribution of preinvasive and invasive squamous cell carcinomas in the lower genital tract is related to a common carcinogenic stimulus (11). This "field-effect" theory attempts to account for the development of multiple sequential or simultaneous carcinomas involving tissue derived from a shared anlage. The demonstration of HPV DNA sequences in cervical, vaginal, and vulvar neoplasms is consistent with this view. Another cause of VAIN is radiation because a prior history of pelvic irradiation for benign uterine disease has been reported in most series (2,8,9,23). It is possible that HPV and radiation are synergistic in some cases.

Gross Findings. Like its cervical counterpart, intraepithelial lesions of the vagina are best appreciated by colposcopic examination after application of 3 to 5 percent acetic acid. Colposcopic examination reveals well-circumscribed, white, slightly elevated lesions with epithelial and vascular patterns similar to those of CIN.

Microscopic Findings. Microscopically, VAIN is similar to CIN, and the criteria for grading intraepithelial lesions are the same as those for the cervix (figs. 185–187).

Differential Diagnosis. Atrophy in older women, immature squamous metaplasia in women with adenosis, and reactive atypia are the lesions most commonly confused with VAIN. Although both atrophy and immature squamous metaplasia display a high nuclear-cytoplasmic ratio they lack nuclear atypia, which is the hallmark of VAIN. The squamous (reactive) atypias are characterized by prominent nucleoli, retention of cell membranes and cellular polarity, and an absence of marked cellular crowding and abnormal mitotic figures. Because vaginal adenosis may be extensive in the diethylstilbestrol (DES)-exposed patient, complete replacement of the glands by immature squamous metaplasia may, under low power, resemble invasive squamous cell carci-

noma. If attention is directed to the degree of cytologic atypia, the distinction between immature squamous metaplasia and invasive squamous cell carcinoma should not be difficult.

Clinical Behavior and Treatment. Squamous intraepithelial lesions of the vagina are typically diagnosed by abnormal cytology in patients who have had a hysterectomy for cervical neoplasia or benign uterine disease. The presence of VAIN should also be considered in a patient with an intact uterus who has abnormal cytology that is inconsistent with the findings on cervical colposcopy, and in whom a cone biopsy shows no lesion. Progression to invasive vaginal carcinoma occurs in approximately 5 percent of the cases and has been documented by serial biopsies showing changes from VAIN 1 through VAIN 2 and 3 to invasive cancer (23).

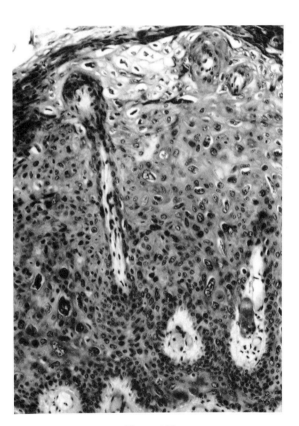

Figure 186
VAIN 2

Compared with VAIN 1, there is greater proliferation, crowding, loss of polarity, and cytologic atypia in the basal and parabasal layers involving the lower half of the epithelium. Koilocytotic atypia, characterized by irregularly shaped pyknotic nuclei, is present in the upper third of the epithelium.

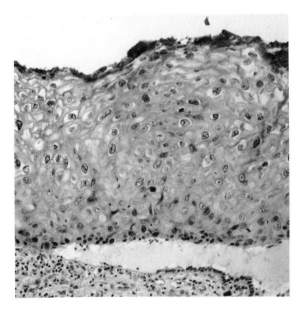

Figure 185
VAIN 1

There is minimal proliferation in the basal layers. Prominent koilocytotic atypia characterized by cells with enlarged, slightly pleomorphic, atypical nuclei and vacuolated cytoplasm occupy the upper two thirds of the epithelium. As in the cervix, flat vaginal lesions with bona fide koilocytotic atypia, even with minimal proliferation in the basal layers, are classified VAIN 1.

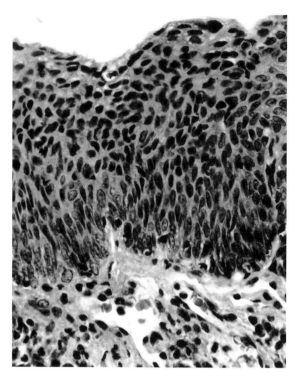

Figure 187
VAIN 3
The full thickness of the epithelium is replaced by abnormal basal and parabasal cells with a high nuclear-cytoplasmic ratio. The nuclei are oval and the cells have their longitudinal axis perpendicular to the basement membrane, except for the superficial layers where they are horizontal.

Similar lesions may follow radiation treatment for carcinoma of the cervix. These lesions are designated *postirradiation dysplasia* (14). The sooner they become evident, the more likely they are to be neoplastic. Those that develop within 3 years are associated with recurrent cervical carcinoma in 71 percent of patients, compared to 44 percent in women in whom dysplasia develops 3 years after radiation (25).

Finally, VAIN may develop in women with adenosis who have been exposed to DES in utero. Vaginal adenosis in the DES-exposed woman corresponds somewhat to benign glandular epithelium of the cervical transformation zone in unexposed women. Accordingly, some investigators regard vaginal adenosis in the DES-exposed woman as an extension of the cervical transformation zone from the cervix to the vagina. Because preinvasive and invasive squamous neoplasms of the cervix develop within the transformation zone, there has been concern that squamous cell carcinoma will develop in a large proportion of the DES-exposed population because of the large transformation zone. The National Cooperative Diethylstilbestrol Adenosis (DESAD) Project reported an increased incidence of CIN and VAIN in the DES-exposed group compared with matched controls (22). The majority of these intraepithelial lesions, however, were low-grade lesions. The findings suggest that the DES-exposed patient, because of the large transformation zone, may be at a greater risk of HPV infection, which leads in turn to the development of VAIN. At this point, an increase in the number of squamous cell carcinomas in the DES-exposed population has not been demonstrated, but further follow-up of this cohort is necessary for a final answer.

Treatment of VAIN is excisional biopsy for small lesions. Partial vaginectomy, laser vaporization (24), or intravaginal application of 5-fluorouracil cream (26) is reserved for more extensive lesions.

Squamous Cell Carcinoma

Definition. This neoplasm is composed of malignant squamous cells and is often associated with squamous cell carcinomas of the cervix and vulva. It may be difficult to distinguish the site of origin of the tumor in cases involving more than one organ.

General Features. Invasive squamous cell carcinoma of the vagina accounts for 1 to 2 percent of all malignant tumors of the female genital tract. Cervical squamous cell carcinoma is 50 times more prevalent than vaginal squamous cell carcinoma (12). According to the convention established by the International Federation of Gynecologists and Obstetricians (FIGO), a primary vaginal carcinoma must not involve the cervix; if there is cervical involvement the tumor is considered a cervical carcinoma with extension to the vagina. In addition, in patients with a history of prior preinvasive or invasive cervical or vulvar carcinoma, a 5- to 10-year disease-free interval is considered necessary to rule out recurrent disease (16,19). Approximately 85 percent of recurrent cervical and vulvar cancers occur within the first 3 years after treatment, but it is not unusual for a vaginal tumor to develop 20 years after treatment of a primary cervical carcinoma (1). From a practical

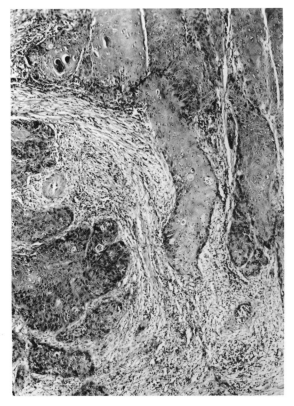

Figure 188
SQUAMOUS CELL CARCINOMA
This tumor is characterized by nests of squamous epithelium surrounded by a dense fibroblastic stroma with extensive inflammatory cell infiltration. There is no keratinization.

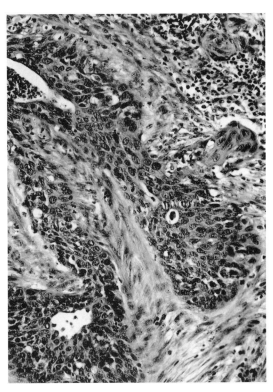

Figure 189
SQUAMOUS CELL CARCINOMA
This nonkeratinizing squamous cell carcinoma shows a relatively uniform population of cells.

standpoint, patients treated for cervical cancer must be carefully followed for the remainder of their lives. Most vaginal carcinomas are secondary, either by direct extension from the cervix or vulva or by metastasis from such sites as the endometrium, urinary bladder, ovary, or rectum.

Clinical Features. Patients range in age from the teens through the 80s, with a mean age of 64 years. They are approximately 10 years older than women with cervical carcinoma. Nearly 75 percent of them present with painless bleeding or urinary tract symptoms. The cytology smear is useful in detecting tumors in asymptomatic women.

Gross Findings. Vaginal carcinoma is commonly located in the upper third of the vagina, often involving the posterior wall. The tumors are ulcerative in half the cases, exophytic in a third, and annular and constricting in the remainder.

Microscopic Findings. Squamous cell carcinoma of the vagina displays a variety of histologic patterns similar to those of cervical squamous cell carcinoma. The majority of the vaginal neoplasms are nonkeratinizing (4) and moderately differentiated (figs. 188, 189) (20). There appears to be no correlation between the grade of the tumor and the outcome (6).

Invasive squamous cell carcinomas are recognized occasionally at a microinvasive stage characterized by tongues of tumor invading the stroma to a depth of 3 mm or less, as in microinvasive carcinoma of the cervix. When invasion is 3 mm or less measured from the basement membrane, metastasis is unlikely if lymphatic/vascular space invasion is not identified (17). There may be a subset of patients with minimal disease that can be treated conservatively, but additional cases must be studied to justify microinvasive squamous carcinoma of the vagina as a distinct entity.

Staging. The FIGO staging for vaginal carcinoma is as follows:

Stage 0	Intraepithelial carcinoma
Stage I	Carcinoma limited to the vaginal wall
Stage II	Carcinoma involving subvaginal tissue but not extending to the pelvic wall
Stage III	Carcinoma extending to the pelvic wall or pubic symphysis
Stage IV	Carcinoma extending beyond the true pelvis or involving the mucosa of bladder or rectum
Stage IV-A	Carcinoma involving adjacent organs
Stage IV-B	Carcinoma at distant sites

Clinical Behavior and Treatment. Squamous cell carcinomas spread by direct extension into the bladder, rectum, broad ligament, and rectovaginal septum. They also invade lymphatics and blood vessels, metastasizing to regional lymph nodes and distant sites including the lungs, liver, and brain. Recurrence is typically local and usually develops within 2 years after treatment.

Surgical treatment is similar to that of cervical and vulvar cancer and is based on the location of the vaginal neoplasm relative to the cervix or vulva. Radiation therapy, however, is the primary form of treatment for vaginal carcinoma. Tumors in the upper portion of the vagina, like cervical carcinomas, gain access to lymphatics that drain to the pelvic sidewall whereas tumors involving the lower portion of the vagina, like vulvar carcinomas, invade lymphatics that drain to the inguinal-femoral nodes. The prognosis had been poor in the past because of late detection and because the rich vascular and lymphatic supply of the vagina permits early invasion. Survival in recent years, however, has improved, with reported 5-year survival for stage I tumors of 70 to 90 percent and for tumors of all stages of 50 percent (10,15).

Verrucous Carcinoma

Verrucous carcinoma has the same appearance as in the cervix and vulva and is described in greater detail in those chapters. In the lower female genital tract, verrucous carcinoma occurs most often in the vulva, followed by the cervix and vagina. Because of the confusion in terminology,

it is difficult to ascertain the precise number of cases reported (3). The tumor characteristically recurs locally and can be successfully treated by wide local excision. In view of their large size, some tumors must be treated by exenteration, abdominoperineal resection, and vaginectomy. The 5-year survival is 70 percent. Invasive squamous cell carcinoma occasionally accompanies or follows verrucous carcinoma.

Warty (Condylomatous) Carcinoma

Squamous cell carcinomas with striking condylomatous features microscopically are designated *warty carcinomas* (21). Like verrucous carcinomas, warty carcinomas appear to have a less aggressive behavior than typical well-differentiated squamous cell carcinoma, although the experience with warty carcinoma is extremely limited. Microscopically, warty carcinoma has the features of a squamous cell carcinoma at the deep margin, but has striking condylomatous features (figs. 190–192).

Unlike verrucous carcinoma, the exophytic papillary growths in warty carcinoma contain fibrovascular cores. In addition, many of the malignant cells display koilocytotic atypia and greater nuclear atypia than verrucous carcinoma (figs. 191, 192).

GLANDULAR LESIONS

Adenosis

Definition. Adenosis is the presence of glandular epithelium or its secretory products in the vagina.

General Features. The vagina is lined entirely by squamous epithelium and is normally devoid of glands. The abnormal presence of glands in the vagina was first described by von Preuschen (62), and was designated *adenomatosis vaginae* by Bonney and Glendining (28). Subsequently, Plautt and Dreyfuss (52) coined the term *adenosis*.

In 1971 adenosis was related to prenatal DES exposure (43), occurring in approximately one third of the exposed offspring (39). In these women the frequency of detection of adenosis has depended on several factors. These include the manner in which the patient presents for examination, the dosage of DES during pregnancy, the time in pregnancy when DES was first given, and the age of the patient at the time of examination

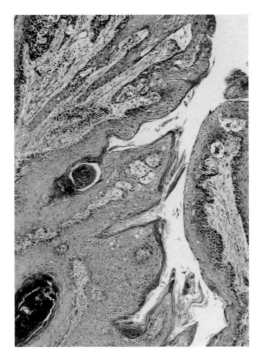

Figure 190
WARTY CARCINOMA
Here a condylomatous growth pattern is shown on the surface. Unlike verrucous carcinoma, the squamous papillae contain fibrovascular cores.

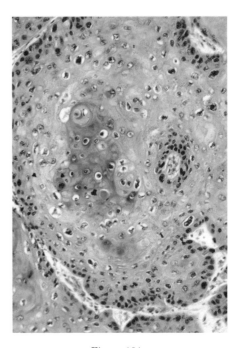

Figure 191
WARTY CARCINOMA
Unlike verrucous carcinoma warty carcinoma has many squamous cells displaying koilocytotic atypia.

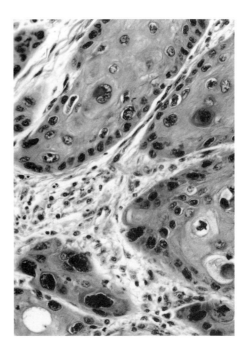

Figure 192
WARTY CARCINOMA
This example has irregularly shaped nests of squamous epithelium invading the stroma. The cytologic atypia is greater than in verrucous carcinoma.

(50). Before 1971 adenosis was rarely reported. In an autopsy study of 100 fetuses, children, and young women not exposed to DES in whom the vaginas were extensively sampled, adenosis was detected in only 8 cases (47). Because adenosis is usually asymptomatic, it occurs more commonly than is generally recognized in the absence of careful vaginal examination.

The embryologic basis for the development of adenosis in the DES-exposed woman is described in the chapter Embryology of the Lower Female Genital Tract. Briefly, during gestation DES inhibits the urogenital-derived squamous epithelium destined to become the vaginal epithelium from normally growing up to the junction of the ectocervix and endocervix and replacing the preexisting müllerian-derived columnar epithelium. The embryonic müllerian epithelium that is not replaced persists and develops into adenosis. Similar findings have been reported in animals including mice and rhesus monkeys treated with DES during pregnancy (31,46,51). In unexposed women, adenosis probably also arises on a congenital basis. In these individuals it remains latent throughout childhood, becoming evident after puberty perhaps as a result of the influence of steroid hormones (45,47). Adenosis in unexposed and DES-exposed women is microscopically identical (54).

Gross structural abnormalities of the cervix occur in about 25 percent of the DES-exposed population and are rare in women who are unexposed. The structural abnormalities include cervical hypoplasia, cervical hoods, transverse vaginal septa, pseudopolyps, and obliteration of the vaginal fornices (38).

Recently, adenosis characterized by the presence of glands lined by mucinous or endometrial-type epithelium has been described in the vagina after laser vaporization or intravaginal application of topical 5-fluorouracil for treatment of extensive vaginal condylomas. The development of adenosis in these patients is probably related to the extensive denuding of the epithelium, but the precise etiology of the lesion in this setting is unknown (59).

Clinical Features. Most women with adenosis are asymptomatic; some, however, present with a mucous discharge or bleeding. Areas of adenosis and associated squamous metaplasia are usually visible by colposcopy and iodine staining. In nearly 75 percent of the cases adenosis is found in the upper third of the vagina, although it may be found at any level. The anterior wall is most commonly involved.

Gross Findings. Adenosis may present as multiple cysts from 0.5 to 4 cm in diameter or as a diffusely red granular appearance of the mucosa. Colposcopic examination reveals columnar and metaplastic squamous epithelium.

Microscopic Findings. Adenosis is characterized by the presence of glands in the lamina propria or replacement or covering of the surface squamous epithelium by glandular epithelium. The glands may be lined by three types of epithelium. The most common is mucinous epithelium resembling endocervical epithelium (fig. 193). The second type is composed of simple or pseudo-stratified, cuboidal or columnar cells, at least some of which are ciliated (figs. 194,195), resembling the

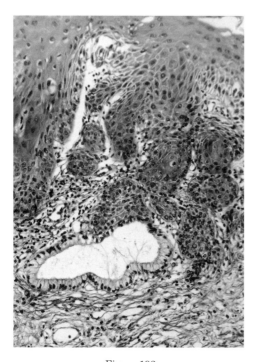

Figure 193
ADENOSIS, MUCINOUS TYPE
The gland is lined by endocervical-type epithelium; there is extensive squamous metaplasia.

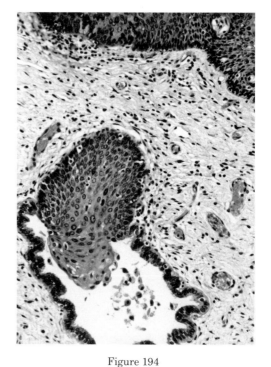

Figure 194
ADENOSIS, TUBAL TYPE
Metaplastic squamous epithelium fills a portion of the gland lumen.

epithelium of the fallopian tube or endometrium (tuboendometrial type). The third type of epithelium, which is only rarely encountered, is composed of cuboidal embryonic type cells with relatively scant cytoplasm lining tiny glands that lie at the junction of the squamous epithelium and the lamina propria (fig. 196). Mixtures of the various types of adenosis may occur.

The distribution of adenosis is correlated with its cellular composition. Adenosis on the surface is almost always of the mucinous type whereas the glands may be of the mucinous or tuboendometrial type in the lamina propria. In the upper vagina mucinous epithelium is more common than tuboendometrial epithelium. In the distal vagina, adenosis is less frequently encountered, and tuboendometrial-type adenosis is more common than mucinous adenosis.

Squamous metaplasia, replacing the glandular epithelium of adenosis to some extent, is typically present (see figs. 193, 194). At first the metaplasia is immature, but later it matures, becomes glycogenated, and eventually replaces the gland lumens. In the final stages of the replacement of glands by squamous metaplasia, the only vestige of adenosis may be intercellular pools of mucin or mucin droplets within the squamous epithelial cells (fig. 197).

A lymphocytic and plasma cell infiltrate frequently surrounds glands of adenosis or is present beneath the columnar epithelium on the surface. Neutrophils are less commonly observed.

Microglandular hyperplasia identical to that occurring in the cervix may develop in women with adenosis who are on oral contraceptives (figs. 198, 199). The microscopic features are described in the chapter Tumors of the Cervix.

Differential Diagnosis. Mesonephric (Gartner duct) remnants, particularly when they are hyperplastic, may be confused with adenosis. Unlike adenosis, which tends to be superficial in the anterior wall, mesonephric remnants are present mostly deep in the lateral walls. At their

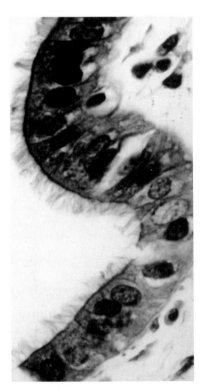

Figure 195
ADENOSIS, TUBAL TYPE
In this high magnification of tubal-type adenosis the epithelium is ciliated and resembles the epithelium lining the fallopian tube. (Fig. 4.64 from Sedlis A, Robboy SJ. Diseases of the vagina. In: Kurman RJ, ed. Blaustein's pathology of the female genital tract. 3rd ed. New York: Springer-Verlag, 1987:97–140.)

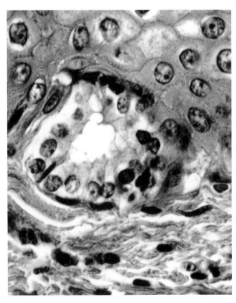

Figure 196
ADENOSIS, EMBRYONIC TYPE
The glands are at the junction of the squamous epithelium and the lamina propria. They are lined by nondescript cuboidal epithelium. (Fig. 6 from Robboy SJ, et al. Vaginal adenosis in women born prior to the diethylestrol era. Hum Pathol 1986;17:488–92.)

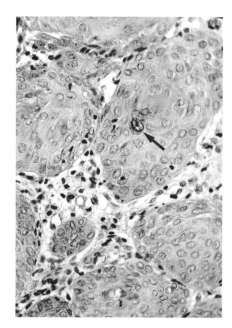

Figure 197
SQUAMOUS METAPLASIA
REPLACING ADENOSIS
This squamous metaplasia is completely replacing vaginal adenosis. A small droplet of mucin (arrow) in the center of one of the squamous epithelial nests is the only vestige of mucin-secreting epithelium.

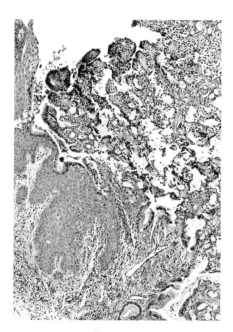

Figure 198
MICROGLANDULAR HYPERPLASIA
INVOLVING ADENOSIS
On low power microglandular hyperplasia within vaginal adenosis shows a marked proliferation of small crowded glands which may be confused with clear cell carcinoma.

terminations, however, they may be superficial. Mesonephric structures are composed of closely grouped tubules, often clustered around a duct, and are lined by a single layer of cuboidal cells containing uniform, round nuclei with granular chromatin. Dense, eosinophilic, PAS-positive nonmucinous material is characteristically found in the lumens, and a loose vascular stroma, distinctly different from the fibromuscular stroma of the vagina, often surrounds the tubules (figs. 200–202).

Endometriosis may also be confused with adenosis. Unlike adenosis, the glands of endometriosis are surrounded by endometrial stroma and may be associated with old or recent hemorrhage.

Extensive vaginal adenosis that is replaced by immature metaplastic squamous epithelium may simulate invasive squamous cell carcinoma. However, the absence of significant cytologic atypia and the uniform rounded outlines of the nests, in contrast to the more irregular contours of the nests of squamous cell carcinoma, facilitates the differential diagnosis.

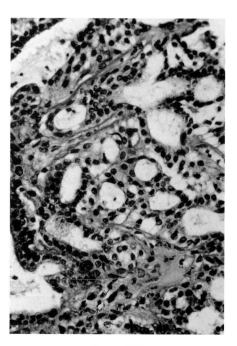

Figure 199
MICROGLANDULAR HYPERPLASIA
INVOLVING ADENOSIS
High magnification of microglandular hyperplasia illustrated in figure 198. Note that the small glands are lined by a single layer of cells with bland nuclei. Mitoses are not evident.

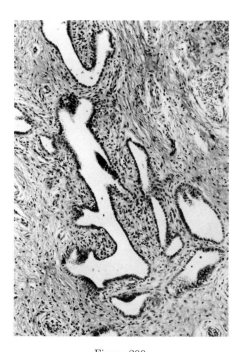

Figure 200
MESONEPHRIC REMNANT
This mesonephric remnant consists of a mesonephric duct lined by a single layer of cuboidal cells.

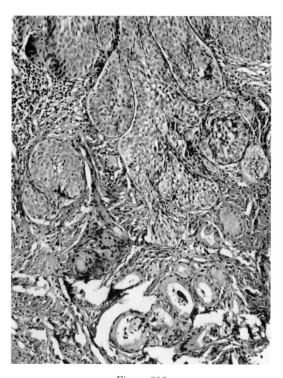

Figure 202
MESONEPHRIC HYPERPLASIA
High magnification showing mesonephric tubules lined by cuboidal epithelium with minimal nuclear atypia.

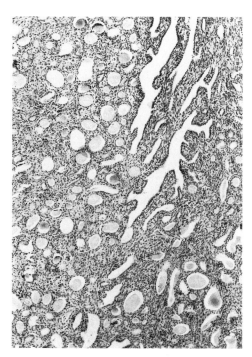

Figure 201
MESONEPHRIC HYPERPLASIA
Segments of mesonephric duct are surrounded by crowded tubules, most of which contain an eosinophilic coagulum in their lumen.

Cytology. Detection of columnar or metaplastic squamous cells from the middle and upper third of the vagina is helpful in the diagnostic evaluation of women suspected of having been exposed to DES in utero. However, similar findings occur in 10 percent of unexposed women probably as result of contamination of the vaginal specimen by columnar or metaplastic squamous cells from the cervix (55).

Clinical Behavior and Treatment. Followup studies indicate that adenosis spontaneously regresses in the majority of patients (27,49). Because of the risk of the development of clear cell carcinoma, these patients should be carefully followed, but treatment of the adenosis is unnecessary.

Atypical Adenosis

Atypical adenosis occurs in tuboendometrial epithelium. The atypical glands tend to be more complex than the glands of typical adenosis and are lined by enlarged cells with atypical nuclei, which are pleomorphic, hyperchromatic, and contain prominent nucleoli (figs. 203, 204). Mitotic

151

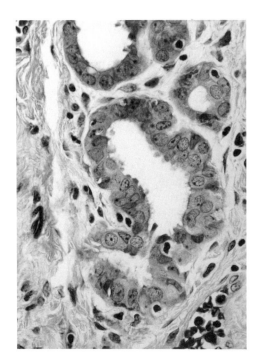

Figure 203
ATYPICAL ADENOSIS
Cells with enlarged nuclei containing prominent nucleoli. (Fig. 2D from Robboy SJ, et al. Atypical vaginal adenosis and cervical ectropion. Association with clear cell adenocarcinoma in diethylstilbestrol-exposed offspring. Cancer 1984; 54:869–75.)

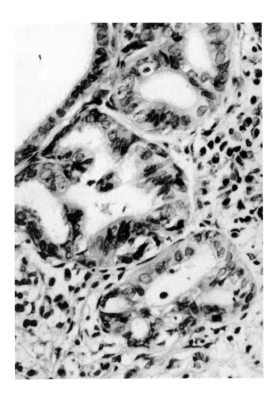

Figure 204
ATYPICAL ADENOSIS
Complex glands with a cribriform arrangement. There is loss of cellular polarity, nuclear enlargement, and atypia. (Fig. 1B from Robboy SJ, et al. Atypical vaginal adenosis and cervical ectropion. Association with clear cell adenocarcinoma in diethylstilbestrol-exposed offspring. Cancer 1984;54:869–75.)

figures are relatively infrequent and hobnail cells may be present. Whereas benign-appearing tuboendometrial adenosis is euploid or polyploid, the cells in atypical adenosis are aneuploid (34).

The frequent finding of atypical adenosis lined by tuboendometrial, in contrast to mucinous, epithelium immediately adjacent to clear cell adenocarcinoma suggests that atypical adenosis may be the precursor of clear cell carcinoma (56,57). Although clear cell carcinoma has been shown to develop in 10 patients with adenosis (58), no case of atypical adenosis has been reported to progress to clear cell carcinoma, and therefore, definitive proof that atypical adenosis is premalignant is lacking.

Müllerian Papilloma

The müllerian papilloma may arise in the vagina and cervix of infants and young girls. It is a benign papillary tumor composed of connective tissue fronds covered by cuboidal or mucinous epithelium. Occasionally, some of the cells

may have a hobnail appearance, suggesting a clear cell carcinoma; however, there are no clear cells and cytologic atypia and mitotic activity are absent (fig. 205). The origin of the tumor is not clear, although reports suggest a müllerian origin (61).

Endometrioid, Endocervical, and Intestinal-Type Adenocarcinomas

Before 1971, when the association between in utero DES exposure and clear cell adenocarcinoma was first made (42), adenocarcinoma of the vagina accounted for only 5 to 10 percent of vaginal carcinomas (33). With the increased number of clear cell adenocarcinomas recognized after 1971, the frequency rose to nearly 25 percent of all vaginal carcinomas in 1988. It is likely that this figure will decline, in view of the discontinuation of DES in pregnancy.

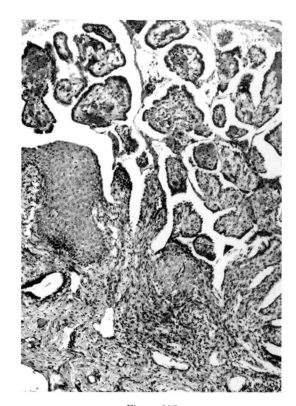

Figure 205
MÜLLERIAN PAPILLOMA
This lesion is composed of arborizing connective tissue fronds covered by flat cuboidal epithelium.

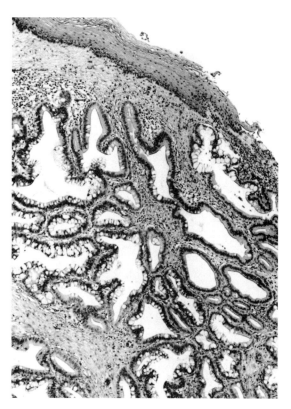

Figure 206
MUCINOUS CARCINOMA,
INTESTINAL TYPE
The tumor is composed of glands lined by columnar cells, many of which are of the goblet type seen in the intestine. (Fig. 1 from Fox H, et al. Enteric tumors of the lower female genital tract: a report of three cases. Histopathology 1988;12:167–76.)

Before the müllerian derivation of clear cell carcinoma was established (42), adenocarcinomas were classified as either adenocarcinoma not otherwise specified or mesonephroma. It is now recognized that the former group was composed of endometrial-type (endometrioid) and mucinous carcinomas and the latter mesonephroma group, of clear cell carcinomas, rare yolk sac tumors, and a few examples of true mesonephric carcinomas. There have been only a few cases of endometrioid carcinoma reported. Almost all have been recorded in the older American and foreign literature specifically to cite their relationship to vaginal adenosis. These tumors have the same histologic appearance as their more common counterparts in endometrium. A few cases of endometrioid carcinoma associated with adenosis have occurred in DES-exposed offspring. In addition, others have risen in vaginal endometriosis (35,48). Mucinous carcinomas may resemble typical endocervical (29) or intestinal (32) adenocarcinomas (figs. 206, 207). The histologic appearance of these tumors in the vagina is similar to that of their counterparts in the cervix. In view of the rarity of endometrioid, endocervical, and intestinal carcinomas, little is known of their etiology and behavior.

Clear Cell Adenocarcinoma

Definition. An adenocarcinoma displaying solid, tubulocystic, or papillary patterns in which most of the cells are clear cells or hobnail cells.

General Features. In 1971 the association of clear cell adenocarcinoma of the vagina and prenatal exposure to DES was reported (43). Since 1987, 535 patients with clear cell adenocarcinoma have been identified, with a history of DES exposure in approximately two thirds of them. DES and other chemically related nonsteroidal estrogens, such as dienestrol or hexestrol, were used in the treatment of threatened and repeated abortions from the mid-1940s through the early 1970s; approximately 2 million women were exposed in utero to these drugs in the United States. A smaller number of patients with documented DES exposure are known to have been born in Canada, western Europe, Australia, Mexico, and Africa.

The risk of development of this form of cancer in the exposed woman up to the age of 24 years is 0.014 to 0.14 percent (37). Thus, although DES is a carcinogen in humans and many other species, the rarity of clear cell carcinoma in the exposed population suggests that it is an incomplete carcinogen and that other factors are necessary to produce neoplastic transformation. Factors that appear to increase the risk of clear cell carcinoma are exposure to DES before the 12th week of pregnancy, maternal history of a prior spontaneous abortion, and conception in the fall (36). Since most of the carcinomas are first detected around the time of puberty or within the decade thereafter, endogenous steroid hormones have been suspected to play a role. There is substantial experimental evidence that DES is a teratogen that leads to congenital anomalies of the upper and lower female genital tract such as vaginal adenosis, cervical ectropion, and a variety of gross structural abnormalities of the cervix. In patients with clear cell carcinoma, adenosis is found immediately adjacent to the tumor in over 90 percent of the cases and is thought to be its likely precursor (39).

Clinical Features. Women with clear cell carcinoma range in age from 6 to 42 years with a peak age of 19 to 20 years; the majority of women are under the age of 30. Vaginal bleeding and discharge are the most common complaints, but a significant number of women are asymptomatic. Abnormal vaginal cytology may lead to detection, but is negative in a substantial number of cases (60).

Approximately 50 percent of clear cell carcinomas involve the vagina, usually in the upper third of the anterior wall. Any part of the vagina, however, may be involved. Vaginal clear cell carcinoma may also involve the cervix.

Gross Findings. Most clear cell carcinomas are polypoid, nodular, or papillary, but some are flat or ulcerated. Small tumors, particularly those

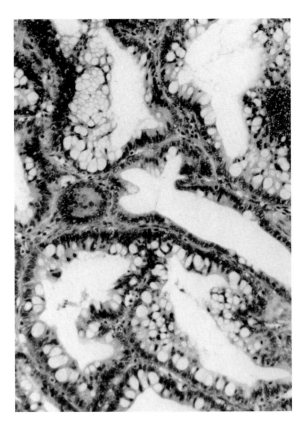

Figure 207
MUCINOUS CARCINOMA,
INTESTINAL TYPE
High magnification of tumor shown in figure 206 showing glands lined by goblet cells. (Fig. 1 from Fox H, et al. Enteric tumors of the lower female genital tract: a report of three cases. Histopathology 1988;12:167–76.)

confined to the lamina propria, may be invisible on gross or even colposcopic examination and are only detected by palpation. Large tumors may be up to 10 cm in greatest dimension.

Microscopic Findings. Clear cell carcinoma of the vagina has an appearance similar to clear cell carcinoma arising in the cervix, endometrium, and ovary. Although the tumor is named on the basis of the clear cell, the predominant cell type is usually the hobnail cell characterized by inconspicuous cytoplasm, and a bulbous nucleus which protrudes into glandular lumens (figs. 208–210). In contrast, the presence of abundant intracytoplasmic glycogen accounts for the clear cytoplasm in the clear cell (figs. 211, 212). The tumor cells may be flat with bland nuclei and scant cytoplasm. Nonglycogenated cells that are neither flat nor hobnail have granular eosinophilic cytoplasm and

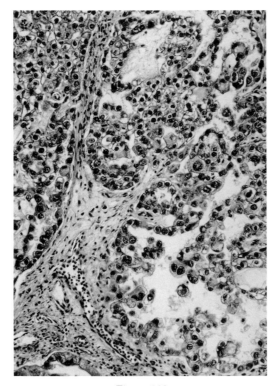

Figure 208
CLEAR CELL CARCINOMA
Neoplastic clear cells are arranged in tubulopapillary configurations.

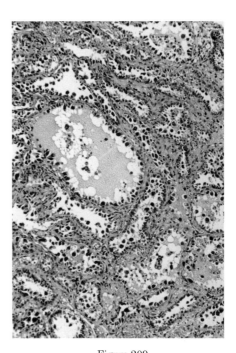

Figure 209
CLEAR CELL CARCINOMA
This clear cell carcinoma shows a tubulocystic pattern in which the tubules and cysts are lined by hobnail cells.

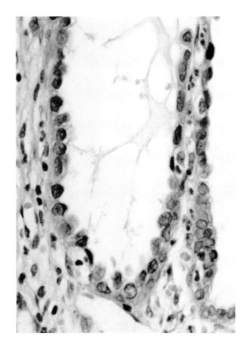

Figure 210
CLEAR CELL CARCINOMA
This figure shows high magnification of hobnail cells (left) and flattened cells (top right). The hobnail cells are characterized by protrusion of the nucleus into the lumen and scant cytoplasm. (Courtesy of Dr. Stanley J. Robboy, Newark, NJ.)

are usually intermingled with the other cell types. The nuclei vary considerably in their appearance. Significant enlargement and atypia may be present in clear and hobnail cells, but flat cells are typically bland (see fig. 210). Mitotic activity is also variable but is usually low.

Clear cell carcinomas may display a variety of patterns described as solid, tubulocystic, and papillary. Of these, the tubulocystic pattern is the most common (see fig. 209). Solid areas tend to be composed of sheets of clear or eosinophilic cells (see fig. 211). The tubulocystic areas are usually lined by any of the four types of cells. Tumors displaying a tubulocystic pattern, in which the predominant cell is the flattened cell, appear bland and may be erroneously interpreted as benign or atypical adenosis (see fig. 210). Unlike this bland pattern of clear cell carcinoma, adenosis is not composed of flattened cells; instead the glands are lined by cuboidal or columnar epithelium. Papillary areas of clear cell carcinoma are usually lined by clear or hobnail cells.

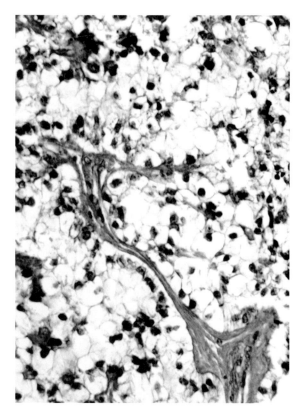

Figure 211
CLEAR CELL CARCINOMA
This example of clear cell carcinoma shows a solid pattern. (Fig. 2 from Scully RE, et al. Vaginal and cervical abnormalities, including clear cell adenocarcinoma, related to prenatal exposure to stilbestrol. Ann Clin Lab Sci 1974;4: 222–53.)

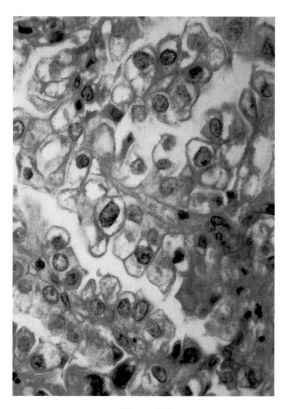

Figure 212
CLEAR CELL CARCINOMA
High magnification of clear cell carcinoma to demonstrate atypical nuclei and abundant vacuolated cytoplasm.

Psammoma bodies and intracellular hyaline bodies may be encountered. Although mucin is present within gland lumens, it is rarely found intracytoplasmically.

Ultrastructural Findings. The presence of abundant glycogen, even in cells in which it is not apparent on light microscopy, is the most prominent feature. The presence of numerous short, blunt microvilli is also characteristic. Golgi apparatuses and numerous mitochondria are less consistently observed (30). Ultrastructurally, the malignant cells, regardless of their variable appearance on light microscopy, are all of the same basic type. Electron microscopy is not helpful diagnostically.

DNA Ploidy Patterns. Four patterns of nuclear DNA distribution have been described: 1) peridiploid stem cell lines (2N to 3N), 2) peritetraploid stem cell lines (3N to 5N), 3) hypertetraploid stem cell lines (5N), and 4) highly aneuploid without detectable stem cell lines (63). The first two patterns are associated with stage I and II tumors, whereas the last two patterns are more often associated with stage III and IV disease. Although these findings suggest that ploidy may have prognostic significance, they are inconclusive because only a few high-ploidy–low-stage tumors were examined. Clinically advanced tumors have a poor prognosis, regardless of ploidy level.

Cytology. In cellular preparations the malignant cells occur singly or in clumps and resemble large endocervical cells. Typically, the nuclei are large with a prominent nucleolus. Occasionally, nuclear atypia is only minimal; bizarre nuclei may be present. The cytoplasm is delicate (60). Although clear cell carcinomas can be detected cytologically, the results have been reported as "positive" or "suspicious" in only 74 percent. Part of the problem may be due to the method of collection. A routine smear from the cervix may not detect a vaginal neoplasm. In addition, the bland cytologic features of some tumors, and the presence of a marked inflammatory infiltrate, contribute to the difficulty of cytologic detection.

Clinical Behavior and Treatment. The tumor spreads by local invasion and lymphatic and hematogenous metastasis. Recurrence appears in 25 percent of the patients. Spread to pelvic lymph nodes occurs in 16 percent of patients with stage I disease (40). The risk of lymph node metastasis increases dramatically with invasion beyond 3 mm in depth. Nonetheless, lymph node metastasis occurs in 5 percent of patients with stage I disease with invasion less than 3 mm (41). Pelvic lymph node metastasis occurs in 50 percent of patients with stage II disease. Factors associated with a favorable prognosis are: 1) an absence of symptoms at the time of detection, 2) age of 19 years or older at diagnosis, 3) small tumor size, 4) minimal invasion, and 5) a tubulocystic pattern.

The 5-year survival of patients with tumors of all stages is approximately 80 percent, and is nearly 90 percent for patients with stage I tumors. Although most recurrences occur within 3 years, disease-free intervals of up to 19 years have been observed. Compared with squamous cell carcinoma of the vagina and cervix, clear cell adenocarcinoma has a greater tendency to spread beyond the abdominal cavity. Of the initial recurrences in clear cell carcinoma, 36 percent are in the lungs or supraclavicular lymph nodes, in contrast to less than 10 percent at these sites for squamous cell carcinoma (53). For early-stage disease radical hysterectomy, vaginectomy, and lymphadenectomy are recommended because there is a higher risk of recurrence with local excision. Radiotherapy is equally effective for early disease, but is generally reserved for advanced-stage tumors (40).

Mesonephric Carcinoma

Only a few cases of carcinoma arising from mesonephric remnants in the vagina have been reported (44,64). These tumors are composed of well-formed tubules lined by atypical, mitotically active, cuboidal to columnar epithelium that bears a resemblance to mesonephric duct remnants. In contrast to clear cell carcinoma,

mesonephric carcinoma does not contain clear cells or hobnail cells. Intracellular mucin and glycogen are not present, and the tubules are often surrounded by a basement membrane that can be appreciated with PAS stains. In more poorly differentiated carcinomas the resemblance to mesonephric duct remnants is less obvious because the predominant architecture is that of crowded solid nests and cords of cells.

OTHER EPITHELIAL TUMORS

Adenosquamous Carcinoma

Adenosquamous carcinomas represent about 2 percent of primary vaginal carcinomas. Six were reported in women with a mean age of 55 years from three series of 244 cases of primary epithelial tumors of the vagina (67–69). In none of these cases was adenosis or endometriosis present. However, the possibility that small foci of adenosis or endometriosis were not sampled or were overgrown by tumor cannot be excluded. Adenosquamous carcinomas in the lower third of the vagina may arise from minor vestibular glands or Bartholin glands. An origin from mesonephric ducts is unlikely, because carcinomas of mesonephric differentiation do not undergo squamous differentiation. A cloacogenic origin has been suggested in view of the similar appearance of some adenosquamous carcinomas to cloacogenic carcinomas of the rectum and anus (67).

Microscopically, adenosquamous carcinomas are composed of both squamous and glandular elements and resemble their counterparts in the cervix. Some are mucoepidermoid carcinomas. Some tumors have been locally aggressive (67), and one metastasized to the lungs and was fatal within 19 months of diagnosis (69).

Adenoid Basal Carcinoma

A primary vaginal carcinoma with features of an adenoid basal cell carcinoma has been reported (66). Similar tumors have been described in the cervix and vulva.

Adenoid Cystic Carcinoma

Adenoid cystic carcinomas similar to those in the cervix may occur as primary vaginal tumors (figs. 213, 214).

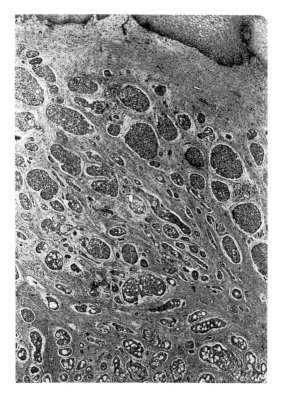

Figure 213
ADENOID CYSTIC CARCINOMA
The tumor is composed of well-circumscribed rounded masses and of cells diffusely infiltrating the lamina propria. (Courtesy of Dr. Robert E. Scully, Boston, MA.)

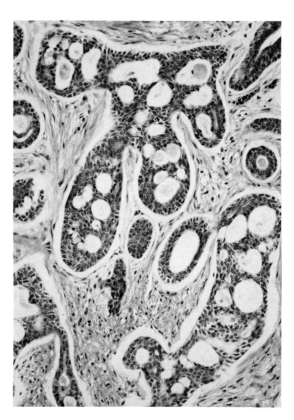

Figure 214
ADENOID CYSTIC CARCINOMA
The tumor is composed of relatively small cells with hyperchromatic nuclei surrounding sharply defined small cystic areas.

Carcinoid Tumor and Small Cell Carcinoma

A single case of a carcinoid tumor of the vagina has been reported (65). The patient did not have the carcinoid syndrome and urinary 5-hydroxyindole acetic acid levels were normal. Microscopically, the tumor had the appearance of a mucinous carcinoid (adenocarcinoid), being composed of mucin-secreting goblet cells and small undifferentiated cells, some of which were positive with argentaffin and argyrophil stains. Widespread metastasis developed, and the patient died 1 year after treatment.

On rare occasions small cell carcinoma may arise as a primary vaginal tumor identical in appearance to small cell carcinoma of the cervix (figs. 215, 216).

Undifferentiated Carcinoma

As in other sites, undifferentiated carcinomas may occur in the vagina.

MESENCHYMAL TUMORS

Leiomyoma

Leiomyomas are the most common mesenchymal tumor of the vagina in adult women (70,95). They occur in women in the reproductive and postmenopausal age groups ranging from 19 to 72 years, with a mean age of 44 years. Tumors detected during early pregnancy may enlarge rapidly. Most leiomyomas are asymptomatic, but depending on their size and position, they may be associated with pain, bleeding, dyspareunia, dystocia, and urinary or rectal symptoms. They may occur at any level of the vagina and tend to be solitary.

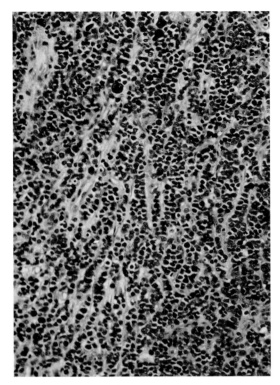

Figure 215
SMALL CELL CARCINOMA
The tumor is characterized by a diffuse infiltration of small round cells with scant cytoplasm and hyperchromatic nuclei.

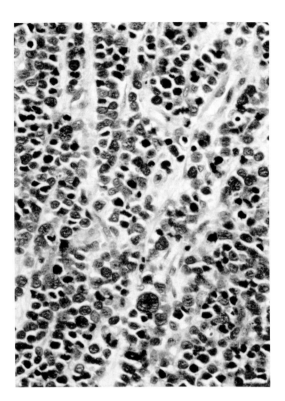

Figure 216
SMALL CELL CARCINOMA
This high magnification of the tumor in figure 215 shows a relatively uniform population of small cells and an occasional cell with a large round nucleus.

Gross Findings. On gross examination the tumor has the same appearance as that of a uterine leiomyoma. Vaginal leiomyomas are well circumscribed and range in size from 0.5 to 15 cm, with a median of 3 cm (93).

Microscopic Findings. Microscopically, vaginal leiomyomas resemble uterine leiomyomas and may display epithelioid and clear cell patterns (93). Mitotic activity is low or absent. Tumors with 5 or more mitotic figures per 10 high-power fields and moderate or marked cellular atypia are classified as *leiomyosarcomas* (see Leiomyosarcoma). In one series of 60 smooth muscle tumors of the vagina (93), 33 had no mitotic activity and 18 had 1 to 4 mitoses per 10 high-power fields; none of these tumors recurred or metastasized. In pregnancy, increased mitotic activity may be observed in some tumors, but in the absence of significant atypia, these tumors should be classified as leiomyomas. Local excision is adequate treatment for vaginal leiomyomas.

Rhabdomyoma

Only 20 cases of vaginal rhabdomyoma have been recorded (76,91) since the initial report by Ceremshak (71). The patients range in age from 34 to 57 years; mean age is 44 years. Rhabdomyomas are solitary and nodular or polypoid, ranging in diameter from 1 to 11 cm. They may arise anywhere in the vagina, and some protrude into the lumen.

Rhabdomyomas are composed of mature, bland rhabdomyoblasts that are oval or racket-shaped with obvious cross striations (figs. 217, 218). Abundant connective tissue stroma surrounds individual muscle cells. Electron microscopy reveals well-organized myofibrils with Z-bands similar to normal striated muscle (79,83).

It is important to distinguish the vaginal rhabdomyoma from sarcoma botryoides (embryonal rhabdomyosarcoma), and from the vaginal polyp. Unlike the rhabdomyoma, sarcoma botryoides of the vagina occurs in young children and not adults. The rhabdomyoma lacks a cambium layer, is composed of primitive mesenchymal cells, and the rhabdomyoblasts are mature with obvious cross striations. There is no nuclear atypia and mitotic figures are absent. Vaginal polyps have a clinical presentation similar to that of rhabdomyomas but are distinguished microscopically by the absence of striated muscle cells. Rhabdomyomas are benign and are treated by local excision.

Other Benign Mesenchymal Tumors

A variety of benign mesenchymal neoplasms of histiocytic, neurogenic, and vascular origin have been reported. These consist largely of single case reports. The tumors have the same histologic appearance and clinical behavior as those in other sites, where they occur more commonly, and are therefore not described in detail. The tumors include granular cell tumor (77,82), neurofibroma (74,78), paraganglioma (89), glomus tumor (92), and hemangioma (80).

Leiomyosarcoma

Smooth muscle tumors with 5 or more mitotic figures per 10 high power fields exhibiting moderate or marked cytologic atypia are classified as *leiomyosarcomas* (93). The behavior of smooth muscle tumors with more than 5 mitotic figures per 10 high power fields but lacking atypia is unknown. Because older reports in the literature have used variable criteria, it is difficult to be certain of the prevalence of these tumors. Peters et al. (88), in reviewing the literature, found that 41 (60 percent) of 68 vaginal sarcomas in adults were leiomyosarcomas. The patients ranged in age from 25 to 86 years. The most common presenting symptom was bleeding.

On gross examination leiomyosarcomas are usually bulky, ranging in size from 3 to 10 cm (73). Microscopically, they are identical to leiomyosarcomas elsewhere.

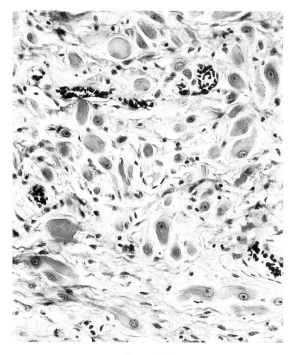

Figure 217
RHABDOMYOMA
The tumor is composed of mature bland rhabdomyoblasts that are predominantly round or oval.

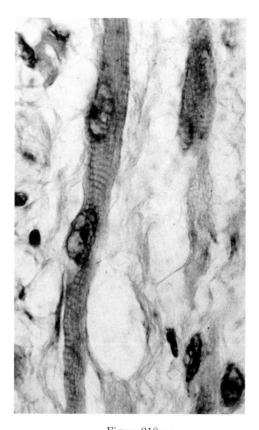

Figure 218
RHABDOMYOMA
Two cells displaying obvious cross striations. (Courtesy of Dr. Thomas Bonfiglio, Rochester, NY.)

Leiomyosarcomas invade locally and also metastasize via the bloodstream to distant sites. In one review, the 5-year survival was 36 percent (88). Partial vaginectomy may suffice for small neoplasms, but because of the difficulty in obtaining adequate margins between the vagina and bladder and rectum, pelvic exenteration may be necessary for large tumors.

Sarcoma Botryoides (Embryonal Rhabdomyosarcoma)

Definition. Embryonal rhabdomyosarcoma arising in organs with a mucosal lining has the appearance of a bunch of grapes, and hence the term *botryoid* has been used. In the vagina the tumor has distinctive pathologic features justifying the term *sarcoma botryoides*.

General Features. Sarcoma botryoides, although rare, is the most common vaginal sarcoma (73). It occurs almost exclusively in children and infants. Nearly 90 percent are encountered in children less than 5 years old; the mean age is 2.5 years (75). Four cases have been reported in women after puberty; the oldest patient was 41 years old (84).

The histogenesis is not known. The tumor develops from mesenchymal cells in the lamina propria that differentiate to some degree into striated muscle.

Clinical Features. Typically, sarcoma botryoides presents as a mass filling the vagina and often protruding from it. Small lesions present as translucent nodules. The overlying mucosa may be intact or ulcerated. Patients may present with bleeding and discharge. Bladder and rectal symptoms are associated with local extension of the tumor. On rare occasions the patient presents with metastasis to the lungs or bone (81). The tumor may arise anywhere in the vagina but most frequently involves the anterior wall.

Gross Findings. The tumor is pedunculated or sessile and is composed of multiple polypoid masses, each of which measures 3 to 4 cm. The entire tumor ranges from 0.2 to 15 cm in greatest dimension. Sectioning reveals a gray, translucent, myxoid tissue with areas of hemorrhage.

Microscopic Findings. The tumor is covered by an attenuated layer of squamous epithelium, beneath which is a compact, highly cellular cambium layer of small, round to spindle-shaped, undifferentiated cells with hyperchromatic nuclei and scant cytoplasm (figs. 219, 220) (86). These cells occasionally invade into the overlying squamous epithelium (fig. 221). Beneath the cambium layer there is a more sparsely cellular region containing a similar population of cells more widely separated by an edematous or myxomatous stroma. In this region, and in the cambium layer, rhabdomyoblasts are recognized as round, racquet-shaped or strap cells with prominent eosinophilic cytoplasm. Cross striations may be difficult to identify but do not need to be identified to make the diagnosis (figs. 222, 223). The neoplastic cells tend to condense around blood vessels. Mitotic activity is generally brisk. Heterologous elements such as bone and cartilage are not present.

Immunohistochemical and Ultrastructural Findings. Immunohistochemistry and electron microscopy may be helpful in identifying striated muscle differentiation that is not evident by conventional light microscopy. Although not specific for striated muscle, commercially available desmin (fig. 224) and muscle-specific actin are far more sensitive in detecting

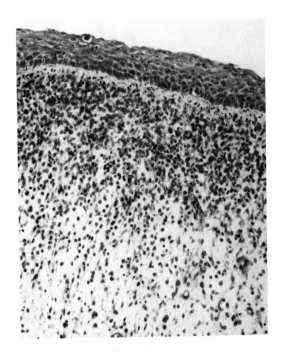

Figure 219
SARCOMA BOTRYOIDES
The tumor shown here has attenuated squamous epithelium and an underlying cambium layer characterized by a band-like distribution of small cells with hyperchromatic nuclei.

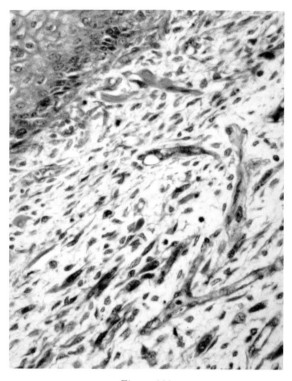

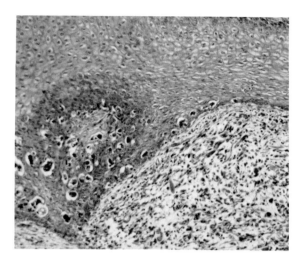

Figure 221
SARCOMA BOTRYOIDES
This figure shows invasion of the overlying squamous epithelium by malignant cells.

Figure 220
SARCOMA BOTRYOIDES
The tumor contains undifferentiated cells with hyperchromatic nuclei and scant cytoplasm in the stroma. A portion of overlying squamous epithelium is visible in the upper left.

muscle (smooth and striated) differentiation than myoglobin which is specific for striated muscle. Muscle-specific actin antibody is not specific for muscle because it may react with myoepithelial cells and myofibroblasts as well. A positive reaction for desmin or muscle-specific actin in a tumor suspected of being a sarcoma botryoides versus a benign vaginal polyp is helpful, but must be interpreted in the context of the light microscopic findings. Electron microscopic examination may reveal myofibrils consisting of thin and thick filaments in the more differentiated cells (85).

Differential Diagnosis. Sarcoma botryoides should be distinguished from benign vaginal polyps, rhabdomyomas, and müllerian papillomas. In contrast to sarcoma botryoides, which is covered by squamous epithelium, and contains hyperchromatic, undifferentiated spindle cells in the stroma, the müllerian papilloma is covered by columnar epithelium and the stroma is bland. The müllerian papilloma also lacks a cambium

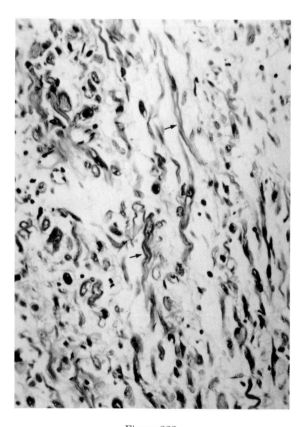

Figure 222
SARCOMA BOTRYOIDES
In this figure strap cells (arrows) are demonstrated.

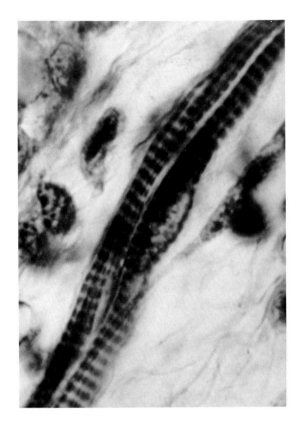

Figure 223
SARCOMA BOTRYOIDES
Shown here is a high magnification of two typical strap cells with cross striations from a sarcoma botryoides. Phosphotungstic acid hematoxylin stain. (Fig. 61 from Fascicle 33, First Series.)

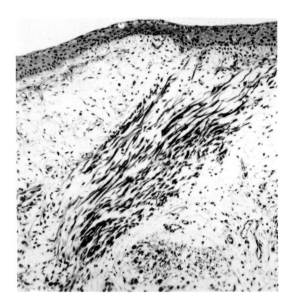

Figure 224
SARCOMA BOTRYOIDES
The tumor has a myxomatous stroma and a group of cells that appear to be strap cells that are positive for desmin in the center of the field. Desmin with hematoxylin counterstain.

layer. The diagnosis of sarcoma botryoides must be considered when dealing with a polypoid lesion of the vagina in a child. Attention should be directed to the small undifferentiated cells under high magnification because they may be incorrectly interpreted as inflammatory cells under low magnification.

Clinical Behavior and Treatment. The tumor grows primarily by local invasion. Depending on its location in the vagina, it invades anteriorly into the bladder or posteriorly into the rectum. Distant metastasis occurs later in the course of the disease and involves inguinal, pelvic, retroperitoneal, and mediastinal lymph nodes, lungs, liver, pericardium, kidneys, and bones.

Sarcoma botryoides is a very aggressive tumor. Pelvic exenteration was advocated in the past because of the high local recurrence rate.

More recently, extended surgery combined with chemotherapy has led to a dramatic improvement in survival. This surgery is less radical and spares the bladder and rectum. In a study in which vincristine, actinomycin D, and cyclophosphamide were used immediately after a biopsy, and followed by a hysterectomy and partial or total vaginectomy, there were only 3 deaths out of a group of 28 patients (81).

Endometrioid Stromal Sarcoma

Both low-grade and high-grade endometrioid stromal sarcomas have been encountered in the vagina (88). In two reports, the tumors appeared to have arisen from endometriosis. Before concluding that such a neoplasm is primary in the vagina, an origin in the uterus should be excluded.

Other Malignant Mesenchymal Tumors

Malignant schwannoma (73), fibrosarcoma (87), malignant fibrous histiocytoma (94), angiosarcoma (90), alveolar soft-part sarcoma (72), alveolar rhabdomyosarcoma, and unclassifiable sarcomas have all been described in the vagina, but they do not exhibit unique clinical or pathologic features in this region.

MIXED EPITHELIAL AND MESENCHYMAL TUMORS

Mixed Tumor

This tumor is composed of epithelial and mesenchymal cells and simulates to some extent a mixed tumor (pleomorphic adenoma) of the salivary gland. The origin may be from müllerian-derived epithelium, but its frequent location in the hymenal region suggests an origin from minor or major vestibular glands. Most reports of this unusual neoplasm have been individual cases (96,97), except for a series of eight cases reported by Sirota et al. (101). The patients range in age from 20 to 53 years, with a mean age of 31 years. The tumors arise on the lateral, posterior, and anterior walls, but have a predilection for the hymenal area. They range in size from 1.5 to 5 cm and are usually located just beneath the mucosal surface presenting as an asymptomatic mass.

On gross examination mixed tumors are discrete, gray, and soft. Microscopically, a mixture of epithelial and mesenchymal tissues is observed. The bulk of the tumor is composed of nondescript spindle cells, probably representing fibroblasts, although some investigators have suggested they are myoepithelial cells (101). These cells are arranged in bundles but characteristically display a whorled pattern. The cells display little if any cytologic atypia, and mitotic figures are uncommon (fig. 225). Nests of glycogenated stratified squamous epithelium, which may demonstrate pearl formation, may be dispersed throughout the stroma. Scattered glands lined by mucinous epithelium may also be present. The glandular epithelium merges with the squamous epithelium. This combination of tissue elements somewhat resembles that in a Brenner tumor of the ovary. The neoplasm of the vagina reported by Chen (98) might be a form of mixed tumor. All the typical mixed tumors of the vagina have behaved in a benign fashion after local excision.

Mixed Tumor Resembling Synovial Sarcoma

Neoplasms occur that display a biphasic pattern arising in the lateral fornix of the vagina (99,100). Regarded as mixed tumors resembling

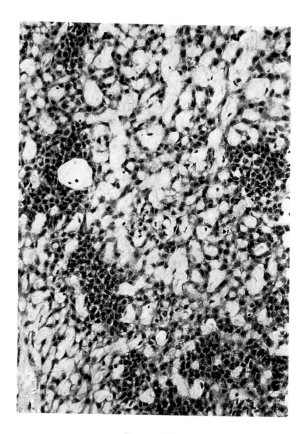

Figure 225
MIXED TUMOR
The tumor is composed of round to spindle-shaped cells with minimal cytologic atypia.

synovial sarcoma, the tumors are composed predominantly of gland-like structures. The glands are lined by flattened epithelial cells that abut spindle-shaped cells, suggesting sarcomatous differentiation (figs. 226, 227). The biphasic differentiation suggests a synovial sarcoma, but the neoplasm does not resemble the typical synovial sarcoma arising in soft tissue. In one study electron microscopic examination demonstrated slender, long microvilli protruding into the acinar lumens, reminiscent of synovial cells (99). In another study, although the light and ultrastructural findings were suggestive of synovial sarcoma, electron microscopy did not reveal telolysomes which are seen in synovial sarcoma (100). Moreover, because the tumor was closely associated with mesonephric remnants and was located in the lateral fornix, the authors concluded that it probably arose from mesonephric nests.

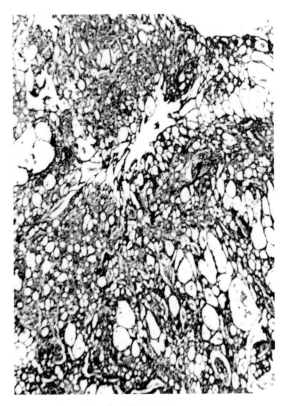

Figure 226
MIXED TUMOR RESEMBLING
SYNOVIAL SARCOMA
The tumor is composed of rounded epithelial-like cells and flattened spindle-shaped cells in an acinar pattern. The tumor does not resemble the typical synovial sarcoma of soft tissue. (Courtesy of Dr. Takashi Okagaki, Minneapolis, MN.)

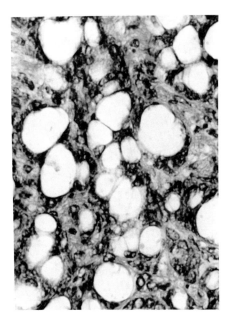

Figure 227
MIXED TUMOR RESEMBLING
SYNOVIAL SARCOMA
High magnification of mixed tumor resembling synovial sarcoma with epithelial-like cells lining acini. (Fig. 4.41 from Sedlis A, Robboy R. Diseases of the vagina. In: Kurman RJ, ed. Blaustein's pathology of the female genital tract. New York: Springer-Verlag, 1987:97–140.)

Adenosarcoma

The vagina may be the site of recurrence of a uterine adenosarcoma or the site of a primary adenosarcoma. It has gross features similar to those of sarcoma botryoides, but microscopically is similar to adenosarcomas arising in the uterine corpus. The leaf-like pattern, characterized by clefts lined by bland epithelium overlying a hypercellular spindle-cell stroma, is typical (figs. 228, 229).

Malignant Mixed Mesodermal Tumor

There have been seven reports of primary malignant mixed mesodermal tumors of the vagina (88). In four there was a history of prior radiation. The histologic appearance is similar to that of mixed mesodermal tumors of the uterine corpus.

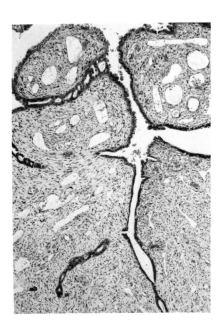

Figure 228
ADENOSARCOMA
The tumor is characterized by a leaf-like pattern. Clefts are lined by bland epithelium overlying a hypercellular stroma.

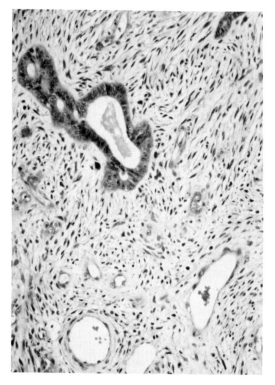

Figure 229
ADENOSARCOMA
Bland epithelium and hypercellular stroma with only minimal cytologic atypia characterize this tumor.

MISCELLANEOUS TUMORS

Melanocytic Nevus

Nevi identical to those on the skin may occur in the vagina.

Blue Nevus

This lesion occurs rarely in the vagina (115). In the female genital tract it occurs more frequently in the cervix and vulva. It has a histologic appearance similar to that of its counterpart in the skin.

Malignant Melanoma

General Features. Primary melanoma of the vagina accounts for less than 0.3 percent of all melanomas and less than 3 percent of malignant tumors of the vagina (110). Approximately 115 cases have been reported (114). The tumor is thought to arise from melanocytes, which are present in the vaginal epithelium in 3 percent of normal women (112). These tumors occur predominantly in white postmenopausal women with a mean age of 62 years. The most common symptom is vaginal bleeding. Melanoma may occur anywhere in the vagina, but most often involves the lower third (fig. 230) (114).

Gross Findings. Typically, melanomas project above the surface and are blue or black and soft. They are usually ulcerated (113). They range in size from 0.5 cm in diameter to a large tumor involving the entire vaginal wall (104).

Microscopic Findings. Microscopically, vaginal melanomas do not have a distinctive pattern. The tumor cells are usually pigmented, but may be amelanotic. The tumor can be composed predominantly of small or spindle-shaped cells (figs. 231, 232). Cellular pleomorphism may be marked and mitotic activity is often high. Junctional activity can almost always be demonstrated (fig. 233) and frequently there is lateral junctional spread of tumor cells. Junctional activity identifies the vagina as the primary site of the tumor. Melanocytes in the vagina near melanoma are often angulated and atypical, reminiscent of those in lentiginous melanoma of the skin (104). Their presence is useful in distinguishing melanoma from a benign nevus.

Because the vagina does not have a papillary and reticular dermis, Chung et al (104) modified Clark levels and Breslow thickness measurements. Among 31 patients in whom the level of invasion could be determined, only 4 had tumors that invaded less than 2 mm (114). The deep invasion of these tumors at the time of diagnosis probably accounts for their poor prognosis. Accordingly, the depth of invasion in millimeters should be indicated in order to provide an estimate of prognosis.

Differential Diagnosis. As in other sites, it is important to maintain a high index of suspicion for melanoma when faced with a poorly differentiated neoplasm that is difficult to classify. Because of their rarity in the vagina, and the frequent associated ulceration with loss of areas of junctional activity, melanomas may be confused with lymphomas or squamous cell carcinoma. Immunoperoxidase reactions for S-100, melanoma-specific antigen (HMB-45), keratin, and leukocyte common antigen are very useful in the differential diagnosis with melanomas positive for the first two and negative for the second two.

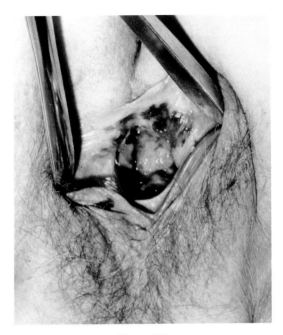

Figure 230
PRIMARY MALIGNANT MELANOMA
OF THE VAGINA
The tumor involves the distal third of the vagina. (Fig. 1
from Norris HJ, Taylor HB. Melanomas of the vagina. Am
J Clin Path 1966;46:420–6.)

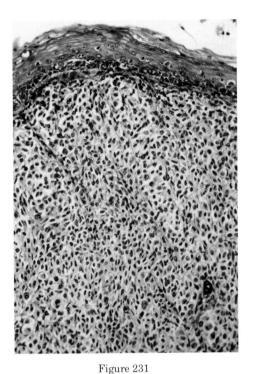

Figure 231
MALIGNANT MELANOMA
This is the small cell variant that is a relatively common
pattern in the vagina.

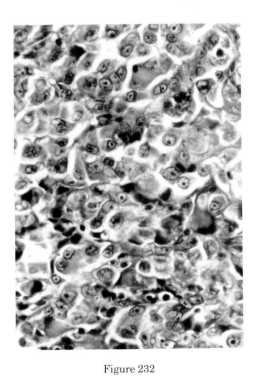

Figure 232
MALIGNANT MELANOMA
This tumor is composed of epithelioid-type cells with
rounded nuclei and prominent nucleoli.

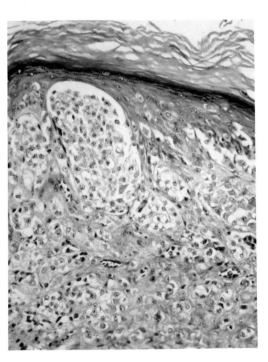

Figure 233
MALIGNANT MELANOMA
Prominent junctional activity is evident in this figure.

Clinical Behavior and Treatment. The prognosis is much worse than for cutaneous melanomas, with the 5-year crude survival rate ranging from 5 to 20 percent. Like cutaneous melanomas, vaginal melanomas may recur long after 5 years. The prognosis appears to be influenced by tumor size, with lesions greater than 3 cm having a significantly worse prognosis (114). Although patients with tumors that invade 1 mm or less appear to have a better survival, the numbers of cases are too few to draw firm conclusions. Age, mitotic count, stage, and location of lesion do not influence survival. No difference in survival has been demonstrated whether radical surgery or wide local excision followed by radiotherapy is chosen.

Yolk Sac Tumor

Yolk sac tumors (endodermal sinus tumors) resembling those found in the ovary and testis may arise in the vagina. Of those originating in the lower genital tract, the vast majority arise in the vagina, with an occasional example arising in the cervix or vulva. At least 56 yolk sac tumors of the vagina have been reported (105). They may arise from displaced germ cells arrested during embryonic migration from the yolk sac to the gonadal ridge. Aberrant differentiation from somatic cells is an alternative mode of origin (116).

Vaginal yolk sac tumors have been reported exclusively in children 3 years of age or younger. The patients present with bleeding or discharge and have polypoid or sessile tumors 1 to 5 cm in greatest dimension. Gross examination discloses a gray-white, soft, friable tumor that may be focally hemorrhagic. Microscopically, the tumor displays the various patterns encountered in the more common ovarian yolk sac tumor, the most frequent being the microcystic or reticular pattern (fig. 234).

Schiller-Duval bodies (figs. 235, 236) and hyaline droplets are characteristic. As in the ovary, immunohistochemical reactions for alpha-1-fetoprotein, alpha-1-antitrypsin, and albumin are typically positive (116).

In the past, the outlook was grave, with the majority of patients succumbing despite radical surgery. Since 1970, the use of multiagent chemotherapy, usually consisting of vincristine, actinomycin D, and cyclophosphamide (VAC) combined with surgery, has resulted in an excellent cure rate (106). A novel approach utilizing primary

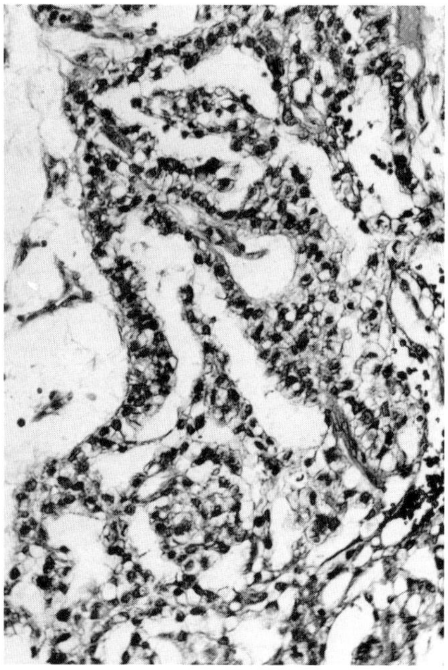

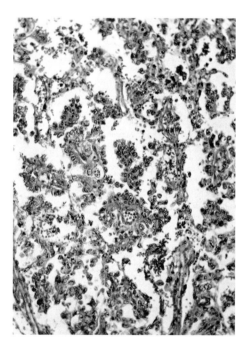

Figure 234
YOLK SAC TUMOR
The tumor is composed of cells with primitive nuclei forming microcystic spaces.

Figure 235
YOLK SAC TUMOR
This tumor demonstrates a festooned pattern with Schiller-Duval bodies.

chemotherapy (VAC) followed by local excision without pelvic irradiation has resulted in long-term cure. By preserving reproductive and sexual function, the latter approach appears to be the treatment of choice (102).

Mature Cystic Teratoma

Five teratomas of the vagina and an unusual ectopia composed exclusively of thyroid and parathyroid tissue have been reported (109). The five teratomas were all mature and cystic, lined by squamous epithelium and containing hair and sebaceous material. Neural tissue and teeth have been reported in three cases (109). Primary immature (malignant) teratomas, embryonal carcinomas, and dysgerminomas have not been reported in the vagina.

Adenomatoid Tumor

A primary vaginal adenomatoid tumor has been reported (111). The microscopic appearance was that of a typical adenomatoid tumor.

Villous Adenoma

A case of a villous adenoma of the vagina of a 59-year-old woman has been reported (108), and we have seen additional examples. The tumors present as polypoid lesions (fig. 237). Sigmoidoscopy and barium enema are negative. Microscopically, the lesions are identical to villous adenomas of the large intestine (figs. 238, 239). Because the vagina is, at least in part, of urogenital sinus origin, it is likely that these tumors arise from cells with endodermal potential for differentiation.

Malignant Lymphoma and Other Lymphohistiocytic Lesions

Malignant lymphoma may involve the vagina as part of a systemic disease or is sometimes localized to it (103). In the lower genital tract, lymphoma more often involves the cervix, which is discussed in greater detail in the chapter Tumors of the Cervix.

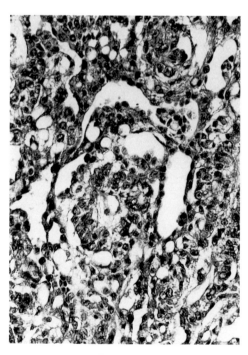

Figure 236
YOLK SAC TUMOR

The microcystic pattern with a Schiller-Duval body in the center of the field is characterized by a central vessel surrounded by a mantle of primitive cells protruding into a space. (Fig. 5 from Norris HJ, et al. Carcinoma of the infant vagina. A distinctive tumor. Arch Pathol 1970;90:473–9.)

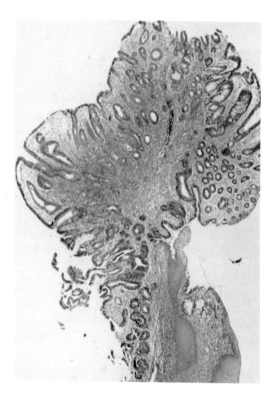

Figure 237
VILLOUS ADENOMA

Villous adenoma presenting as a polypoid mass in the vagina. (Courtesy of Dr. Robert E. Scully, Boston, MA.)

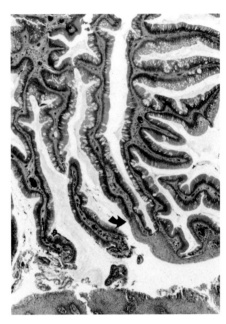

Figure 238
VILLOUS ADENOMA

The tumor has delicate papillary fronds lined by columnar epithelial cells and goblet cells similar to villous adenomas of the large intestine. Transition from squamous epithelium to columnar epithelium is shown (arrow).

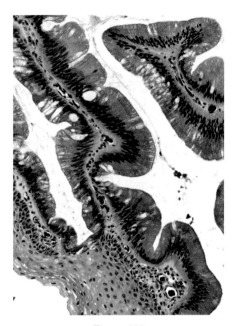

Figure 239
VILLOUS ADENOMA

High magnification of the lesion shown in figure 238. The columnar epithelium resembles that of a villous adenoma of the large intestine.

Plasmacytomas may be primary in the vagina (107). Of the five reported cases in this location, one recurred locally, and in another case local recurrence and multiple bone metastases occurred. Finally, eosinophilic granuloma has also been described in the vagina (117). This lesion may be associated with some or all of the other features in the syndrome, i.e., diabetes insipidus, pituitary hypofunction, and abnormal chest and skeletal films.

SECONDARY TUMORS

Neoplasms of the vagina are much more often metastatic than primary. Spread to the vagina is either by direct extension, vascular or lymphatic embolization, or infrequently, direct implantation. In a review of 355 carcinomas involving the vagina, Fu and Reagan (118) reported that 84 percent were secondary and 16 percent primary. Among secondary squamous carcinomas, the most common primary site was the cervix (79 percent) followed by the vulva (17 percent). Among adenocarcinomas, 92 percent were secondary. The most frequent primary site was the endometrium (32 percent) (fig. 240),

followed by the rectum and colon (26 percent), and ovary (17 percent). Other less commonly encountered neoplasms metastatic to the vagina include transitional cell carcinoma from the urinary bladder and urethra, renal cell carcinoma, uterine mixed mesodermal tumors, malignant melanoma, breast carcinoma (fig. 241), choriocarcinoma, carcinoma of the Bartholin gland, and cloacogenic carcinoma of the anus.

TUMOR-LIKE LESIONS

Vaginal Polyp
(Mesodermal Stromal Polyp)

This lesion is a fibroepithelial polyp that has also been referred to as *pseudosarcoma botryoides* (122). Patients range in age from newborn to 71 years, with the vast majority over the age of 20 years. The median age in the largest series was 35 years (124). Nearly one third of the patients are pregnant at the time of diagnosis. Although occasionally presenting with abnormal bleeding, most of the polyps are incidental findings. The majority are single and occur on the lateral wall in the lower third of the vagina.

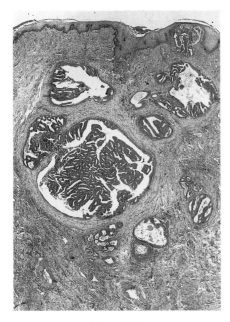

Figure 240
METASTATIC ENDOMETRIAL
ADENOCARCINOMA
The tumor is present beneath an intact vaginal epithelium. (Fig. 55 from Fascicle 33, First Series.)

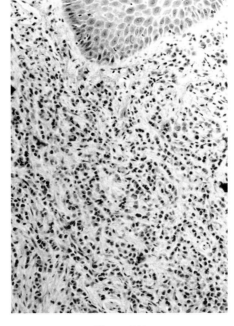

Figure 241
METASTATIC BREAST CARCINOMA
The tumor demonstrates the characteristic Indian-file pattern.

Vaginal polyps range in size from 0.5 to 4 cm, with a median diameter of 1.7 cm. They are usually polypoid or pedunculated and, on section, gray-white, soft, and rubbery. Microscopically, they are well circumscribed and composed of edematous fibrous tissue covered by benign squamous epithelium (fig. 242).

The loose fibrous tissue stroma contains numerous dilated blood vessels. Scattered enlarged fibroblasts with plump hyperchromatic or vesicular nuclei and delicate cytoplasmic processes are seen in a background of relatively acellular stroma. In approximately half the cases, the fibroblasts are atypical with large, pleomorphic, and often hyperchromatic multiple nuclei (fig. 243). Neither a cambium layer nor heterologous elements are present and mitotic activity is low. Although edema may be present focally, it is not a striking feature.

The pathogenesis of vaginal polyps is not clear. Because approximately a third of the patients are pregnant at the time of diagnosis, it is possible that these lesions are hormone induced. They may represent focal hyperplasia of subepithelial stromal cells that form a myxoid stromal matrix extending from the endocervix to the vulva in mature women (123). Atypical stromal cells may also be seen in nasal polyps (120), giant cell cystitis, radiation cystitis, and nodular fasciitis (124). It is likely, therefore, that these cells are reactive in nature.

The importance of recognizing vaginal polyps lies in distinguishing them from sarcoma botryoides. A number of clinical and pathologic features facilitate the differential diagnosis. Vaginal polyps almost always occur in adults, whereas vaginal sarcoma botryoides rarely occurs beyond the age of 8 years. The rare botryoid-type sarcomas occurring in teenagers or adults arise higher in the genital tract, most commonly the cervix. Unlike sarcoma botryoides, which grows rapidly, polyps pursue an indolent course (125). Microscopically, in contrast to sarcoma botryoides, vaginal polyps lack a cambium layer, small undifferentiated stromal cells, invasion of the overlying squamous epithelial cells, and rhabdomyoblasts. Immunoperoxidase reactions for desmin, muscle-specific actin, and myoglobin are negative in vaginal polyps.

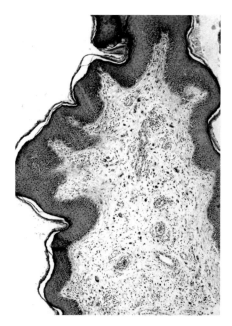

Figure 242
VAGINAL POLYP
The lesion is composed of edematous fibrous tissue and covered by benign squamous epithelium. Numerous blood vessels are present in the loose fibrous tissue stroma.

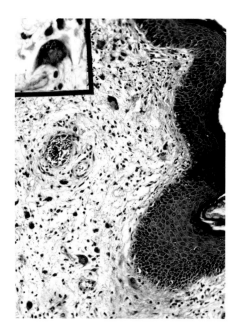

Figure 243
VAGINAL POLYP
Higher magnification shows enlarged fibroblasts and plump hyperchromatic enlarged nuclei in a relatively acellular stroma. Inset shows high magnification of an atypical stromal cell with delicate cytoplasmic processes.

Treatment consists of local excision. Local recurrence may occur if the lesion is incompletely removed. There has been no evidence of malignant behavior.

Postoperative Spindle Cell Nodule

This benign spindle cell lesion develops just beneath the surface squamous epithelium and is characteristically discovered shortly after a surgical procedure such as hysterectomy (126). The lesion is composed of actively proliferating plump spindle cells arranged in intersecting fascicles that infiltrate the adjacent tissue in irregular tongues (fig. 244). A storiform pattern is not evident. The cells contain abundant eosinophilic or amphophilic cytoplasm. The nuclei are oval and relatively uniform, with delicate chromatin and one or two distinct nucleoli (fig. 245). Mitotic figures can range from 1 to 25 per 10 high-power fields. A delicate network of blood vessels is present within the lesion, and there is typically ulceration of the overlying epithelium accompanied by an acute inflammatory infiltrate. The proliferating cells are mostly fibroblasts and myofibroblasts, or smooth muscle cells in a vascular ma-

trix. Similar to granulation tissue, these lesions only rarely recur despite incomplete excision.

Postoperative spindle cell nodules are most often confused with leiomyosarcoma, but in contrast are smaller in overall dimension. Their nuclei are relatively uniform in size, with delicate chromatin and one or two prominent nucleoli. Most important, they follow a recent surgical procedure. Other reactive sarcoma-like processes that have been described in the vagina are postoperative fibrohistiocytic proliferation (reparative granuloma) (128) and nodular fasciitis (119). The former lesion has a storiform pattern and contains foamy histiocytes and foreign-body giant cells. It may be related to the spindle cell nodule, differing in its appearance because of a longer time interval between the operation and the diagnosis. In contrast to the spindle cell nodule, nodular fasciitis is composed of more densely collagenized, less vascular tissue. Also, nodular fasciitis is associated with local nonsurgical trauma, in contrast to the spindle cell nodule, which typically develops after a surgical procedure. Finally, nodular fasciitis usually arises in subcutaneous tissue of an extremity and rarely in mucosal locations.

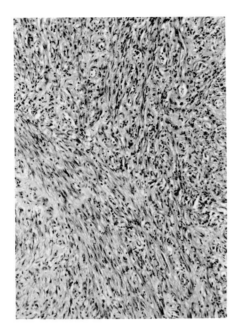

Figure 244
POSTOPERATIVE SPINDLE CELL NODULE
The lesion is composed of spindle-shaped cells arranged in intersecting fascicles. (Courtesy of Dr. Robert E. Scully, Boston, MA.)

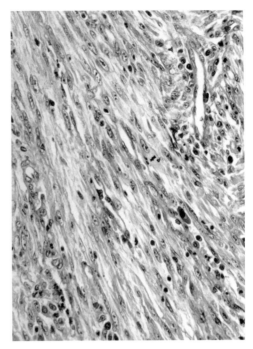

Figure 245
POSTOPERATIVE SPINDLE CELL NODULE
The nodule is composed of proliferating plump spindle cells with abundant eosinophilic or amphophilic cytoplasm. The nuclei are oval with delicate uniform chromatin and distinct nucleoli. (Courtesy of Dr. Robert E. Scully, Boston, MA.)

Vault Granulation Tissue

Granulation tissue, typically showing an acute and chronic inflammatory infiltrate, often develops at the vaginal cuff after hysterectomy. Plump fibroblasts and numerous capillaries are characteristic.

Prolapsed Fallopian Tube

After hysterectomy, typically vaginal hysterectomy, a portion of the fallopian tube may prolapse through the vaginal cuff. Clinically, prolapsed fallopian tube is exquisitely tender on palpation and may be associated with dyspareunia. On gross examination, the prolapsed tube may appear as a red granular polypoid mass. Microscopically, it is usually not difficult to recognize the architecture of the fallopian tube, although it usually is partially obscured by granulation tissue and inflammation (fig. 246) (127). Prolapsed tube should not be confused with adenosis, endometriosis, or papillary adenocarcinomas. The location of the lesion, history of prior hysterectomy, architecture, and recognition of tubal epithelial cell types facilitate the diagnosis.

Endometriosis

The combination of endometrial glands and stroma is diagnostic. Sometimes hemorrhage, macrophages filled with hemofuscin, hemosiderin, or both, and granulation tissue obscure the picture. In particular, because endometrial-type stroma may be scant in endometriotic lesions in this location, confusion with adenocarcinoma or adenosis may occur. The absence of significant cytologic atypia and mitotic activity permits distinction from a malignant process; the glands are generally deeper than those of adenosis.

Decidua

Decidua may be confused with a nonkeratinizing squamous cell carcinoma. Patients are either pregnant or on high-dose progestational drugs. Immunoperoxidase reactions for keratin aid in the differential diagnosis. Decidua is negative for cytokeratin, whereas squamous cell carcinoma is diffusely positive.

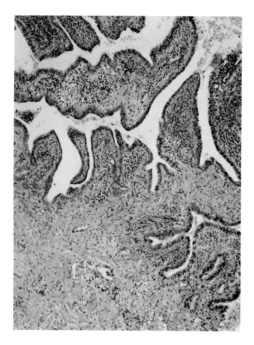

Figure 246
PROLAPSED FALLOPIAN TUBE
Prolapsed fallopian tube retains its normal architecture.
(Fig. 4.16 from Sedlis A, Robboy SJ. Diseases of the vagina.
In: Kurman RJ, ed. Blaustein's pathology of the female genital
tract, 3rd ed. New York: Springer-Verlag 1987:97–140.)

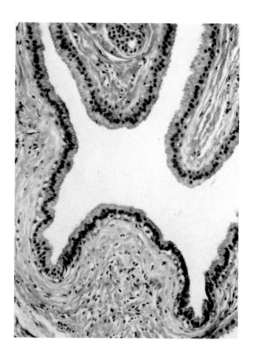

Figure 247
MUCINOUS CYST
This cyst is lined by columnar endocervical-type epithelium.

Cysts

Vaginal cysts are not common and usually do not present a problem in the differentiation from tumors. Cysts are classified according to their epithelial lining (121). Most of them are *squamous epithelial inclusion cysts* resulting from surgical trauma with implantation of squamous epithelium beneath the surface. This type of cyst is usually single and located in the posterior or lateral wall of the vagina at the site of a previous episiotomy.

Müllerian-derived cysts are lined by columnar, mucin-secreting, endocervical-type epithelium (fig. 247). Ciliated tubal-type epithelium and squamous metaplasia may also be encountered. These cysts should be distinguished from adenosis, which may also be focally cystic. In contrast to adenosis, a müllerian cyst is a single large structure that is typically visible on gross examination and may be associated with pain and dyspareunia. Vaginal adenosis does not present clinically as a single large cyst but as

multiple small cysts and on microscopic examination with numerous microscopic glands in the lamina propria.

Mesonephric cysts, also termed *Gartner duct cysts*, are rare. They tend to be smaller than müllerian cysts, usually not exceeding 2 cm, and are located in the lateral vaginal wall. Microscopically, they are lined by nonmucin-secreting cuboidal or low columnar epithelium. Cilia are absent and foci of squamous metaplasia are very unusual. Less commonly, *mesonephric remnants* in the form of a mesonephric duct and tubules are encountered. These structures may be confused with adenosis (see figs. 200–202).

Urothelial cysts are usually less than 1 cm, and are typically found in the distal vagina in a suburethral location. Microscopically, they are lined by transitional epithelium, but stratified cuboidal or columnar epithelium may be admixed; cilia are not present.

Lymphoma-Like Lesion

These lesions are similar to their counterparts in the cervix.

REFERENCES

Squamous Lesions

1. Anderson ES. Primary carcinoma of the vagina: a study of 29 cases. Gynecol Oncol 1989;33:317–20.
2. Benedet JL, Sanders BH. Carcinoma in situ of the vagina. Am J Obstet Gynecol 1984;148:695–700.
3. Crowther ME, Lowe DG, Shepherd JH. Verrucous carcinoma of the female genital tract: a review. Obstet Gynecol Surv 1988;43:263–80.
4. Fu YS, Reagan JW. Pathology of the uterine cervix, vagina, and vulva. Philadelphia: WB Saunders, 1989:213.
5. Henson D, Tarone R. An epidemiologic study of cancer of the cervix, vagina, and vulva based on the Third National Cancer Survey in the United States. Am J Obstet Gynecol 1977;129:525–32.
6. Herbst AL, Green TH Jr, Ulfelder H. Primary carcinoma of the vagina. An analysis of 68 cases. Am J Obstet Gynecol 1970;106:210–8.
7. Hummer WK, Mussey E, Decker DG, Dockerty MB. Carcinoma in situ of the vagina. Am J Obstet Gynecol 1970;108:1109–16.
8. Kanbour AI, Klionsky B, Murphy AI. Carcinoma of the vagina following cervical cancer. Cancer 1974;34:1838–41.
9. Lenehan PM, Meffe F, Lickrish GM. Vaginal intraepithelial neoplasia: biologic aspects and management. Obstet Gynecol 1986;68:333–7.
10. Manetta A, Pinto JL, Larson JE, Stevens CW Jr, Pinto JS, Podczaski ES. Primary invasive carcinoma of the vagina. Obstet Gynecol 1988;72:77–1.
11. Marcus SL. Multiple squamous cell carcinoma involving the cervix, vagina, and vulva. The theory of multicentric origin. Am J Obstet Gynecol 1961;80:802–12.
12. Murad TM, Durant JR, Maddox WA, Dowling EA. The pathologic behavior of primary vaginal carcinoma and its relationship to cervical cancer. Cancer 1975;35:787–94.
13. Nuovo GJ, Blanco JS, Silverstein SJ, Crum CP. Histologic correlates of papillomavirus infection of the vagina. Obstet Gynecol 1988;72:770–4.
14. Patten SF, Reagan JW, Obenauf M, et al. Postirradiation dysplasia of the uterine cervix and vagina. An analytical study of the cells. Cancer 1963;16:173–82.
15. Perez CA, Camel HM. Long-term follow-up in radiation therapy of carcinoma of the vagina. Cancer 1982; 49:1308–15.
16. Peters WA III, Kumar NB, Morley GW. Carcinoma of the vagina. Factors influencing treatment outcome. Cancer 1985;55:892–7.
17. _____, Kumar NB, Morley GW. Microinvasive carcinoma of the vagina: a distinct clinical entity? Am J Obstet Gynecol 1985;153:505–7.
18. Potkul RK, Lancaster WD, Kurman RJ, Lewandowski G, Weck PK, Delgado G. Vulvar condylomas and squamous vestibular micropapilloma. Differences in appearance and response to treatment. J Reprod Med 1990; 35:1019–22.
19. Pride GL, Buchler DA. Carcinoma of the vagina 10 or more years following pelvic irradiation therapy. Am J Obstet Gynecol 1977;127:513–7.
20. _____, Schultz AE, Chuprevich TW, Buchler DA. Primary invasive squamous carcinoma of the vagina. Obstet Gynecol 1979;53:218–25.
21. Rastkar G, Okagaki T, Twiggs LB, Clark BA. Early invasive and in situ warty carcinoma of the vulva: clinical, histologic, and electron microscopic study with particular reference to viral association. Am J Obstet Gynecol 1982;143:814–20.
22. Robboy SJ, Noller KL, O'Brien P, et al. Increased incidence of cervical and vaginal dysplasia in 3,980 diethylstilbestrol-exposed young women. Experience of the National Collaborative Diethylstilbestrol Adenosis Project. JAMA 1984;252:2979–83.
23. Rutledge F. Cancer of the vagina. Am J Obstet Gynecol 1967;97:635–55.
24. Stuart GC, Flagler EA, Nation JG, Duggan M, Robertson DI. Laser vaporization of vaginal intraepithelial neoplasia. Am J Obstet Gynecol 1988;158:240–3.
25. Wentz WB, Reagan JW. Clinical significance of postirradiation dysplasia of the uterine cervix. Am J Obstet Gynecol 1970;106:812–7.
26. Woodruff JD, Parmley TH, Julian CG. Topical 5-fluorouracil in the treatment of vaginal carcinoma in-situ. Gynecol Oncol 1975;3:124–320.

Glandular Lesions

27. Antonioli DA, Burke L, Friedman EA. Natural history of diethylstilbestrol-associated genital tract lesions. Cervical ectopy and cervicovaginal hood. Am J Obstet Gynecol 1980;137:847–53.
28. Bonney V, Glendining B. Adenomatosis vaginae: a hitherto undescribed condition. Proc Soc Med 1911;4:18–25.
29. Clement PB, Benedet JL. Adenocarcinoma in situ of the vagina: a case report. Cancer 1979;43:2479–85.
30. Dickersin GR, Welch WR, Erlandson R, Robboy SJ. Ultrastructure of 16 cases of clear cell adenocarcinoma of the vagina and cervix in young women. Cancer 1980;45:1615–24.
31. Forsberg JG. Late effects in the vaginal and cervical epithelia after injections of diethylstilbestrol into neonatal mice. Am J Obstet Gynecol 1975;121:101–4.
32. Fox H, Wells M, Harris M, McWilliam LJ, Anderson GS. Enteric tumors of the lower female genital tract: a report of three cases. Histopathol 1988;12:167–76.
33. Frick HC II, Jacox HW, Taylor HC. Primary carcinoma of the vagina. Am J Obstet Gynecol 1968;101:695–703.
34. Fu YS, Reagan JW, Richart RM, Townsend DE. Nuclear DNA and histologic studies of genital lesions in diethylstilbestrol-exposed progeny. II. Intraepithelial glandular abnormalities. Am J Clin Pathol 1979;72:515–20.

35. Haskel S, Chen SS, Spiegel G. Vaginal endometrioid adeno-carcinoma arising in vaginal endometriosis: a case report and literature review. Gynecol Oncol 1989;34:232–6.

36. Herbst AL, Anderson, Hubby MM, Haenszel WM, Kaufman RH, Noller KL. Risk factors for the development of diethyl-stilbestrol-associated clear cell adenocarcinoma: a case-control study. Am J Obstet Gynecol 1986; 154:814–22.

37. _____, Cole P, Colton T, Robboy SJ, Scully RE. Age-incidence and risk of diethylstilbestrol-related clear cell adenocarcinoma of the vagina and cervix. Am J Obstet Gynecol 1977;128:43–8.

38. _____, Kurman RJ, Scully RE. Vaginal and cervical abnormalities after exposure to stilbestrol in utero. Obstet Gynecol 1972;40:287–98.

39. _____, Kurman RJ, Scully RE, Poskanzer DC. Clear-cell adenocarcinoma of the genital tract in young fe-males. Registry report. N Eng J Med 1972;287:1259–64.

40. _____, Norusis MJ, Rosenow PJ, Welch WR, Scully RE. An analysis of 346 cases of clear cell adenocarcinoma of the vagina and cervix with emphasis on recurrence and survival. Gynecol Oncol 1979;7:111–22.

41. _____, Robboy SJ, Scully RE, Poskanzer DC. Clear cell adenocarcinoma of the vagina and cervix in girls: analysis of 170 registry cases. Am J Obstet Gynecol 1974;119:713–24.

42. _____, Scully RE. Adenocarcinoma of the vagina in adolescence. A report of 7 cases including 6 clear-cell carcinomas (so-called mesonephromas). Cancer 1970;25:745–57.

43. _____, Ulfelder H, Poskanzer DC. Adenocarcinoma of the vagina. Association of maternal stilbestrol therapy with tumor appearance in young women. N Engl J Med 1971;284:878–81.

44. Hinchey WW, Silva EG, Guarda LA, Ordonez NG, Wharton JT. Paravaginal wolffian duct (mesonephros) adeno-carcinoma: a light and electron microscopic study. Am J Clin Pathol 1983;80:539–44.

45. Johnson LD, Driscoll SG, Hertig AT, Cole PT, Nickerson RJ. Vaginal adenosis in stillborns and neonates exposed to diethylstilbestrol and steroidal estrogens and progestins. Obstet Gynecol 1979;53:671–9.

46. _____, Palmer AE, King NW, Hertig AT: Vaginal adenosis in cebus apella monkeys exposed to DES in utero. Obstet Gynecol 1981;57:629–35.

47. Kurman RJ, Scully RE. The incidence and histogenesis of vaginal adenosis. An autopsy study. Hum Pathol 1974;5:265–76.

48. Mostoufizadeh M, Scully RE. Malignant tumors arising in endometriosis. Clin Obstet Gynecol 1980;23:951–63.

49. Noller KL, Townsend DE, Kaufman RH, et al. Matura-tion of vaginal and cervical epithelium in women ex-posed to diethylstilbestrol (DESAD project). Am J Obstet Gynecol 1983;146:279–85.

50. O'Brien PC, Noller K, Robboy SJ, et al. Vaginal epithelial changes in young women enrolled in the national coop-erative diethylstilbestrol adenosis (DESAD) project. Ob-stet Gynecol 1979;53:300–8.

51. Plapinger L, Bern HA. Adenosis-like lesions and other cervicovaginal abnormalities in mice treated prenatally with estrogen. JNCI 1979;63:507–18.

52. Plaut A, Dreyfuss ML. Adenosis of vagina and its rela-tion to primary adenocarcinoma of the vagina. Surg Gynecol Obstet 1940;71:756–65.

53. Robboy SJ, Herbst AL, Scully RE. Clear-cell adenocarci-noma of the vagina and cervix in young females: analysis of 37 tumors that persisted or recurred after primary therapy. Cancer 1974;34:606–14.

54. _____, Hill EC, Sandberg EC, Czernobilsky B: Vagi-nal adenosis in women born prior to the diethylstilbes-trol era. Hum Pathol 1986;17:488–92.

55. _____, Szyfelbein WM, Goellner JR, et al. Dysplasia and cytologic findings in 4,589 young women enrolled in diethylstilbestrol-adenosis (DESAD) project. Am J Ob-stet Gynecol 1981;140:579–86.

56. _____, Welch WR, Young RH, Truslow GY, Herbst AL, Scully RE. Topographic relation of cervical ectropion and vaginal adenosis to clear cell adenocarcinoma. Obstet Gynecol 1982;60:546–51.

57. _____, Young RH, Welch WR, et al. Atypical vaginal adenosis and cervical ectropion. Association with clear cell adenocarcinoma in diethylstilbestrol-exposed off-spring. Cancer 1984;54:869–75.

58. Sander R, Nuss RC, Rhatigan RM. Diethylstilbestrol-as-sociated vaginal adenosis followed by clear cell adeno-carcinoma. Int J Gynecol Pathol 1986;5:362–70.

59. Sedlacek TV, Riva JM, Magen A, Morgen CE, Cunnane MG. Vaginal and vulvar adenosis. An unsuspected side effect of CO_2 laser vaporization. J Reprod Med 1990; 35:995–1001.

60. Taft PD, Robboy SJ, Herbst AL, Scully RE. Cytology of clear-cell adenocarcinoma of genital tract in young fe-males: review of 95 cases from the registry. Acta Cytol 1974;18:279–90.

61. Ulbright TM, Alexander RA, Fraus FT. Intramural pap-illoma of the vagina: evidence of the müllerian histogen-esis. Cancer 1981;48:2260–6.

62. von Preuschen. Ueber cystenbildung in der vagina. Arch Pathol Anat 1877;70:111–28.

63. Welch WR, Fu YS, Robboy SJ, Herbst AL. Nuclear DNA content of clear cell adenocarcinoma of the vagina and cervix and its relationship to prognosis. Gynecol Oncol 1983;15:230–8.

64. Yousem HL. Adenocarcinoma of Gartner's duct cyst pre-senting as a vaginal lesion. A case report. Sinai Hosp J 1961;112–4.

Other Epithelial Tumors

65. Fukushima M, Twiggs LB, Okagaki T. Mixed intestinal adenocarcinoma-argentaffin carcinoma of the vagina. Gynecol Oncol 1986;23:387–94.

66. Naves AE, Monti JA, Chichoni E. Basal cell-like carci-noma of the upper third of the vagina. Am J Obstet Gynecol 1980;137:136–7.

67. Rhatigan RM, Mojadidi Q. Adenosquamous carcinomas of the vulva and vagina. Amer J Clin Pathol 1973;60:208–17.

68. Sheets JL, Dockerty MD, Decker DG, Welch JS. Primary epithelial malignancy in the vagina. Am J Obstet Gynecol 1964;89:121–8.

69. Sulak P, Barnhill D, Heller P, et al. Nonsquamous cancer of the vagina. Gynecol Oncol 1988;29:309–20.

Mesenchymal Tumors

70. Bennett HG, Ehrlich MM. Myoma of the vagina. Am J Obstet Gynecol 1941;42:314–20.

71. Ceremsak RJ. Benign rhabdomyoma of the vagina. Am J Clin Pathol 1969;52:604–6.

72. Chapman GW, Benda JO, Williams T. Alveolar soft part sarcoma of the vagina. Gynecol Oncol 1984;18:125–9.

73. Davos I, Abell MR. Sarcomas of the vagina. Obstet Gynecol 1976;47:342–50.

74. Dekel A, Avidan D, Bar-Ziv J, Ben David M, Goldman JA. Neurofibroma of the vagina presenting with urinary retention. Review of the literature and report of a case. Obstet Gynecol Surv 1988;43:325–7.

75. Friedman M, Peretz BA, Nissenbaum M, Paldi E. Modern treatment of vaginal embryonal rhabdomyosarcoma. Obstet Gynecol Surv 1986;41:614–8.

76. Gad A, Eusebi V. Rhabdomyoma of the vagina. J Pathol 1975;115:179–81.

77. Geschicter CF. Tumors of muscle. Am J Cancer 1934;22:378–410.

78. Gold BM. Neurofibromatosis of the bladder and vagina. Am J Obstet Gynecol 1972;113:1055–6.

79. Gold JH, Bossen EH. Benign vaginal rhabdomyoma: a light and electron microscopic study. Cancer 1976;37:2283–94.

80. Gompel C, Silverberg SG. Pathology in gynecology and obstetrics. Philadelphia: Lippincott, 1977.

81. Hays DM, Shimada H, Raney RB, et al. Clinical staging and treatment results in rhabdomyosarcoma of the female genital tract among children and adolescents. Cancer 1988;61:1893–903.

82. Koskela O. Granular cell myoblastoma of the vagina. Ann Chir Gynecol Fenn 1964;53:270–3.

83. Leone PG, Taylor HB. Ultrastructure of a benign polypoid rhabdomyoma of the vagina. Cancer 1973;31:1414–7.

84. Levene M. Congenital retinoblastoma and sarcoma botryoides of the vagina. Cancer 1960;13:532–7.

85. Morales AR, Fine G, Horn RC. Rhabdomyosarcoma: an ultrastructural appraisal. In: Sommers SC, ed. Pathology Annual. Norwalk: Appleton-Century-Crofts, 1972;7:81.

86. Ober WB, Edgcomb JH. Sarcoma botryoides in the female urogenital tract. Cancer 1954;7:75–91.

87. Palmer JP, Biback SM. Primary cancer of the vagina. Am J Obstet Gynecol 1954;67:377–97.

88. Peters WA III, Kumar NB, Anderson WA, Morley GW. Primary sarcoma of the adult vagina: a clinicopathologic study. Obstet Gynecol 1985;65:699–704.

89. Pezeshkpour G. Solitary paraganglioma of the vagina--report of a case. Am J Obstet Gynecol 1981;139:219–21.

90. Prempree T, Tang CK, Hatef A, et al. Angiosarcoma of the vagina: a clinicopathologic report. A reappraisal of the radiation treatment of angiosarcomas of the female genital tract. Cancer 1983;51:618–22.

91. Schmidt WA. Pathology of the vagina. In: Fox H, ed. Haines and Taylor Obstetrical and Gynaecological Pathology. London: Churchill Livingstone, 1987;1:146–216.

92. Spitzer M, Molho L, Seltzer VL, et al. Vaginal glomus tumor: case presentation and ultrastructural findings. Obstet Gynecol 1985;66:86–8S.

93. Tavassoli FA, Norris HJ. Smooth muscle tumors of the vagina. Obstet Gynecol 1979;53:689–93.

94. Webb MJ, Symmonds RE, Weiland LH. Malignant fibrous histiocytoma of the vagina. Am J Obstet Gynecol 1974;119:190–2.

95. Wharton LR. Gynecology. Philadelphia: WB Saunders, 1947:452–6.

Mixed Epithelial and Mesenchymal Tumors

96. Buntine DW, Henderson PR, Biggs JSG. Benign müllerian mixed tumor of the vagina. Gynecol Oncol 1979;8:21–6.

97. Chen KTK. Benign mixed tumor of the vagina. Obstet Gynecol 1981;57:89–90S.

98. Chen KTK. Brenner tumor of the vagina. Diag Gynecol Obstet 1981;3:255–8.

99. Okagaki T, Ishida T, Hilgers RD. A malignant tumor of the vagina resembling synovial sarcoma: a light and electron microscopic study. Cancer 1976;37:2306–20.

100. Shevchuk MM, Fenoglio CM, Lattes R, Frick HC, Richart RM. Malignant mixed tumor of the vagina probably arising in mesonephric nests. Cancer 1978;42:214–33.

101. Sirota RL, Dickerson GR, Scully RE. Mixed tumors of the vagina. A clinicopathologic analysis of eight cases. Am J Surg Pathol 1981;5:413–22.

Miscellaneous Tumors

102. Andersen WA, Sabio H, Durso N, Mills SE, Levien M, Underwood PB Jr. Endodermal sinus tumor of the vagina. The role of primary chemotherapy. Cancer 1985;56:1025–7.

103. Chorlton I, Karnei RF, King FM, Norris HJ. Primary malignant reticuloendothelial disease involving the vagina, cervix, and corpus uteri. Obstet Gynecol 1974;44:735–48.

104. Chung AF, Casey MJ, Flannery JT, Woodruff JM, Lewis JL. Malignant melanoma of the vagina--report of 19 cases. Obstet Gynecol 1980;55:720–7.

105. Clement PB, Young RH, Scully RE. Extraovarian pelvic yolk sac tumors. Cancer 1988;62:620–6.

106. Copeland LJ, Sneige N, Ordonez NG, et al. Endodermal sinus tumor of the vagina and cervix. Cancer 1985;55:2558–65.

107. Doss LL. Simultaneous extramedullary plasmacytomas of the vagina and vulva: a case report and review of the literature. Cancer 1978;41:2468–74.

108. Fox H, Wells M, Harris M, McWilliam LJ, Anderson GS. Enteric tumors of the lower female genital tract: a report of three cases. Histopathology 1988;12:167–76.

109. Kurman RJ, Prabha AC. Thyroid and parathyroid glands in the vaginal wall: report of a case. Am J Clin Pathol 1973;59:503–7.

110. Levitan Z, Gordon AN, Kaplan AL, Kaufman RH. Primary malignant melanoma of the vagina: report of four cases and review of the literature. Gynecol Oncol 1989;33:85–90.

111. Lorenz G. Adenomatoid tumor of the ovary and vagina (author's trans). Zentral Gynakol Gynakkol 1978;100:1412–6.

112. Nigogosyan G, de la Pava S, Pickren JW. Melanoblasts in vaginal mucosa. Cancer 1964;17:912–3.

113. Norris HJ, Taylor HB. Melanomas of the vagina. Am J Clin Pathol 1966;46:420–6.

114. Reid GC, Schmidt RW, Roberts JA, Hopkins MP, Barrett RJ, Morley GW. Primary melanoma of the vagina: a clinicopathologic analysis. Obstet Gynecol 1989;74:190–9.

115. Tobon H, Murphy AI. Benign blue nevus of the vagina. Cancer 1977;40:3174–6.

116. Young RH, Scully RE. Endodermal sinus tumor of the vagina: a report of nine cases and review of the literature. Gynecol Oncol 1984;18:380–92.

117. Zinkham WH. Multifocal eosinophilic granuloma. Natural history, etiology, and management. Am J Med 1976;60:457–63.

Secondary Tumors

118. Fu YS, Reagan JW. Pathology of the uterine cervix, vagina and vulva. Philadelphia: WB Saunders, 1989:374.

Tumor-Like Lesions

119. Allen PW. Nodular fasciitis. Pathology 1972;4:9–26.

120. Compagno J, Hyams VJ, Lepore ML. Nasal polyposis with stromal atypia. Review of follow-up study of 14 cases. Arch Pathol Lab Med 1976;100:224–6.

121. Deppisch LM. Cysts of the vagina: classification and clinical correlations. Obstet Gynecol 1975;45:632–7.

122. Elliott GB, Reynolds HA, Fidler HK. Pseudo-sarcoma botryoides of cervix and vagina in pregnancy. J Obstet Gynaecol Br Commonw 1967;74:728–33.

123. _____, Elliott JDA. Superficial stromal reactions of lower genital tract. Arch Pathol 1973;95:100–1.

124. Norris HJ, Taylor HB. Polyps of the vagina. Cancer 1966;19:227–32.

125. Ostör AG, Fortune DW, Riley CB. Fibroepithelial polyps with atypical stromal cells (pseudosarcoma botryoides) of vulva and vagina. A report of 13 cases. Int J Gynecol Pathol 1988;7:351–60.

126. Proppe KH, Scully RE, Rosai J. Postoperative spindle cell nodules of genitourinary tract resembling sarcomas. A report of eight cases. Am J Surg Pathol 1984;8:101–8.

127. Silverberg SG, Frable WJ. Prolapse of fallopian tube into vaginal vault after hysterectomy. Histopathology, cytopathology and differential diagnosis. Arch Pathol 1974;97:100–3.

128. Snover DC, Phillips G, Dehner LP. Reactive fibrohistiocytic proliferation simulating fibrous histiocytoma. Am J Clin Pathol 1981;76:232–5.

129. Ulbright TM, Alexander RA, Fraus FT. Intramural papilloma of the vagina: evidence of müllerian histogenesis. Cancer 1981;48:2260–6.

❖❖❖

TUMORS OF THE VULVA

SQUAMOUS LESIONS

Squamous (Vestibular) Papilloma

Definition. A benign papillary lesion that characteristically occurs within the vulvar vestibule and is composed of a delicate fibrovascular connective tissue core covered by squamous epithelium. Vestibular papillomas may be less than 0.1 cm in length and rarely exceed 0.5 cm. They may be solitary or multiple, occurring in clusters (*vestibular* or *squamous papillomatosis*), and are often associated with pruritus (35). They have been identified in approximately 25 percent of women presenting to a colposcopy clinic (13).

Microscopic Findings. Vestibular papillomas are soft and fleshy. Microscopically, they are covered by either nonkeratinized epithelium, which may be glycogen rich in women of reproductive age, or slightly keratinized epithelium (fig. 248). They lack features of HPV infection such as koilocytosis and parabasal cell proliferation. Molecular biological analysis rarely detects HPV DNA sequences in vestibular papillomas (5,13,48).

Differential Diagnosis. The differential diagnosis includes condyloma acuminatum and hymenal tags. In contrast to a condyloma, the vestibular papilloma lacks koilocytosis. In addition, it typically has a central fibrovascular core and does not show the marked degree of arborization characteristic of the condyloma acuminatum.

No treatment is required if the lesions are asymptomatic. Local ablation by excisional biopsy, topical administration of trichloroacetic acid, or superficial laser ablation can be used for the management of symptomatic lesions.

Fibroepithelial Polyp

Definition. A benign polypoid mass with a prominent fibrovascular core covered by keratinized squamous epithelium. It may be of two distinct morphologic types, one that is predominantly epithelial and another that is primarily stromal. In contrast to the vestibular papilloma, the fibroepithelial polyp occurs on the hair-bearing skin of the vulva.

General Features. The fibroepithelial polyp is rare on the vulva. It is usually solitary and ranges from 1 to 10 cm in diameter. The larger ones are more apt to be pedunculated and may resemble a condyloma acuminatum. The lesion is soft and fleshy, with a prominent fibrovascular stromal component. The epithelium on the surface ranges from highly papillary and acanthotic with hyperkeratosis to thin and atrophic (fig. 249) (56). There is evidence that some lesions are regressing nevomelanocytic nevi.

Differential Diagnosis. The differential diagnosis includes condyloma acuminatum, neurofibroma, aggressive angiomyxoma, leiomyoma, and various polypoid soft tissue tumors. Condylomas usually display koilocytosis, although sometimes this may be focal, and have a more complex branching architecture. Neurofibromas are more cellular and exhibit S-100 immunoreactivity. The aggressive angiomyxoma is deeper, infiltrative,

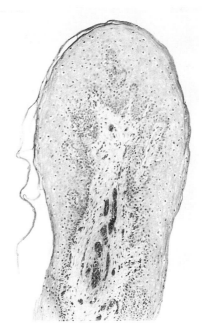

Figure 248
SQUAMOUS (VESTIBULAR) PAPILLOMA
The fibrovascular stalk of the vestibular papilloma has substantially less fibrous tissue than the fibroepithelial polyp. The overlying squamous epithelium is thinly keratinized, and there is no evidence of koilocytosis.

and less polypoid. It also has a more prominent vascular component with muscular arteries scattered throughout. Leiomyomas are more cellular and are composed of smooth muscle cells that are immunoreactive for desmin. Treatment of fibroepithelial polyps is local excision.

Condyloma Acuminatum

Definition. A verrucous lesion characterized by acanthosis with elongation and thickening of the rete ridges and usually displaying cytopathic effects (koilocytosis) caused by HPV infection.

General Features. Condylomas range in frequency from 1 to nearly 50 percent in various populations. They are usually multiple and commonly involve the vulvar vestibule, medial aspects of the labia majora, as well as the hair-bearing skin and perianal area. Because small lesions may be difficult to detect on clinical examination, the use of 3 to 5 percent topical acetic acid and colposcopic examination is necessary.

Gross Findings. Condylomas are typically verrucous, papillary or sessile, but may appear as red, granular areas that turn white after the application of acetic acid.

Microscopic Findings. Although koilocytosis in the upper third of the epithelium is considered pathognomonic, a substantial proportion of condylomas lack koilocytosis. Often additional deeper sections disclose focal areas of koilocytosis. In those instances when koilocytosis cannot be found, other ancillary findings such as acanthosis, parakeratosis, dyskeratosis, hyperkeratosis, and crowding of parabasal cells assist in the diagnosis of an exophytic papillary lesion. The complex branching papillae are an important architectural feature of condylomas (fig. 250). The koilocyte is characterized by nuclear enlargement, wrinkling of the nuclear membrane, and cytoplasmic cavitation. Near the surface, in the granular layer, the nucleus may be shrunken. The nuclear chromatin is hyperchromatic or smudgy. Mitotic figures are characteristically normal in appearance but may be increased in number as compared with adjacent normal epithelium. Condylomas are typically diploid (75). Approximately 10 percent of

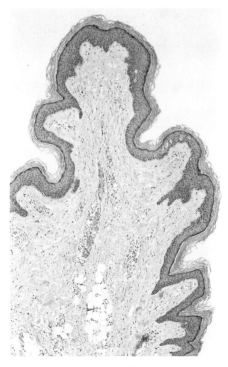

Figure 249
FIBROEPITHELIAL POLYP

The lesion has a broad fibrovascular stalk with some fat tissue at its base. The surface epithelium is thin and hyperkeratotic. (Courtesy of Dr. K. Kendall Pierson, Gainesville, FL.)

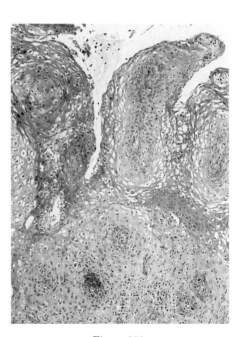

Figure 250
CONDYLOMA ACUMINATUM

This lesion shows branching papillae with fibrovascular cores. Many of the papillae are tangentially cut. Koilocytosis is present in the overlying epithelium.

condylomas show nuclear atypia of varying degrees. Depending on their severity, such lesions should be classified as condylomas with vulvar intraepithelial neoplasia (VIN) 2 or 3.

Differential Diagnosis. The differential diagnosis of a condyloma acuminatum includes squamous cell carcinoma, particularly the verrucous type (45), keratoacanthoma, vulvar intraepithelial neoplasia, and epidermolytic acanthoma (20).

Condylomas may become quite large, particularly in pregnancy. These lesions should be classified as condylomas without the adjective giant to avoid confusion with verrucous carcinoma.

Verrucous carcinoma has broad rete ridges and a pushing border and, unlike condyloma acuminatum, may be deeply infiltrative and locally destructive; koilocytosis is absent (see Verrucous Carcinoma). Another type of squamous cell carcinoma designated *warty (condylomatous) carcinoma* may be confused with condyloma acuminatum showing cytologic atypia. This neoplasm is infiltrative, with moderate to marked nuclear pleomorphism. The infiltrating tumor typically has cells with large nuclei and cytoplasmic vacuolization consistent with koilocytosis. In contrast to a condyloma, the base of this tumor has the appearance of an invasive squamous cell carcinoma. The keratoacanthoma has a central keratin plug and an irregular dermal interface. Condyloma acuminatum, especially one that has recently been treated with podophyllin, may have nuclear changes that might suggest VIN. However, VIN has variable degrees of cellular crowding, nuclear pleomorphism, abnormal mitotic figures, and other features that distinguish it from condyloma acuminatum (81).

Epidermolytic acanthoma is a rare benign vulvar neoplasm which presents as multiple verrucoid, slightly pigmented, circumscribed nodules usually 5 mm or less in diameter. In one case several lesions were present on the medial aspect of the labia majora (20). Microscopically, there is prominent acanthosis and hyperkeratosis with a prominent granular layer and granular degeneration of all but the basal and parabasal layers (fig. 251). Within the granular layer, numerous irregularly-shaped keratohyaline bodies are present. Electron microscopic examination demonstrates intact basal and parabasal cells. Within the more superficial epithelium, tonofilaments and desmosomal junc-

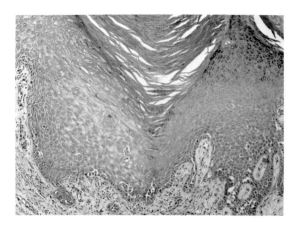

Figure 251
EPIDERMOLYTIC ACANTHOMA
The surface epithelium is thickened and hyperkeratotic. In areas of the parabasal epithelium acantholysis is present. (Courtesy of Dr. F. Mack Sexton, Charlotte, NC.)

tions are disrupted and perinuclear aggregates of tonofilaments can be identified.

Immunohistochemical Findings. The capsid protein of HPV is an antigen shared by all papillomaviruses. Approximately 50 percent of typical condylomas, regardless of their site, are immunoreactive with the commercially available antibody to the capsid antigen. The immunoreactivity is found within the nucleus of the koilocyte, and its presence requires approximately 200 viral copies per nucleus. False negative results in typical vulvar condylomas are related to the presence of insufficient viral antigen, the age of the lesion, prior therapy, or tissue fixation. Because of this lack of sensitivity, immunohistochemistry is not useful clinically. In situ hybridization kits are more sensitive and can be of value in confirming the histologic diagnosis of a condyloma; it should be remembered that even with this technique not all condylomas are positive.

Ultrastructural Findings. Electron microscopy has demonstrated HPV particles within the nucleus of the koilocyte in 25 to 50 percent of cases (60,61). The virus is approximately 55 nm in diameter and is occasionally present in the form of filaments. The number of viral particles reaches a peak within 6 to 12 months after inoculation and decreases within 24 to 36 months (60,61).

Clinical Behavior and Treatment. Condylomas are sexually transmitted. They may regress spontaneously but usually persist or increase in size and number. There is an increased frequency of condylomas in pregnancy, among oral contraceptive users, in women with diabetes mellitus and patients who are immunosuppressed. Regression of vulvar condylomas may occur after pregnancy (60). Approximately 30 percent of women with vulvar condylomas have associated cervical or vaginal condylomas or intraepithelial neoplasia (60,83). Consequently, before therapy, examination of the entire lower genital tract is necessary to determine the extent of disease. Small lesions are treated by ablation with topical administration of bi- or trichloroacetic acid or podophyllin. Large lesions may be surgically excised, whereas multiple small lesions with diffuse involvement are usually treated by laser vaporization.

Malignant transformation is rare. This phenomenon occurs most often in immunosuppressed individuals (14,90). Concurrence of vulvar condyloma acuminatum and squamous cell carcinoma has been observed (22,73). The giant condyloma of Buschke-Lowenstein is now considered a verrucous carcinoma and reports of this tumor arising within vulvar condylomas may represent examples of malignant transformation. The risk of progression of a typical condyloma to VIN or squamous carcinoma probably depends on the type of HPV it contains and the immunocompetence of the host.

Seborrheic Keratosis

Definition. A benign epithelial growth characterized by an elevated acanthotic epidermis associated with papillomatosis, hyperkeratosis, and epithelial invaginations forming horn cysts.

General Features. Multiple seborrheic keratoses are common on the hair-bearing skin of the vulva, especially in the elderly. When the superficial portions of lesions are pulled from the skin surface, small punctate bleeding sites may be seen beneath them. The Leser-Trelat syndrome, characterized by the rapid development of multiple seborrheic keratoses, may herald the appearance of a malignant tumor in an internal organ.

Gross Findings. Seborrheic keratoses are typically raised, waxy, and brown to black. There is a sharp delineation between the lesion and the dermis, creating the appearance that it is "tacked on."

Microscopic Findings. On microscopic examination a nearly straight line can be drawn below the keratosis, with the line intersecting the deep rete of the normal epithelium on both sides of the lesion (fig. 252). Hyperkeratosis, papillomatosis, and intraepithelial keratin cysts are characteristic. The squamous cells include basal and parabasal cell types. No significant nuclear atypia is present. Hyperpigmentation, due to the presence of melanin within the basal and lower parabasal cells, is frequently seen.

Differential Diagnosis. Condyloma acuminatum, vulvar intraepithelial neoplasia, basal cell carcinoma, superficial spreading melanoma, and other focally hyperplastic epithelial disorders should be considered in the differential diagnosis. Condyloma acuminatum has koilocytosis and dyskeratosis, but keratin cysts are rarely seen. Vulvar intraepithelial neoplasia is characterized by nuclear pleomorphism and hyperchromasia and may involve skin appendages. Basal cell carcinoma has smaller cells with dense nuclear chromatin and is typically locally infiltrative in a trabecular or pushing manner. Malignant melanoma has nuclear pleomorphism and contains melanoma antigen (HMB-45) and S-100 antigen demonstrated by immunohistochemical staining. Squamous cell hyperplasia does not contain keratin pearls or exhibit papillomatosis.

Usually no therapy is needed unless the lesion is a cosmetic concern or the clinical diagnosis is uncertain. Under such circumstances, a superficial or shave biopsy is recommended. Cryotherapy is also effective.

Keratoacanthoma

Keratoacanthoma is a benign tumor composed of well-differentiated squamous epithelium with a central keratin-filled crater and an infiltrative border that typically regresses spontaneously within 6 months. Keratoacanthomas are very rare on the vulva (68). Typically, they are rapidly growing solitary tumors with hard, raised, rough, irregular, nonulcerated surfaces. They may be up to 4 cm in diameter and are usually not tender or inflamed. A central keratinous plug may protrude in a horn-like manner

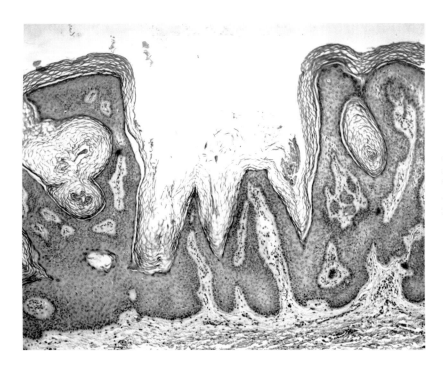

Figure 252
SEBORRHEIC KERATOSIS
A nearly straight line can be drawn between the base of the keratosis and the underlying dermis. There is epithelial maturation with a hyperkeratotic surface. Keratin plugs are seen near the surface.

from the surface. On microscopic examination the base of the lesion is a symmetrical, cup-like mass of keratin surrounded by squamous cells. A dense inflammatory infiltrate is usually present at the border of the lesion, and a foreign body reaction may also be evident (figs. 253, 254).

Keratoacanthoma may be difficult to distinguish from squamous cell carcinoma. Squamous cell carcinoma generally lacks a keratin crater and has a more irregular infiltrating margin. Treatment of keratoacanthoma is an excisional biopsy.

Squamous Intraepithelial Lesions

Definition. Proliferative intraepithelial squamous lesions which display abnormal maturation, nuclear enlargement, and atypia. The latter is characterized by pleomorphism, coarse chromatin clumping, and irregular nuclear contours. These lesions have been designated *dysplasia* (mild, moderate, severe) and *carcinoma in situ* or *vulvar intraepithelial neoplasia* (VIN) (grades 1,2,3) (69,89). In this Fascicle flat lesions with koilocytotic atypia and minimal evidence of proliferation are included in the category of VIN 1.

General Features. The most common sites of VIN are on the labia minora and the perineum. Perianal involvement occurs in approximately one third of cases of VIN and may extend into the anus. Approximately 70 percent of VIN lesions are multifocal, whereas the remainder are unifocal (11,12,18,32,33,64,65,89,93). Vulvar pruritus is the most common symptom of VIN but one third of the patients are asymptomatic.

The clinical appearance is variable. Over 50 percent of the lesions are white, with the remainder brown, black, or red. They may be plaque-like (pl. III), but are often macular or papular.

Microscopic Findings. VIN is characterized by a proliferation of cells with nuclear enlargement, hyperchromasia, and pleomorphism. Chromatin is coarse with radial dispersion toward the nuclear membrane. In addition, there is infolding of the nuclear membrane and abnormal mitotic figures. The cells are crowded with disordered maturation. The radial growth of VIN may result in replacement of the epithelium of the skin appendages by VIN. Skin appendage involvement occurs in approximately 20 percent of the cases in which the lesion is confined to a nonhair-bearing area, and 30 percent of the cases in which the hair-bearing skin is involved.

Microscopic Grading and Subtyping. The grading of VIN depends upon the extent of replacement of the epithelium by abnormal cells in the most severely involved areas. In VIN 1 abnormal cellular changes are present mainly in

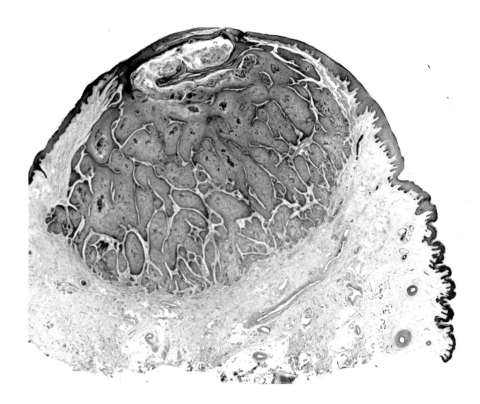

Figure 253
KERATOACANTHOMA

A surface keratotic plug is present that is cup-like and surrounded by squamous epithelium. The keratin plug may protrude as a horn-like mass. Although the deeper portions of this keratoacanthoma appear somewhat irregular and infiltrative, the tumor-stromal interface is well defined and symmetric. There is minimal inflammatory infiltrate within the dermis. Strict criteria should be applied when making this diagnosis, to distinguish it from squamous cell carcinoma. (Courtesy of Dr. Ronald Rhatigan, Jacksonville, FL.)

Figure 254
KERATOACANTHOMA

The dermis at the tumor-dermal interface has a mild chronic inflammatory infiltrate. Tongues of epithelium extend into the dermis. The tumor cells are well differentiated. (Courtesy of Dr. Ronald Rhatigan, Jacksonville, FL.)

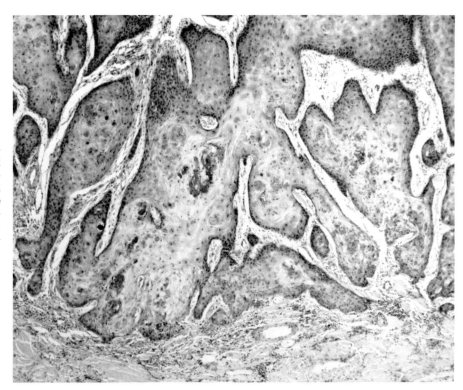

PLATE III

CLINICAL APPEARANCE OF VULVAR INTRAEPITHELIAL NEOPLASIA

There are numerous pigmented macules on the vulva, some of which have a central depigmented area. Nonpigmented red areas are present on the labia minora which are also VIN. On the perineal body, anterior to the rectum, red and pigmented VIN lesions are seen. (Courtesy of Dr. I. Keith Stone, Gainesville, FL.)

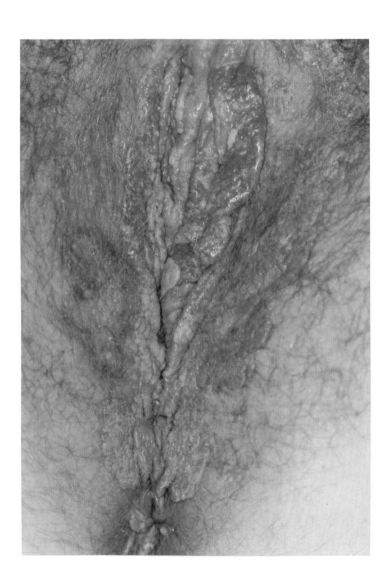

the lower third of the epithelium (figs. 255, 256) with maturation of the surface epithelium. Koilocytosis may be present. Pure VIN 1 is rare; typically it is adjacent to a high-grade VIN lesion. As indicated previously, vulvar condylomas that are flat, and have nuclear atypia as described above, are included in this group whereas exophytic condylomas are classified as condylomata acuminata (see Condyloma Acuminatum).

The cellular changes of a VIN 2 lesion extend into the middle third of the epithelium (figs. 257, 258). Abnormal mitotic figures are generally easily found. Surface maturation may include a granular layer and a variable degree of hyperkeratosis. Pure VIN 2 is less commonly seen than VIN 3, and is often found associated with VIN 3.

VIN 3 shows considerable morphologic heterogeneity. Studies suggest that the different morphologic patterns may reflect differing etiologies (62,79). Accordingly, VIN 3 is subdivided into three types: *warty (condylomatous), basaloid (usual type),* and *differentiated (simplex type).*

Warty VIN is characterized by marked proliferation, parakeratosis, and hyperkeratosis. The epithelium typically displays an undulating or spiked surface creating a "warty" or "condylomatous" appearance (fig. 259). Although there is marked proliferation, as evidenced by acanthosis and numerous mitotic figures, including abnormal mitotic figures, the cells show evidence of maturation, albeit abnormal. Individual cells often have well-defined cell membranes with

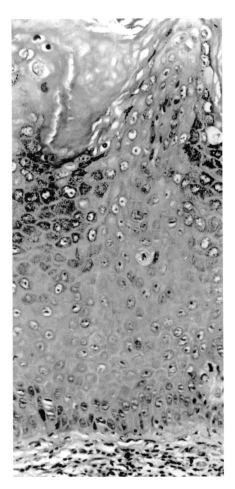

Figure 256
VIN 1

This lesion has a micropapillary, or spiked, surface pattern with hyperkeratosis. Koilocytosis is noted in the upper third. There is abnormal maturation; nuclear pleomorphism and mitotic activity are confined to the lower one third of the epithelium.

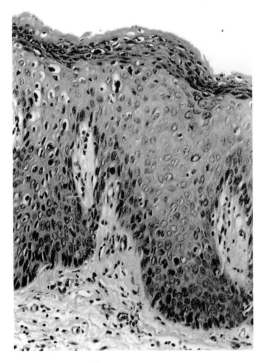

Figure 255
VIN 1

Normal epithelium is seen on the right side and VIN 1 with koilocytosis is seen on the left side. There is lack of maturation in the lower third and maturation with koilocytosis in the upper two thirds of the epithelium. Flat lesions with koilocytosis, proliferation, and nuclear hyperchromasia in the deeper layers of the epithelium are classified as VIN 1.

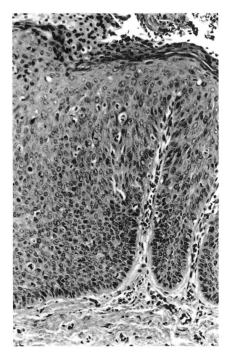

Figure 257
VIN 2, WARTY TYPE
In this lesion an abnormal mitotic figure is seen in the lower one third of the epithelium. There is a lack of epithelial maturation involving the lower half of the epithelium.

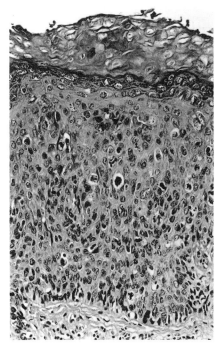

Figure 258
VIN 2, WARTY TYPE
This lesion lacks maturation of the lower half of the epithelium. Mitotic figures and moderate nuclear pleomorphism are seen in the lower third of the epithelium.

Figure 259
VIN 3, WARTY TYPE
The surface has an undulating and spiked appearance. There is abnormal cellular maturation manifested by cells with hyperchromatic, pleomorphic nuclei and abundant cytoplasm distributed throughout the full thickness of the epithelium.

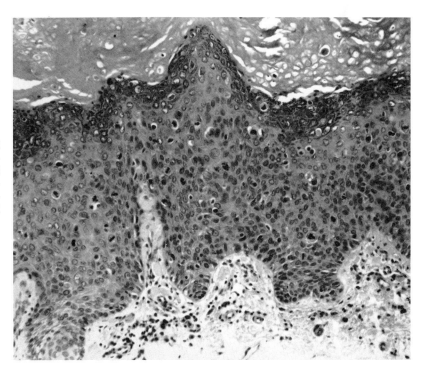

prominent eosinophilic cytoplasm. Individual cell keratinization is often observed. The nuclei are enlarged, with coarsely granular chromatin, and there is an increased nuclear-cytoplasmic ratio. Cells with hyperchromatic, shrunken nuclei surrounded by clear cytoplasm are characteristic. Koilocytotic atypia involving the surface epithelium may be present. Multinucleated giant cells are another frequently observed feature. Rete pegs are typically wide, extend deeply into the stroma, and are separated by thin stromal papillae often penetrating close to the surface (fig. 260).

Basaloid VIN is characterized by thickened epithelium with a smooth, relatively flat surface lacking the undulated and spiked appearance of warty VIN (fig. 261). Hyperkeratosis is variably present, but not to the extent observed in warty VIN. The epithelium is either entirely, or almost entirely, composed of atypical immature parabasal type cells, similar to the classic appearance of carcinoma in situ of the cervix (CIN 3). Individual cells have poorly defined cell membranes, scant cytoplasm, and enlarged hyperchromatic nuclei. Koilocytosis involving the surface occurs, but it is less frequently encountered than in warty VIN. Mitotic figures, including abnormal mitotic figures, are numerous. As with warty VIN, extension of the intraepithelial process into hair follicles and adnexal structures is frequently present. Basaloid and warty VIN may be present adjacent to invasive squamous cell carcinomas of the basaloid or warty types respectively, although basaloid VIN may also occur adjacent to warty carcinoma and conversely

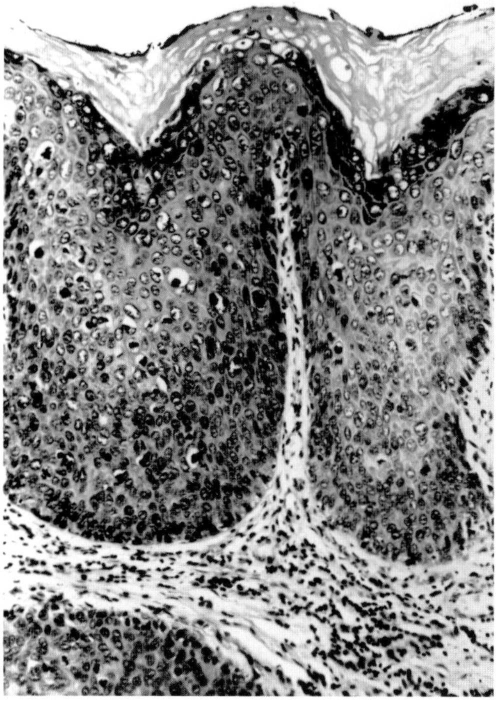

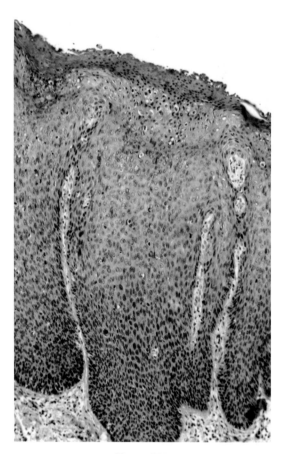

Figure 261
VIN 3, BASALOID TYPE
This lesion has thickened epithelium with prominent acanthosis with mild hyperkeratosis and parakeratosis. The nuclei are pleomorphic and hyperchromatic and lack maturation, appearing as atypical immature parabasal type cells. The cells have poorly defined cell membranes and scant cytoplasm. (From Toki T, et al. Int J Gynecol Pathol 1991;10: 107–125.)

Figure 260
VIN 3, WARTY TYPE
The surface has an undulating appearance. Epithelial maturation is abnormal. Multinucleated epithelial cells are seen.

warty VIN may be adjacent to basaloid carcinoma (see Invasive Squamous Cell Carcinoma).

The differentiated type of VIN 3 (simplex type) is characterized by abnormal cells confined to the basal and parabasal portions of the rete pegs (1). The superficial layers show normal maturation, although mild nuclear atypia may be present (figs. 262, 263). In the basal areas the epithelial cells have prominent eosinophilic cytoplasm, and keratin pearl formation may be present. The nuclei have dispersed chromatin and usually prominent nucleoli. This type of VIN 3 is often present adjacent to the typical type of keratinizing squamous cell carcinoma (fig. 262). The differentiated type of VIN 3 is distinguished from VIN 1 by the presence of cells with prominent increased eosinophilic cytoplasm and nuclear chromatin changes, including radial dispersion of chromatin and prominent nucleoli. In addition,

pearl formation is seen in the well-differentiated type of VIN 3 but not in VIN 1.

Although each of these types of VIN 3 exists in a pure form, mixtures of warty and basaloid VIN are common. In these instances the lesion is classified according to the predominant type. The differentiated type of VIN is rarely associated with the other types. Unless otherwise specified, the term VIN without further specification in this Fascicle includes both the warty and basaloid forms.

Immunohistochemical and Ultrastructural Findings. The cells of VIN are immunoreactive for some low– and high–molecular-weight keratins. They are not immunoreactive for carcinoembryonic antigen (CEA), S-100, or melanoma antigen. Ultrastructurally, the nuclei of high-grade VIN show chromatin granularity and clumping (53).

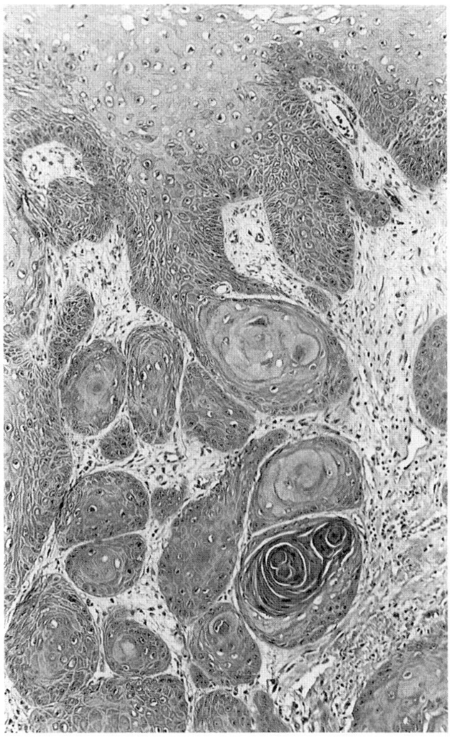

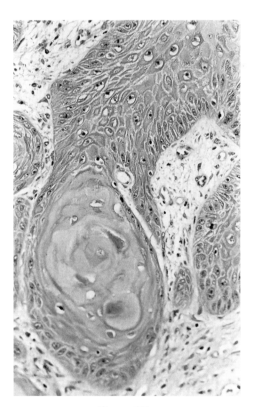

Figure 262
VIN 3, DIFFERENTIATED TYPE AND
INVASIVE SQUAMOUS CELL CARCINOMA

The intraepithelial lesion is above a well-differentiated keratinizing invasive squamous cell carcinoma. The surface epithelium shows normal maturation. Invasive nests of epithelium with squamous pearls appear to be "dropping" from the rete ridges.

Figure 263
VIN 3, DIFFERENTIATED TYPE

In this high power view of figure 262, abnormal keratinocytes, with an increased amount of cytoplasm, are present within the rete ridges. Some nuclei in the basal layer have prominent nucleoli but lack the hyperchromatism characteristic of other VIN lesions.

Differential Diagnosis. Some investigators have recommended distinguishing a multifocal, pigmented, papular lesion with features of VIN, designated bowenoid papulosis, from VIN 3 (82). Studies have shown, however, that microscopically bowenoid papulosis and VIN 3 are indistinguishable (6,86). Furthermore, these multifocal papular lesions, like VIN 3, contain HPV 16 (6,17,34). Accordingly, the term bowenoid papulosis is not acceptable as a histopathologic diagnosis (69,89). The differential diagnosis of VIN also includes invasive squamous cell carcinoma, Paget disease, superficial spreading melanoma, basal cell carcinoma, seborrheic keratosis and condyloma acuminatum, including condyloma acuminatum with podophyllin effect.

Skin appendage involvement by VIN is distinguished from invasive squamous cell carcinoma by preservation of a distinct epithelial stromal junction, lack of stromal desmoplasia, and absence of isolated small clusters of neoplastic squamous cells which usually are differentiated in the stroma of invasive carcinoma. Furthermore, in vulvar nonhair-bearing epithelium, VIN involvement of the sebaceous or vestibular gland epithelium rarely exceeds 1 mm in depth below the basement membrane of the overlying surface epithelium. In hair-bearing skin, VIN involvement of the hair follicles rarely exceeds 2.5 mm, being confined within the basement membrane of the hair follicle epithelium (74). Therefore, nests of malignant cells beyond these depths are highly suggestive of invasion. The presence or absence of invasion requires meticulous evaluation of the entire specimen.

Paget disease has distinctive large atypical cells occurring in clusters, and as single cells within otherwise normal-appearing squamous epithelium. Paget cells are immunoreactive for CEA and almost always contain stainable mucin.

Superficial spreading malignant melanoma has large atypical cells within the epithelium that are immunoreactive for S-100 and melanoma antigen (HMB-45). It must be emphasized that some VIN lesions contain melanin within the neoplastic cells.

Basal cell carcinoma characteristically has smaller cells than VIN, and the invasive nests show peripheral palisading of nuclei. A desmoplastic or fibrotic reaction usually surrounds the invasive nests of basal cell carcinoma.

Seborrheic keratosis is composed of a uniform population of cells with prominent hyperkeratosis and intraepithelial keratin pearl formation. Significant nuclear pleomorphism, hyperchromasia, and abnormal mitotic figures are absent in this lesion.

Condyloma acuminatum typically grows in an exophytic, papillomatous, or verrucous pattern and lacks marked nuclear pleomorphism, hyperchromasia, or abnormal mitotic figures. It should be emphasized that VIN and condyloma may coexist. VIN may be present within, or adjacent to, condyloma acuminatum and in such cases both terms should be included in the diagnosis.

Topical podophyllin results in mitotic arrest. With mitoses arrested in metaphase, abnormal mitoses may be seen. Nuclear disruption, dispersion of nuclear chromatin, and cellular swelling are common with podophyllin effect but rarely found with VIN. Nuclear pleomorphism is typically present in VIN, however, with podophyllin effect the nuclei remain relatively uniform. Unlike VIN, the cellular changes associated with podophyllin effect regress within 2 weeks of discontinuing the applications (81), and therefore podophyllin should not be used for at least 2 weeks before biopsy.

Clinical Behavior and Treatment. Women with VIN have synchronous vulvar invasive squamous cell carcinoma in approximately 10 percent of the reported cases, although higher rates have been reported (15,95). In our experience warty or basaloid VIN is adjacent to the corresponding types of invasive carcinoma in approximately 80 percent of cases (49). The prognosis in these cases is favorable because the majority of the carcinomas are superficial. VIN is found adjacent to superficially invasive carcinoma in 55 to 80 percent of cases (27,70,95). Women with invasive carcinoma and coexistent VIN 3 are young, with a mean age of 54 years (79). In contrast, VIN 3 of the differentiated type is usually found adjacent to typical squamous cell carcinomas; the mean age of these women is 77 years (79).

The progression of VIN to invasive carcinoma appears to be low. It should be noted, however, that the "natural history" of VIN is not known because it is usually treated by complete excision. In one study in which VIN 3 lesions in five women were biopsied, but not completely excised, progression to invasive squamous cell carcinoma occurred in all five patients (43). Spontaneous regression of VIN, however, has been documented (31,32). When local surgical excision is employed, the recurrence or persistence rate depends on the status of the resection margins. When the lesion extends to the margin, the rate is approximately 20 percent; when the margins are free the rate is under 6 percent (32). If multiple lesions are present more than one lesion should be biopsied because the microscopic features may vary from lesion to lesion (88). As in women with condylomas, approximately 30 percent of women with VIN have synchronous or metachronous cervical or vaginal intraepithelial neoplasia, and therefore, examination and subsequent follow-up must include colposcopic examination of the cervix and vagina and cytological screening for these lesions.

Local excision is the most common method of therapy for VIN, and is especially effective in the treatment of small solitary lesions. It has the advantage of providing tissue for microscopic examination to exclude invasion. This is especially important in postmenopausal women with solitary lesions, immunosuppressed patients, and women with Fanconi anemia because of a higher frequency of associated invasive carcinoma (14,15,90). Local excision is also preferred when the lesion is in hair-bearing skin because of the common involvement of skin appendages (74). When multiple or extensive lesions involve nonhair-bearing areas, the treatment can be more superficial therapy, if invasive carcinoma has been excluded by multiple biopsies, because VIN in these instances is generally not deeper than 1 mm. Superficial laser ablation is effective in such cases and preserves normal vulvar anatomy (74). Total or partial vulvectomy is rarely necessary for the treatment of VIN. Observation only, after biopsy to establish the diagnosis, may be considered in young women and pregnant women, because regression of VIN may occur (31,32).

Squamous Cell Carcinoma

Definition. An invasive tumor showing exclusive differentiation into squamous cells. These tumors can be divided into two categories: 1) superficially invasive squamous cell carcinoma, and 2) frankly invasive carcinomas that invade to a depth beyond the limits used to define

superficially invasive carcinoma. There is no consensus on the method of measuring depth of invasion. However, the method that is used should be specified in the pathology report. Superficially invasive squamous cell carcinoma is discussed separately from frankly invasive squamous carcinoma in this presentation.

Superficially Invasive
Squamous Cell Carcinoma

Definition. A carcinoma with a depth of invasion of 1 mm or less and a diameter of 2 cm or less (a solitary carcinoma fulfilling these criterion could be staged as ISSVD stage IA) (46). The rare presence of vascular space invasion does not increase the stage above 1A if the ISSVD stage system is used.

General Features. A superficially invasive squamous cell carcinoma of the vulva may present as an ulcer, a red macule or papule, a white hyperkeratotic plaque, or within an area of vulvar intraepithelial neoplasia that may be brown or black. No specific findings on clinical examination definitively separate VIN from VIN with superficial invasion (15).

Microscopic Findings. The depth of invasion is measured from the epithelial-stromal junction of the most superficial adjacent normal dermal papilla to the deepest point of invasion. The thickness of the tumor is defined as the measurement from the surface, or the granular layer, if a keratinized surface is present, to the deepest point of invasion (fig. 264) (27,85,89,91). Some prefer measuring the depth of invasion, whereas others prefer measuring the thickness. Ideally, both should be done when possible. Because these may differ, it is important to specify which measurement was used when reporting either of these features. Microscopic features that assist in distinguishing superficially invasive squamous carcinoma from VIN include the following: 1) invasion is characterized by isolated squamous cells in the stroma or small irregularly shaped nests of squamous cells; the nests display disorderly orientation of the tumor cells with loss of the usual palisaded arrangement of the basal keratinocytes along the periphery of the nest; 2) invasive squamous cells, in contrast to cells of VIN or pseudoepitheliomatous hyperplasia, often have increased eosinophilic cytoplasm

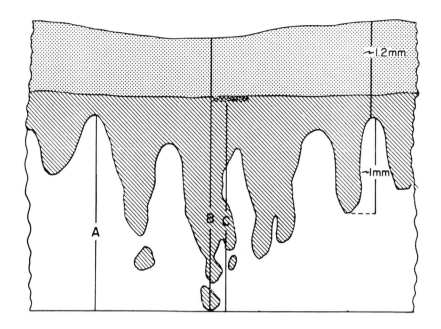

Figure 264
MEASUREMENT
METHODS OF
SQUAMOUS CELL
CARCINOMA
OF THE VULVA

The tumor thickness is defined as the measurement from the granular layer (C) [or surface if nonkeratinized (B)] to the deepest point of invasion. The depth of invasion is defined as the measurement from the epithelial stromal junction of the adjacent most superficial dermal papillae to the deepest point of invasion (A). (Fig. 1 from Wilkinson EJ. Superficially invasive carcinoma of the vulva. Clin Obstet Gynecol 1991;34:651–661.)

and prominent nucleoli; 3) in invasive carcinoma there often is dyskeratosis and keratin pearl formation; 4) an invasive carcinoma has a stromal reaction in the dermis characterized by fibrosis or edema localized to the area of invasion (figs. 265–267) (85); 5) immunoreactive laminin surrounds nests of VIN whereas it is discontinuous around invasive nests of epithelium (28). Although this may facilitate the recognition of invasion, too few cases have been studied to recommend it for clinical use at the present time.

Clinical Behavior and Treatment. The risk of lymph node metastasis in women with superficially invasive squamous cell carcinomas (depth of invasion ≤1.0 mm) is zero in large series where the depth of invasion has been well defined (4,10,27,36,37,40,70,85,91). Therapy for women with superficially invasive squamous cell carcinoma (ISSVD stage IA vulvar carcinoma) is wide local excision with or without ipsilateral node dissection (23,24,36,85). In the absence of clinically suspicious or palpable regional nodes, vascular space involvement by tumor, or a finger-like pattern of tumor growth, wide local excision of the tumor, without ipsilateral lymph node dissection, would be adequate.

Invasive Squamous Cell Carcinoma

General Features. Squamous cell carcinoma accounts for approximately 95 percent of malignant tumors of the vulva and 3.5 to 8 percent of those of the female genital tract (3,30,94). The incidence in the United States is 1.5/100,000 women per year and increases with age; the mean age at presentation is between 60 and 74 years (37,39). The epidemiology of vulvar carcinoma is not as well delineated as that of cervical carcinoma, but there is a recognized increased risk with advancing age, number of life-time sexual partners, cigarette smoking, immunodeficiency, condyloma acuminatum, and genital granulomatous disease (8,72). An increased risk has been identified in women working in cotton mills, related to exposure to industrial oils, as well as those working in the dyeing and cutlery industries.

Recently it was reported that there are differences between young and older women in the distribution of HPV in invasive squamous cell carcinomas. HPV, generally type 16, is found in only 21 percent of vulvar carcinomas in older women (mean age 77 years), compared to 81 percent of younger women (mean age 50 years). Moreover, the histologic features of the invasive

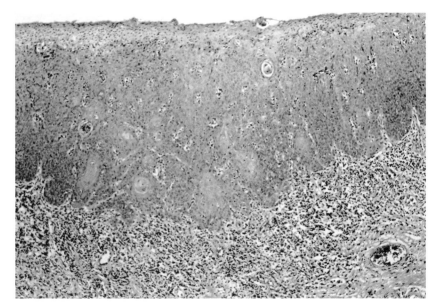

Figure 265
SUPERFICIALLY INVASIVE
SQUAMOUS CELL
CARCINOMA

The invasive focus of squamous cell carcinoma underlies intraepithelial neoplasia. There is a loss of the orderly palisaded arrangement of the epithelial cells at the epithelial-stromal junction. The tumor has a thickness of 1.2 mm and a depth of invasion of 0.9 mm.

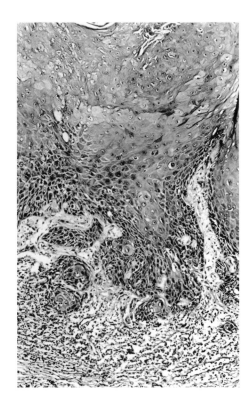

Figure 266
FOCAL SUPERFICIALLY INVASIVE SQUAMOUS
CELL CARCINOMA AND VIN 3,
DIFFERENTIATED TYPE

A focus of invasive carcinoma is at the tip of a rete ridge with VIN. At the point of infiltration there is loss of the palisaded arrangement of the basal cells, and the invasive cells have increased cytoplasm compared with the basal cells.

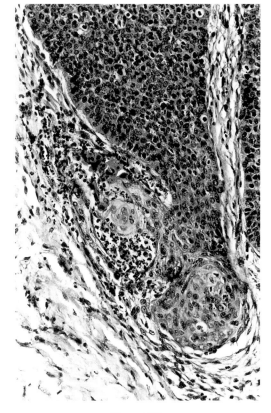

Figure 267
FOCAL SUPERFICIALLY INVASIVE SQUAMOUS
CELL CARCINOMA AND VIN 3,
BASALOID TYPE

The invasive cells have increased cytoplasm. There is a marked inflammatory response.

carcinomas differ. The neoplasms in the older women have the typical appearance of squamous cell carcinomas and are generally well differentiated and highly keratinized, whereas the tumors in the younger women are of the basaloid or warty types (25,49,67,79).

Clinical Features. The most common symptoms are pruritus, pain, discharge, bleeding, dysuria, and foul odor. The tumor may arise anywhere on the vulva but the labia majora, labia minora, and clitoris are the most common sites, with the clitoris the primary site in 5 to 15 percent of the cases (3,36,40,47). The perineal body and posterior fourchette are the primary sites in approximately 15 percent of the cases (94). The carcinoma is solitary in about 90 percent of the cases, and is over 2 cm in diameter in at least 60 percent of them (figs. 268, 269) (27,54,84). VIN is infrequently found adjacent to the typical (keratinized) invasive squamous cell

carcinoma. When present, it is the differentiated (simplex) type of VIN. In contrast, squamous cell hyperplasia is found adjacent to this type of invasive neoplasm more frequently (27,70,94,95). In these cases the adjacent vulvar epithelium is thickened and gray-white due to intraepithelial edema or hyperkeratosis. The invasive carcinoma presents as a focally hyperkeratotic area, ulcer, or mass. Fifteen to 30 percent of women with vulvar squamous cell carcinoma have associated vulvar lichen sclerosis, with the tumor presenting as a nodular or ulcerated mass in an area involved by this disorder (38,95).

Rarely, squamous cell carcinoma may arise in association with a granulomatous lesion of the vulva such as granuloma inguinale (72). Carcinoma also has been reported in young women who are immunosuppressed in association with renal transplantation (14).

Gross Findings. Grossly, invasive squamous carcinoma may be exophytic or a papillomatous mass or ulcer.

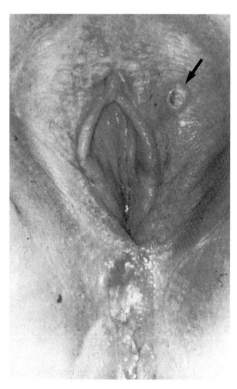

Figure 268
SQUAMOUS CELL CARCINOMA

The tumor (arrow), present on the medial aspect of the left labium majus, has a slightly raised margin and a central ulcer. Such a tumor can be deeply infiltrative, although its surface appearance may suggest otherwise.

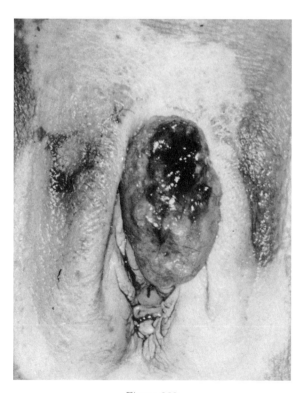

Figure 269
SQUAMOUS CELL CARCINOMA

This large exophytic carcinoma is present within an area of abnormal vulvar epithelium that shows extensive postinflammatory hypopigmentation.

Microscopic Findings. Typical squamous cell carcinomas of the vulva are almost always keratinizing (figs. 270, 271).

Confluent growth of tumor, defined as anastomosing cords of invasive tumor that exceed 1 mm in diameter, is a characteristic of more deeply invasive squamous cell carcinomas (23,24,63,85). In evaluating tumors with a depth of invasion beyond 1 mm, tumor growth pattern appears to have some influence on lymph node metastasis. Tumors with a compact or pushing pattern of growth (fig. 270) are somewhat less likely to metastasize than those with a diffuse or finger-like pattern of infiltrative growth (fig. 271).

Squamous Cell Carcinoma with Tumor Giant Cells. This is a variant of squamous cell carcinoma that is usually nonkeratinizing with multinucleated tumor cells. The tumor cells often show marked nuclear pleomorphism and contain prominent eosinophilic cytoplasm (fig. 272) (87). This tumor may resemble a malignant melanoma but unlike melanoma its cells are not immunoreactive for melanoma antigen or S-100, and it has immunohistochemical and electron microscopic features of typical squamous cell carcinoma.

Spindle Cell Squamous Cell Carcinoma. This tumor is composed of elongated spindle-shaped cells that can mimic a sarcoma (fig. 273). The stroma of these tumors may also contain spindle-shaped cells leading to confusion with carcinosarcoma (77). All

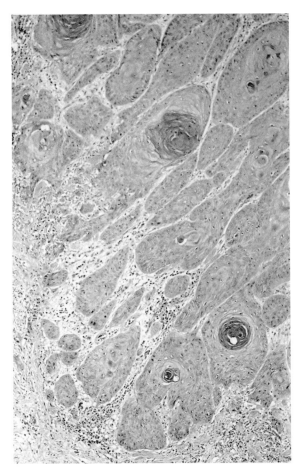

Figure 270
WELL-DIFFERENTIATED KERATINIZING
SQUAMOUS CELL CARCINOMA

Keratin pearls are present in this example. The tumor cells have abundant cytoplasm. Small nests of tumor cells, which have irregular shapes, are present within the dermis. The tumor has a pushing margin.

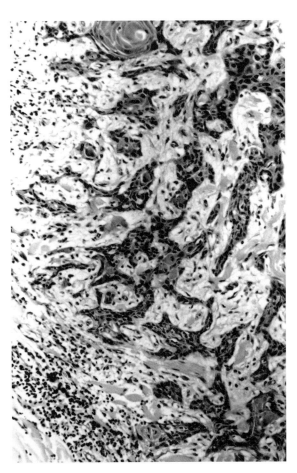

Figure 271
POORLY DIFFERENTIATED KERATINIZING
SQUAMOUS CELL CARCINOMA

A finger-like (or spray) infiltrative pattern is evident. A keratin pearl is present at the top margin. There is stromal desmoplasia with a moderate chronic inflammatory infiltrate.

of the spindle cells are immunoreactive for keratin, reflecting their epithelial origin (16,52,57).

Acantholytic Squamous Cell Carcinoma. This tumor is a variant of squamous carcinoma characterized by areas of pseudoglandular formation, related to cellular acantholysis (fig. 274) (51). Mucin (sialomucin) is characteristically not present. Glycogen, however, is present in the acantholytic cells, and the acellular basophilic material in the pseudoglandular areas has histochemical features of a material with high hyaluronic acid content (42).

Microscopic Grading. The Gynecologic Oncology Group (GOG) has advised grading of squa-

mous cell carcinomas according to the percentage of undifferentiated cells. The latter are small cells with scant cytoplasm showing little or no differentiation and infiltrating the stroma either in elongated cords or small clusters (see fig. 271) (71). This grading system can be reduced to three grades (44). Grade 1 tumors have no undifferentiated cells, grade 2 tumors have undifferentiated cells comprising less than half of the tumor, and grade 3 tumors contain half or more of the poorly differentiated component. Grade 1 tumors have little risk of regional lymph node metastasis; the risk is higher with increasing grade (71). Currently, tumor grading is not routinely performed.

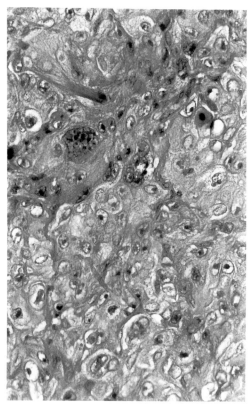

Figure 272
SQUAMOUS CELL CARCINOMA
WITH TUMOR GIANT CELLS

This squamous cell carcinoma has large tumor cells that contain abundant cytoplasm and large nuclei with prominent nucleoli. Multinucleated tumor cells are seen.

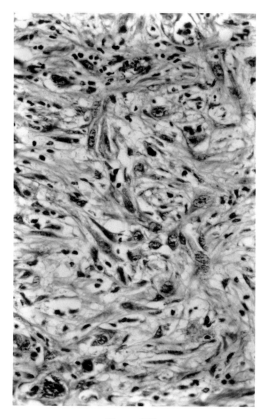

Figure 273
SPINDLE CELL
SQUAMOUS CELL CARCINOMA

The spindle-shaped cells have pleomorphic nuclei. There is moderate stromal desmoplasia with a minimal chronic inflammatory infiltrate.

Clinical pathologic studies have shown that the following features correlate with prognosis and therefore should be included in the surgical pathology report: 1) the depth of invasion in millimeters, 2) the thickness of the tumor in millimeters, 3) the presence or absence of vascular space involvement by the tumor, 4) the diameter of the tumor (as measured from the specimen in the fresh or fixed state), and 5) the clinical measurement of the tumor diameter, when available.

Cytology. Scrapings from the tumor surface show tumor cell groups and single cells displaying nuclear pleomorphism, hyperchromasia, and anisocytosis (21,58). The cytoplasm may be dyskeratotic. These findings are similar to those in fine-needle aspiration specimens from lymph

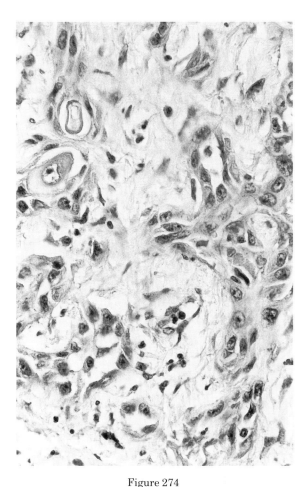

Figure 274
ACANTHOLYTIC SQUAMOUS CELL CARCINOMA
This carcinoma shows focal acantholysis of tumor cells with gland-like formation. The tumor is poorly differentiated with pleomorphic nuclei.

nodes with metastatic vulvar squamous cell carcinoma.

Immunohistochemical Findings. Immunohistochemical studies reveal that most squamous cell carcinomas of the vulva contain both high– and low–molecular-weight keratins (78).

Differential Diagnosis. The differential diagnosis of squamous cell carcinoma includes malignant melanoma, especially those that are amelanotic, metastatic squamous cell carcinoma, epithelioid sarcoma, pseudoepitheliomatous hyperplasia, keratoacanthoma, and skin appendage involvement by VIN.

Malignant melanomas contain immunoreactive S-100 antigen and HMB-45, and lack keratin. In addition, melanomas may have a superficial spreading or intraepithelial melanoma adjacent to the invasive component of tumor. Metastatic squamous cell carcinomas, usually from the cervix or anus, tend to involve deeper tissues and lymphatics without an adjacent intraepithelial component or transition from the adjacent surface epithelium. Epithelioid sarcomas may resemble nonkeratinizing squamous cell carcinoma and have similar immunohistochemical findings. They are distinguished by their granuloma-like appearance, location, which is typically deep and adjacent to fascia, and their lack of an intraepithelial neoplastic component. Pseudoepitheliomatous hyperplasia is composed of nests of bland-appearing squamous cells. At the margin of the nests a palisaded arrangement of the basal cells is often retained. In contrast, carcinomas have more irregularly-shaped jagged edges and tumor nests containing cells with greater nuclear atypia. Granular cell tumors in particular may be associated with overlying pseudoepitheliomatous hyperplasia (92). Prior biopsy sites may also contain embedded epithelium and therefore simulate carcinoma; however, the epithelium is normal-appearing and lacks infiltrative features. In addition, there may be foreign body giant cells containing suture material. Keratoacanthomas have a distinctive hyperkeratotic central core and an infiltrative pattern which converges inwardly or centrally. Despite the infiltrative pattern, the tumor dermal interface of keratoacanthoma is well defined in contrast to the irregular border of squamous cell carcinoma. Skin appendage involvement by VIN may be confused with invasive squamous cell carcinoma, especially if there is tangential sectioning. Unlike squamous cell carcinoma, VIN retains the orderly arrangement of the epithelial cells along the basement membrane, does not have cellular differentiation, and is not associated with stromal desmoplasia or edema. Multiple sections will usually reveal identifiable skin appendage epithelium in continuity with the intraepithelial neoplastic cells (see VIN).

Clinical Behavior. Vulvar squamous cell carcinoma spreads locally and by lymphatics and blood vessels. It commonly extends to the vagina and the distal urethra, and in advanced cases to the base of the bladder, the pelvic bones, and perirectal tissues.

Vascular space invasion increases the probability of lymph node metastasis in vulvar carcinomas when the depth of invasion exceeds 1 mm (10,40,50). The ipsilateral superficial inguinal and femoral nodes are most commonly involved. Contralateral lymph node metastasis may also occur. When the superficial inguinal-femoral nodes are free of tumor there is essentially no risk of deep pelvic lymph node involvement and little risk of deep femoral node metastasis. In contrast, when these superficial nodes contain tumor, approximately 25 percent of the patients have deep pelvic lymph node involvement because these pelvic nodes drain the superficial inguinal nodes (23). Accordingly, the most proximal superficial node, the node of Cloquet (or Rosenmüller), is commonly sampled at the time of vulvectomy since its involvement mandates treatment of the deep pelvic nodes. The medial group of the external iliac nodes drain the superficial inguinal nodes and deep femoral nodes, and are the most common lymph node groups involved when the more superficial nodes contain tumor. The lateral group of the external iliac nodes are infrequently involved. Tumor from the deep pelvic nodes may metastasize to the para-aortic nodes and enter the thoracic duct and the venous circulation, leading to metastasis to the supraclavicular nodes, lungs, liver, and other remote sites. Distant spread also occurs as a result of direct venous invasion.

Staging. The 1989 International Federation of Gynecologists and Obstetricians (FIGO) staging of vulvar carcinoma is shown in Table 5 (29).

Treatment. Squamous cell carcinomas that have a depth of invasion exceeding 5 mm, and those that are stage II to stage IVA, are usually treated by radical vulvectomy with bilateral superficial inguinal-femoral lymph node dissection. If the superficial nodes, including Cloquet node, are free of tumor, no additional therapy is indicated. If the superficial inguinal-femoral nodes, or Cloquet node, are involved by metastatic tumor, the deep pelvic nodes are usually treated by postoperative pelvic radiotherapy. Most superficial stage I tumors may be treated by a more conservative operation, usually wide local excision or partial vulvectomy, with superficial node dissection.

Prognosis. Survival is primarily related to the stage of the disease. Women with tumor of 1 mm in depth of invasion or less are almost always cured, although the occurrence of a second primary vulvar carcinoma has been described in such patients (91). Patients with a stage I carcinoma have a mean 5-year survival of 85 percent, for stage II the 5-year survival is 60 percent, for stage III tumors 40 percent, and for stage IV tumors 10 percent.

Basaloid Carcinoma

Recent studies have shown an elevated prevalence of HPV, mainly type 16, with certain types of invasive squamous carcinomas of the vulva. Among these are basaloid carcinomas, which occur in young women (mean age 54 years), compared with typical keratinizing squamous cell carcinomas (mean age 77 years). Basaloid carcinomas are frequently associated with adjacent VIN, usually of the basaloid type (fig. 275). In contrast to typical squamous cell carcinomas, basaloid carcinomas are associated with synchronous or metachronous squamous neoplasms of the cervix and vagina (49).

On gross examination basaloid carcinomas are similar to typical squamous cell carcinomas. Microscopically, they are characterized by variable-sized nests of immature squamous cells showing little, if any, squamous maturation (fig. 276). Some tumors are composed of small irregularly-shaped clusters and cords of cells surrounded by a densely hyalinized stroma. The basal-type cells within the nests and cords resemble those in the classic type of carcinoma in situ of the cervix. Characteristically, they are

Table 5

The International Federation of Gynecology and Obstetrics (FIGO)
STAGING OF VULVAR CARCINOMA
Union Internationale Contre Le Cancer (UICC) and
American Joint Committee on Cancer (AJCC)

Stage	Description
Stage 0 Tis	Carcinoma in situ, intraepithelial carcinoma
Stage I * T1 N0 M0	Tumor confined to the vulva or vulva and perineum, ≤2 cm in greatest dimension
Stage II T2 N0 M0	Tumor confined to the vulva or vulva and perineum, >2 cm in greatest dimension
Stage III T3 N0 M0 T3 N1 M0 T1 N1 M0 T2 N1 M0	Tumor with: 1. Adjacent spread to the lower urethra and/or the vagina or the anus (T3) and/or 2. Unilateral regional lymph node metastasis (N1)
Stage IVA T1 N2 M0 T2 N2 M0 T3 N2 M0 T4 any N M0	Tumor invades any of the following: Upper urethra, bladder mucosa, rectal mucosa, pelvic bone, (T4) and/or bilateral regional node metastasis (N2)
Stage IVB Any T Any N M1	Any distant metastasis including pelvic nodes

* ISSVD stage IA is defined as a solitary tumor, ≤2 cm in greatest diameter, with a depth of invasion of ≤1 mm (46).

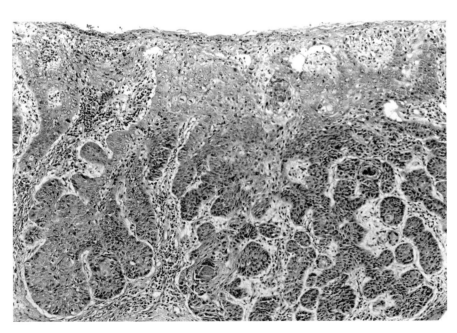

Figure 275
BASALOID CARCINOMA
This tumor lies below an area of vulvar intraepithelial neoplasia.

199

ovoid and relatively uniform in size, with scant cytoplasm and a high nuclear-cytoplasmic ratio, and therefore, they appear undifferentiated. Nuclei contain evenly distributed coarsely granular chromatin creating a stippled appearance. A moderate degree of mitotic activity is usually evident. Occasionally, the cells in the center of a nest show evidence of maturation and contain more abundant cytoplasm. Keratinization may be evident in the center of the nests and keratin pearls are occasionally present. Desmosomes are usually not evident. The behavior of basaloid carcinoma appears to be similar to typical keratinizing squamous carcinomas but there is insufficient experience at this point to draw firm conclusions (49). Basaloid carcinoma may at times be difficult to distinguish from basal cell carcinoma. In contrast to basaloid carcinoma, basal cell carcinomas tend to be more circumscribed and have a lobular appearance. The characteristic palisading of the outermost layer of cells in the nests of basal cell carcinoma is lacking in basaloid carcinoma. The differential diagnosis of basaloid carcinoma also includes metastatic small cell carcinoma and Merkel cell tumor. These tumors have a more diffusely infiltrative pattern characterized by ill-defined nests, trabeculae, and individual cells invading the stroma rather than the broad anastomosing bands and well-defined nests typical of basaloid carcinoma.

Verrucous Carcinoma

Definition. A highly differentiated squamous carcinoma that has a verrucous pattern and invades with a pushing border in the form of bulbous pegs of neoplastic cells (9).

The term *giant condyloma of Buschke-Löwenstein* is considered to be a synonym for verrucous carcinoma. Squamous cell carcinomas having some of the architectural features of verrucous carcinoma but lacking a high degree of differentiation should not be designated verrucous carcinoma (2,45).

Clinical Features. Verrucous carcinoma is a papillary exophytic growth that may distort or completely obscure the vulva. Secondary infection may be associated with a malodorous discharge. Regional lymph nodes are usually not enlarged.

Gross Findings. The tumor has a papillomatous granular appearance, and may be markedly hyperkeratotic (fig. 277).

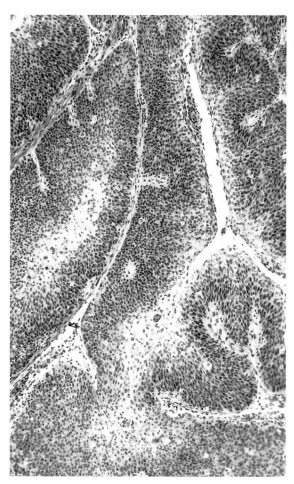

Figure 276
BASALOID CARCINOMA
This tumor is composed of variably-sized masses of immature-appearing and relatively small, squamous cells that show little evidence of maturation. (Fig. 2 from Toki T, et al. Probable nonpapillomavirus etiology of squamous cell carcinoma of the vulva in older women: a clinicopathology study using in situ hybridization and polymerase chain reaction. Int J Gynecol Pathol 1991;10:107–25.)

Microscopic Findings. The microscopic features of verrucous carcinoma include prominent acanthosis with a pushing tumor-dermal interface and bland cytological features (figs. 278, 279). The deep advancing margin is characterized by large bulbous nests of squamous epithelium. There is minimal nuclear pleomorphism, with the greatest degree of nuclear atypia nearest the dermal interface. The nuclei may have coarse chromatin and variable-sized nucleoli, distinguishing them from normal adjacent keratinocytes. Mitotic figures are rare and when

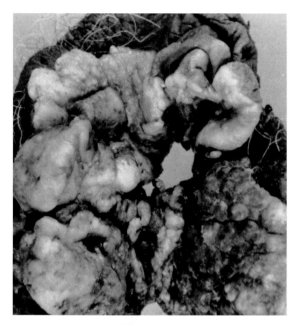

Figure 277
VERRUCOUS CARCINOMA
This large pedunculated and nodular tumor obscures the vulva.

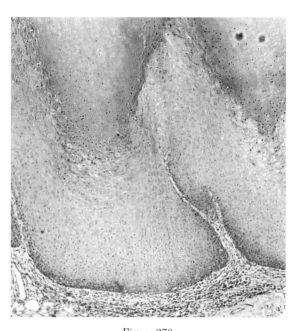

Figure 278
VERRUCOUS CARCINOMA
The tumor-dermal interface is of a pushing type.

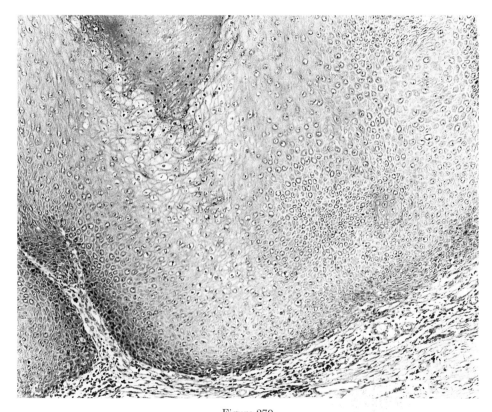

Figure 279
VERRUCOUS CARCINOMA
The epithelium shows surface maturation, parakeratosis, and hyperkeratosis. There is little or no cellular atypia. The stroma shows a mild chronic inflammatory infiltrate.

present are normal. The abundant cytoplasm of the tumor cells is eosinophilic, without dyskeratosis. Koilocytosis is not a feature of this tumor. Parakeratosis and/or hyperkeratosis are usually present, and may be prominent. There is an absence of fibrovascular cores separating the bulbous epithelial downgrowths. An inflammatory infiltrate within the dermis is usually present.

Verrucous carcinoma has been reported to be associated with HPV, typically type 6, or variants of type 6 (59,66,67,73,80). These tumors are typically diploid. Condyloma acuminatum and squamous cell carcinoma may be adjacent to verrucous carcinomas (22,25).

Differential Diagnosis. The differential diagnosis includes the typical variety of squamous cell carcinoma, warty carcinoma, and condyloma acuminatum.

Squamous cell carcinoma of the usual type (keratinizing squamous carcinoma) has greater nuclear pleomorphism and a more irregular type of infiltration of the stroma compared with the bulbous rete pegs of verrucous carcinoma. Warty carcinoma, despite its verruciform appearance, has fibrovascular cores, unlike verrucous carcinoma, within the papillary fronds. In addition, these tumors display greater nuclear atypia, koilocytosis and, at their deep margin invade like typical squamous cell carcinomas. Condyloma acuminatum is characterized by a complex branching papillary architecture with vascular papillae, lacks bulbous downgrowths, and typically shows koilocytosis.

Clinical Behavior and Treatment. Verrucous carcinomas may recur locally after excision. Lymph node metastasis is extremely rare, and its presence should prompt reevaluation of the lesion for areas of the usual type of squamous cell carcinoma. Wide local excision and total vulvectomy without lymph node dissection are the most common methods of therapy. If the tumor is completely excised, the prognosis is excellent.

Warty (Condylomatous) Carcinoma

This is another type of squamous carcinoma that is associated with HPV, particularly type 16, and occurs in younger women (79). The gross appearance may resemble verrucous carcinoma, being large and exophytic with a papillary appearance. Based on the striking verruciform features, the tumor has been designated *warty* or *condylomatous carcinoma* (25,67).

Microscopic Findings. On microscopic examination the surface of the tumor is papillary and covered by hyperkeratotic squamous epithelium that contains fibrovascular cores (fig. 280). At the deep interface between the tumor and the stroma, it is composed of jagged, irregularly-shaped nests of epithelium (fig. 281). Squamous pearls, similar to those found in well-differentiated squamous cell carcinoma, may be present. The individual squamous cells of warty carcinoma, however, display nuclear pleomorphism and cytologic atypia ranging from mild to marked. The nuclear changes are characterized by enlargement, wrinkling of the nuclear membrane, hyperchromasia, and occasionally multinucleation. These changes are typically accompanied by cytoplasmic vacuolization, resulting in an appearance that is consistent with koilocytotic atypia.

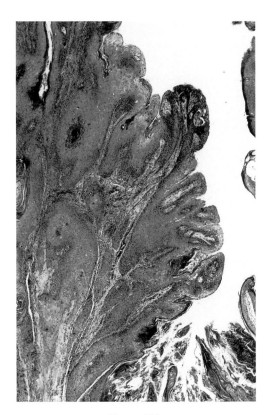

Figure 280
WARTY (CONDYLOMATOUS) CARCINOMA
The tumor has a verruciform appearance with papillae that contain fibrovascular cores. (Fig. 3 from Toki T, et al. Probable nonpapillomavirus etiology of squamous cell carcinoma of the vulva in older women: a clinicopathology study using in situ hybridization and polymerase chain reaction. Int J Gynecol Pathol 1991;10:107–25.)

Differential Diagnosis. The differential diagnosis is mainly that of verrucous carcinoma and the typical keratinizing squamous carcinoma. The presence of large numbers of cells displaying koilocytotic atypia is a characteristic feature of warty carcinoma and assists in the distinction of this tumor from keratinizing squamous cell carcinoma and verrucous carcinoma. Keratinizing squamous cell carcinoma may occasionally contain a few cells showing koilocytotic atypia but not the large numbers seen in warty carcinoma. Verrucous carcinoma does not display koilocytotic atypia.

Clinical Behavior and Treatment. Treatment is the same as for typical (keratinizing) squamous cell carcinoma. Although experience with this tumor is limited, it appears to have a prognosis between verrucous carcinoma and typical squamous carcinoma. The prognosis is generally good, but lymph node metastasis occasionally occurs (49).

Basal Cell Carcinoma

Definition. A locally infiltrative tumor arising in the epidermis or hair follicles in which the peripheral cells simulate the basal cells of the epidermis and are typically palisaded along the margins of the infiltrating nests.

General Features. Basal cell carcinoma of the vulva accounts for 2 to 4 percent of all vulvar cancers (19). It occurs most commonly on the anterior portions of the labia majora of elderly white women (7,76).

Gross Findings. The tumor is usually firm, well circumscribed, granular, and raised or ulcerated. Most basal cell carcinomas of the vulva are 2 cm or less in diameter, but giant forms up to 10 cm in diameter have been described (26).

Microscopic Findings. Like basal cell carcinomas elsewhere on the skin, the tumor can have a variety of growth patterns. Characteristically, the tumor cells are relatively small with hyperchromatic, elongated nuclei, although some pleomorphism may be seen. The cells may be grouped in trabecular or club-shaped masses, with the peripheral cells arranged in a palisaded manner (fig. 282). Squamous differentiation, characterized by enlarged cells with abundant eosinophilic cytoplasm sometimes demonstrating intercellular bridges, may be found within the nests of what is otherwise a typical basal cell carcinoma. Such tumors are still considered basal cell carcinomas. Nests of tumors may be surrounded by a hyalinized reactive stroma.

Subtypes. Variants of basal cell carcinoma may have focal tubular and gland-like differentiation (adenoid basal cell carcinoma) (55). Metatypical basal cell carcinoma (basosquamous carcinoma) is composed of both basal cell carcinoma and squamous cell carcinoma (7). It occurs at a mucocutaneous junction and is composed of relatively small uniform hyperchromatic epithelial cells with a growth pattern typical of basal cell carcinoma. Adjacent to the basal cell component, cells demonstrate more prominent eosinophilic cytoplasm, nuclear enlargement, and pleomorphism, characteristic of squamous cell carcinoma.

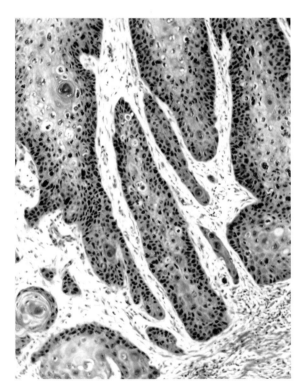

Figure 281
WARTY (CONDYLOMATOUS) CARCINOMA

At the interface with the stroma the tumor is composed of irregularly-shaped nests of epithelium. The squamous cells have abundant eosinophilic cytoplasm and a moderate degree of nuclear enlargement and pleomorphism. (Fig. 4 from Toki T, et al. Probable nonpapillomavirus etiology of squamous cell carcinoma of the vulva in older women: a clinicopathology study using in situ hybridization and polymerase chain reaction. Int J Gynecol Pathol 1991;10:107–25.)

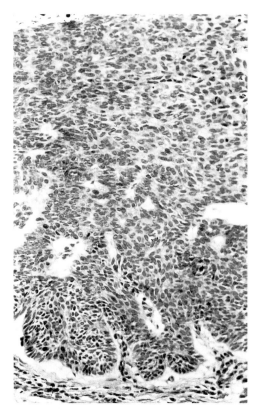

Figure 282
BASAL CELL CARCINOMA
The tumor is composed of relatively small uniform cells with peripheral palisading of nuclei.

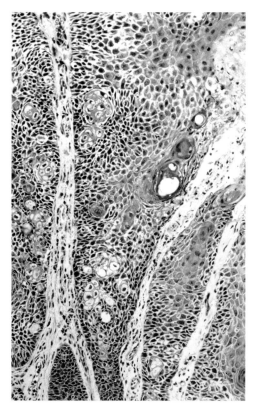

Figure 283
SEBACEOUS CARCINOMA
The tumor has features of squamous cell carcinoma with focal differentiation into groups of vacuolated sebaceous cells.

Sebaceous carcinoma is a tumor with sebaceous differentiation that otherwise has features of basosquamous cell carcinoma (fig. 283). This tumor has been reported in association with VIN (41).

Differential Diagnosis. The differential diagnosis includes squamous cell carcinoma, Merkel cell tumor, and metastatic small cell carcinoma. Squamous cell carcinomas have associated dyskeratosis, with areas of parakeratosis and/or keratin formation. The prominent basal cell component distinguishes metatypical basal cell carcinoma from squamous cell carcinoma.

The nuclei of Merkel cell tumors have stippled chromatin. These tumors, as well as metastatic small cell carcinomas, have a more diffusely infiltrative pattern. Their cells are somewhat smaller with more hyperchromatic nuclei than basal cell carcinoma. They are immunoreactive for neuroendocrine markers and reveal a distinctive perinuclear dot-like immunoreactive cytoplasmic staining with cytokeratin markers.

Clinical Behavior and Treatment. Basal cell carcinomas are characterized by local infiltrative growth. The treatment is local excision. Local recurrence may be as high as 20 percent. Rarely, vulvar basal cell carcinomas metastasize to the inguinal lymph nodes (19).

GLANDULAR LESIONS

Papillary Hidradenoma
(Hidradenoma Papilliferum)

Definition. A benign tumor of apocrine sweat gland origin, composed of epithelial cells lining complex delicate fibrovascular branching stalks. The tumor cells include both secretory and myoepithelial cells.

General Features. This relatively uncommon tumor is seen predominantly in white women, presenting after puberty, when apocrine gland development occurs. Its location ranges

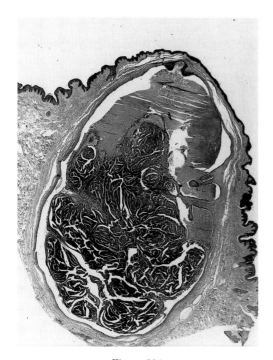

Figure 284
PAPILLARY HIDRADENOMA
This tumor has a complex glandular pattern and is well circumscribed.

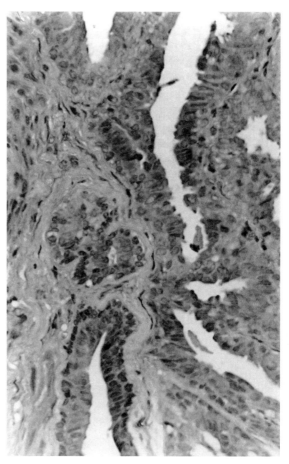

Figure 285
PAPILLARY HIDRADENOMA
A myoepithelial layer is adjacent to the stroma and a secretory epithelial layer lines the glandular spaces

from the lateral aspects of the labia minora to the lateral aspects of the labia majora. Hidradenoma usually presents as an asymptomatic mass but may cause pruritus, ulcerate, bleed, and exude watery fluid.

Gross Findings. The tumor characteristically is a well-circumscribed subcutaneous nodule measuring 0.5 to 1 cm.

Microscopic Findings. The tumor is well circumscribed with compression of the adjacent stroma and pseudocapsule formation (figs. 284, 285). It is composed of complex tubules and acini lined by tall columnar cells that may have an apocrine appearance with underlying myoepithelial cells. The spaces contain PAS-positive diastase-resistant secretion (133). Mild nuclear pleomorphism and minimal mitotic activity may be seen. Electron microscopy confirms the apocrine nature of the cells, which contain secretory granules and lamellar bodies and show evidence of decapitation secretion (124). The tumor cells are CEA negative, supporting their apocrine glandular origin, unlike tumors of eccrine sweat gland origin, which contain CEA (135,136).

Differential Diagnosis. The differential diagnosis includes skin appendage adenocarcinomas (156), metastatic carcinomas, endometriosis, and ectopic breast tissue. Adnexal adenocarcinomas do not have a cystic or papillary configuration and lack a myoepithelial layer. In addition, these tumors are more cellular and display more nuclear atypia. Metastatic carcinomas also lack a two-cell layer, are infiltrating, and have features consistent with their sites of origin. Ectopic breast tissue has a lobular pattern, may show more intraluminal secretion, and often contains ducts.

Clinical Behavior and Treatment. Papillary hidradenoma is a benign tumor that is treated by excisional biopsy.

Nodular (Clear Cell) Hidradenoma

Definition. A benign tumor of eccrine sweat gland origin composed of distinctive small cells with clear cytoplasm. Other terms for this tumor include *clear cell myoepithelioma*, *clear cell nodular hidradenoma*, *solid-cystic hidradenoma*, *eccrine acrospiroma*, and *eccrine sweat gland adenoma of clear cell type*.

General Features. These tumors are rare on the vulva. They form solitary subcutaneous nodules, and may present with pruritus or a burning sensation, but usually are asymptomatic. They may be tender on palpation.

Gross Findings. The tumor is usually 0.5 to 2 cm in diameter, solid, and well circumscribed. On section, it is tan to gray and predominantly solid; cystic or hemorrhagic areas may be present.

Microscopic Findings. The nodular (clear cell) hidradenoma is well circumscribed. It is composed of relatively uniform polygonal cells with small round to irregularly-shaped nuclei and prominent clear cytoplasm (fig. 286). The cells are typically arranged in lobules separated by delicate strands of connective tissue that are rich in collagen. Cystic spaces may be seen within the lobules and tubule formation may occur. Mitotic activity is rare. The surface epithelium is usually unremarkable, but epithelial hyperplasia or thinning, sometimes accompanied by ulceration, may occur. The histochemical and ultrastructural features of the tumor confirm its eccrine sweat gland origin.

Differential Diagnosis. The differential diagnosis includes metastatic clear cell adenocarcinoma, metastatic renal cell carcinoma, clear cell leiomyoma, clear cell carcinoma arising primarily within the skin, including tumors of hair shaft, and clear cell variants of squamous cell carcinoma. Also included in the differential diagnosis are other related benign skin appendage tumors.

Clear cell and renal cell carcinomas are infiltrative and have minimal to marked nuclear pleomorphism. They are often multiple, involve both deep and superficial tissues, and may have vascular space involvement. The clear cell leiomyoma has immunohistochemical features of smooth muscle. Clear cell carcinomas of skin or hair shaft are infiltrative tumors that have nuclear pleomorphism and hyperchromasia. Examination of the adjacent tissues may help to identify their origin. Eccrine acrospiroma and other squamous poroadenomas are morphologically distinctive and are described in the skin Fascicle and other sources.

Clinical Behavior and Treatment. The clear cell hidradenoma is a benign tumor treated by excisional biopsy.

Syringoma

Definition. A benign tumor of eccrine ductal origin characterized by multiple small and relatively uniform epithelial-lined tubules and cysts within a fibrous stroma.

General Features. The syringoma is an uncommon vulvar tumor that typically occurs in young women. The youngest reported case was in a 9-year-old girl (102). It is rare in postmenopausal women (118). Patients may present with

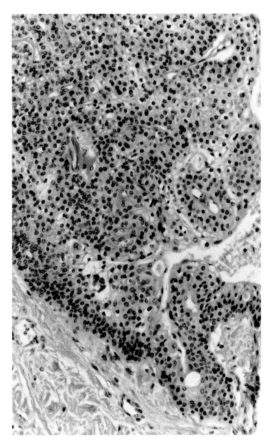

Figure 286
NODULAR HIDRADENOMA
CLEAR CELL TYPE
This tumor is composed of uniform, polygonal cells with small, rounded nuclei. Some of the cells have clear cytoplasm.

pruritus although they are more commonly asymptomatic. The tumors are usually multiple and bilateral and present as symmetrical papules occurring most commonly on the labia majora and less commonly on the lateral aspects of the labia minora. They may also involve the inner thighs (126,159).

Gross Findings. These tumors are typically small, ranging from 1 to 3 mm in diameter, firm and flesh colored.

Microscopic Findings. Syringomas lie within the dermis and are well circumscribed with pushing borders. They are composed of multiple duct-like structures, some of which may be dilated or cystic, and many of which have a distinctive comma shape (fig. 287). Two layers of epithelial cells can be seen. Part of the cyst epithelium may be flattened. Within the cysts,

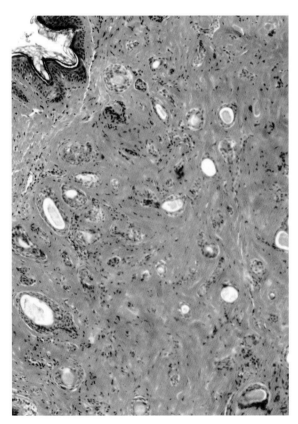

Figure 287
SYRINGOMA

This tumor is within the superficial dermis and contains clusters of small ducts, some of which are comma shaped. Some of the ducts have two cell layers. The stroma of the tumor is densely hyalinized.

the secretory material is PAS positive and diastase resistant. Rupture of cysts may be associated with a chronic inflammatory foreign body reaction and subsequent calcification. A superficial inflammatory reaction may also be seen (118,152). The surrounding stroma is fibrous.

Syringomas have characteristic features of intraepidermal eccrine glands by both immunohistochemical and electron microscopic studies.

Syringomatous differentiation has been described within mixed skin appendage tumors in which chondroid stroma may be present, giving rise to the term *chondroid syringoma*. Mixed tumors have been described on the vulva (145).

Differential Diagnosis. The differential diagnosis includes metastatic and primary adenocarcinoma. Adenocarcinomas are infiltrative, have nuclear pleomorphism, form glands of variable sizes and shapes, and may involve the deep and the superficial dermis. Sweat gland carcinomas may have solid and differentiated areas, but lack the nuclear and structural uniformity of syringoma.

Clinical Behavior and Treatment. Syringomas are usually asymptomatic and treatment is seldom necessary. Surgical excision or other ablative techniques can be used in symptomatic cases.

Trichoepithelioma

This benign hair follicle tumor is rare on the vulva (106). Clinically it may present as single or multiple, firm, nonulcerated nodules. On microscopic examination, the tumor is composed of nests of basaloid cells with small cysts containing keratin (horn cysts) surrounded by stroma (fig. 288). The basal cells may resemble those of basal cell carcinoma. True hair or hair buds are rarely seen.

Trichilemmoma

Trichilemmoma is rare on the vulva, occurring in the dermis of the labium majus, where it presents as a slowly growing solid mass (98). Microscopic examination reveals a lobulated tumor with a pushing border that may show no connection with the overlying epithelium. The tumor cells are palisaded peripherally and have increased cytoplasm as they stratify toward the centers of the nests, which contain amorphous keratin. No

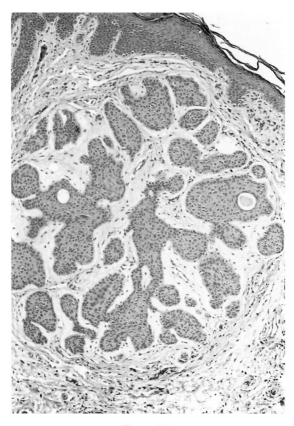

Figure 288
TRICHOEPITHELIOMA
This small vulvar tumor is entirely within the dermis. Small cell nests with radiating buds, two of which contain cystic spaces, are present within a fibrous stroma.

granular layer is formed. Nuclear pleomorphism may be present and calcification may occur. Trichilemmal cysts (pilar tumors) have also been described on the vulva (103,142), as has trichoblastic fibroma (119). Local excision is therapeutic.

Adenoma of Minor Vestibular Glands

This rare benign tumor arises within the vulvar vestibule. It is usually 1 to 2 mm in diameter, and is composed of nodular clusters of small glands lined by mucin-secreting columnar epithelium (99,113). The lesion may be a nodular hyperplasia and not a true neoplasm. In the majority of the cases the lesion is detected as an incidental finding within a specimen excised from the vulvar vestibule in the course of treatment of vulvar vestibulitis (114).

Paget Disease

Definition. A neoplasm characterized by a primary intraepithelial proliferation of atypical glandular-type cells that may invade the dermis, or by intraepithelial proliferation of similar cells secondary to an underlying adenocarcinoma.

General Features. Extramammary Paget disease can develop anywhere along the milk line, from the axilla to the perineal area. It accounts for approximately 2 percent of all vulvar neoplasms. Vulvar Paget disease typically occurs in white postmenopausal women (100, 120). It has, however, been described in a 24-year-old black woman (149). It may also be associated with an underlying adenocarcinoma of the Bartholin gland (155). Perianal Paget disease is associated with a high frequency of rectal adenocarcinoma (125). There have been reports of concurrent vulvar Paget disease and breast adenocarcinoma, but a statistical relationship between these two tumors has not been established (115).

Gross Findings. Paget disease usually is an intraepithelial neoplasm, but can involve the apocrine or eccrine glands and invade the dermis (123,129,141,157). Sometimes it reflects extension from an underlying carcinoma of the Bartholin gland or rectum.

The disease typically presents as an eczematoid pink to red lesion with an irregular margin and weeping surface. Often small foci of white hyperkeratotic epithelium are present (fig. 289).

Microscopic Findings. The early histopathologic findings are usually intraepithelial, where the Paget cells occur singly and in groups. The cells may involve skin appendages and the surface epithelium. Typically, they are grouped predominantly within the basal and parabasal zones, with fewer cells present superficially (figs. 290–292). The cells are generally larger and have paler cytoplasm than the adjacent keratinocytes. Their cytoplasm is finely granular and amphophilic to basophilic, and may be vacuolated, forming signet-ring cells. Occasionally gland spaces are formed within cell groups. The nuclei of the Paget cells are round to oval and may be the same size or larger than those of the adjacent keratinocytes. They vary from vesicular with finely granular to coarsely hyperchromatic chromatin. Generally, one or more enlarged nucleoli are present. Mitotic figures may be found

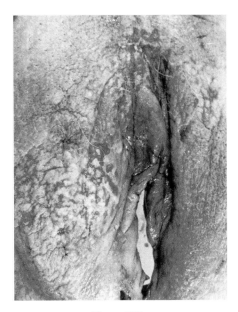

Figure 289
PAGET DISEASE
The lesion is eczematoid with islands of white epithelium. It involves a large area of the right labium majus and a smaller area in the upper left labium majus.

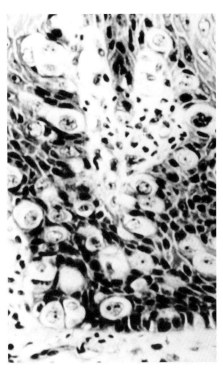

Figure 291
PAGET DISEASE
The Paget cells have abundant clear cytoplasm. The nuclei contain prominent nucleoli and are generally larger than those of the adjacent keratinocytes.

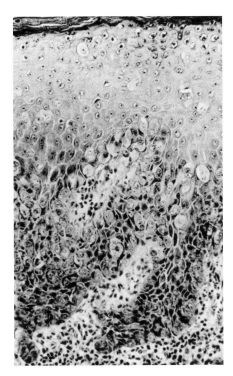

Figure 290
PAGET DISEASE
The large pale Paget cells lie within the basal and parabasal epithelium. A few isolated cells are present more superficially.

but are not frequent. Paget cells can be identified on cytologic examination of scrapings from saline moistened areas (110,139). Adenocarcinoma may be found beneath the Paget disease.

Histochemical and Immunohistochemical Findings. The cytoplasm of some of the Paget cells contains neutral and acid mucopolysaccharide, as reflected in staining with mucicarmine, PAS, aldehyde fuchsin, and alcian blue (125). The mucin stains may be positive in only a small number of cells, and may therefore not be identified in small biopsy specimens. Paget cells may occasionally contain intracytoplasmic melanin, consequently a melanin stain is not useful for differentiating Paget disease from melanoma. The histochemical findings described above, as well as the presence of CEA, are suggestive of eccrine or apocrine duct epithelium (101,132,147).

Immunohistochemical studies have demonstrated the presence of CEA and epithelial membrane antigen (EMA), as well as low–molecular-weight keratin; of these CEA appears to be the

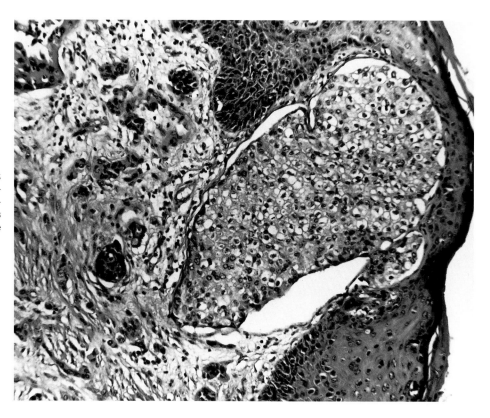

Figure 292
PAGET DISEASE
WITH INVASION
A large mass of Paget cells is present at the epithelial-dermal interface with small clusters of invasive tumor in the dermis.

most sensitive (116). Although useful in diagnosis, these markers do not provide any additional advantages over conventional microscopic analysis in the evaluation of the adequacy of surgical resection margins (116). CEA is also present in normal eccrine and in apocrine ductal epithelium, but absent in apocrine glandular epithelium (132,137). Immunohistochemical stains for S-100 and melanoma antigen (HMB-45) are negative. However, these have not been specifically performed on cases of Paget disease in which melanin pigment has been reported.

Ultrastructural Findings. Electron microscopic studies have generally identified features of adenocarcinoma without cell types that are intermediate between the Paget cells and the adjacent keratinocytes (101,111,138,146).

Differential Diagnosis. Superficial spreading malignant melanoma can mimic Paget disease. Melanoma antigen and S-100 immunohistochemical stains assist in difficult cases. VIN may simulate Paget disease, particularly when there are large, clear dysplastic squamous cells scattered in a background of normal-appearing squamous cells. Histochemical stains for mucin

are helpful in the differential diagnosis, as well as immunohistochemical staining for CEA, which is demonstrable in Paget cells but not in VIN.

Clinical Behavior and Treatment. Paget cells can often be identified microscopically within clinically normal-appearing skin adjacent to Paget disease. This indicates that many cases of "recurrent" vulvar Paget disease represent persistence of clinically unrecognized disease that was not excised at the original procedure (122). The primary treatment of vulvar Paget disease is usually wide excision of the involved area to the fascia. Frozen section examination of the margins of the skin may assist in complete excision. If underlying adenocarcinoma is identified, radical vulvectomy with bilateral inguinal-femoral lymph node dissection is the usual treatment (109,150).

When Paget disease is entirely intraepithelial, the prognosis is excellent. Some patients have been followed many years without evidence of invasion of the dermis. Wide local excision is effective and recurrent or persistent tumor is usually treated effectively by local excision. When an underlying adenocarcinoma is present,

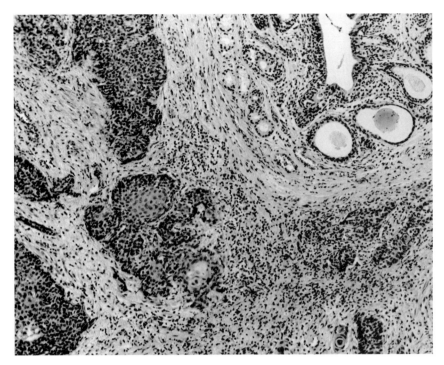

Figure 293
SQUAMOUS CELL
CARCINOMA OF
BARTHOLIN GLAND
Portions of the gland and duct lie adjacent to a squamous cell carcinoma. The tumor is associated with a moderate inflammatory infiltrate in the stroma.

the prognosis is related to the stage of the tumor and the status of the regional lymph nodes. The prognosis is usually poor.

Bartholin Gland Tumors

Definition. The criteria for the diagnosis of a tumor of Bartholin gland origin are that the neoplasm must 1) arise at the site of the Bartholin gland, 2) be consistent histologically with a primary neoplasm of the Bartholin gland, and 3) not be metastatic (104,160).

General Features. A wide variety of tumors may arise from the Bartholin gland. Adenocarcinomas account for approximately 40 percent of them, but others include squamous cell carcinoma (40 percent), adenoid cystic carcinoma (15 percent), transitional cell carcinoma (less than 5 percent), adenosquamous carcinoma (less than 5 percent), and poorly differentiated adenocarcinomas (104,160).

Clinical Features. Carcinoma of Bartholin gland usually presents as an enlargement in the gland area and may be mistaken for a cyst (144). The average age of women with this tumor is 50 years, with a majority of them between 40 and 70 years of age.

Gross Findings. Bartholin gland tumors are typically solid, deeply infiltrative, and occupy the site of the gland, occasionally obscuring its presence. They range in size from 1 to 7 cm in diameter.

Microscopic Findings. Adenocarcinomas of Bartholin gland are usually nonspecific in appearance, but mucinous and papillary types have been described (104). The tumors usually contain intracytoplasmic mucin and are immunoreactive for CEA (135,137). The differential diagnosis of the Bartholin gland adenocarcinoma includes adenocarcinoma of skin appendage origin and metastatic adenocarcinoma. These tumors typically do not involve the Bartholin gland and the tumor type may not be consistent with a primary tumor of the Bartholin gland.

Squamous cell carcinomas arising in the Bartholin gland have the same microscopic appearance as those arising elsewhere in the vulva (fig. 293). These tumors typically contain immunoreactive CEA (136).

Adenoid cystic carcinomas arising in the Bartholin gland are similar to those occurring in salivary glands, the upper respiratory tract, and skin. The tumor is composed of uniform, small cells arranged in cords and nests with a cribriform pattern. Variable-sized cysts filled with an amphophilic or eosinophilic acellular basement membrane–like material (96) may also be encountered (figs. 294, 295). Keratin and S-100 antigen are detectable by immunohistochemical techniques (135). The S-100 reactivity may demonstrate a myoepithelial cell element. Ultrastructural features include basement membrane–like material within the cysts (128). The differential diagnosis of adenoid cystic carcinomas includes adenocarcinoma, basal cell carcinoma, metastatic atypical carcinoid, and small cell carcinoma. Adenocarcinomas lack the uniform acinar arrangement and intraluminal basement membrane material of adenoid cystic carcinoma. Basal cell carcinomas are more solid, and lack the cystic spaces and the intracystic basement membrane–like material. Metastatic carcinoids and small cell carcinomas are more solid, have fewer lumens, contain argyrophil cells, and stain for neuron-specific enolase in most cases. Carcinoids almost always react with antibodies against chromogranin and other neuroendocrine markers.

Adenosquamous carcinomas of Bartholin gland contain a mixture of squamous cells identified by keratin formation and intracellular bridges and glandular cells that typically contain mucin (127,154).

Transitional cell carcinomas arising in the Bartholin gland are composed of uniform polyhedral or rounded epithelial cells often lining broad papillary fronds. Rare areas of glandular or squamous differentiation may be found. The differential diagnosis includes poorly differentiated squamous cell carcinoma and adenocarcinoma. If more than rare foci contain glands or show keratinization, the tumor is of mixed cell types and should be so designated with a listing of the different tumor types.

Clinical Behavior and Treatment. Approximately 20 percent of carcinomas of Bartholin gland are associated with metastases to the inguinal-femoral lymph nodes.

The primary treatment for a Bartholin gland carcinoma is wide excision to the fascia, radical

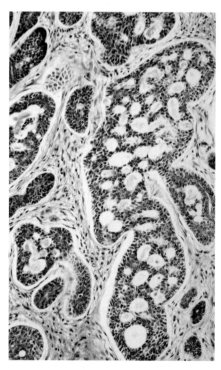

Figure 294
ADENOID CYSTIC CARCINOMA
OF BARTHOLIN GLAND
The tumor is composed of groups of tumor cells with a cylindromatous pattern.

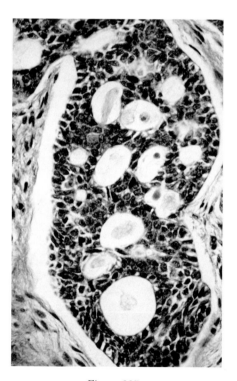

Figure 295
ADENOID CYSTIC CARCINOMA
OF BARTHOLIN GLAND
The tumor cells are small and uniform. Acellular material is seen within the rounded spaces.

hemivulvectomy, or total vulvectomy. Ipsilateral or bilateral inguinal-femoral lymph node dissection is necessary, regardless of the type of primary excision (107,130,155). Adjunctive radiation therapy to the vulva and regional lymph nodes has also been advocated (107).

The 5-year survival of patients with Bartholin gland carcinomas is approximately 50 percent when the groin nodes are free of tumor, but decreases to 18 percent when two or more nodes are involved (104,130,155). If the groin nodes are involved there is a 20 percent probability that pelvic lymph node metastasis will also be present, but if they are free of metastasis, there is essentially no risk of pelvic node metastasis (104).

Therapy for adenoid cystic carcinoma of Bartholin gland is wide local excision with ipsilateral inguinal-femoral lymphadenectomy (108). There is sufficient evidence to state that survival is better with adenoid cystic carcinoma than with other forms of carcinoma of Bartholin gland.

The treatment of vulvar adenosquamous carcinoma is similar to that of squamous cell carcinoma (154). Adenosquamous carcinomas have a poorer prognosis than squamous cell carcinomas, with a reported 5-year survival of 66 percent. The poorer prognosis is in part related to the higher frequency of lymph node metastasis.

Breast Carcinoma and Other Tumors Arising in Ectopic Mammary Tissue

Ectopic breast tissue within the vulva is infrequent even though the vulva is within the milk line (fig. 296). The ectopic breast tissue is usually identified during pregnancy when enlargement due to lactational changes occurs (fig. 297). Occasionally a neoplasm develops in otherwise clinically unnoticed breast tissue (117). Both benign and malignant tumors, as well as fibrocystic disease, have been described within the ectopic breast tissue (105,143).

Fibroadenomas are distinguished from hidradenomas of sweat gland origin by the findings of adjacent ectopic breast tissue and the characteristic features of a fibroadenoma (112). Intraductal papillomas may mimic hidradenoma to the degree that the two cannot be distinguished (143). Lactating adenomas have also been described (140).

Only a few cases of adenocarcinoma of ectopic vulvar breast tissue have been reported (105, 121,148). These tumors have histopathologic features identical to those of breast adenocarcinomas and have been associated with breast adenocarcinoma (121). Most of them are infiltrating ductal carcinomas. In some cases an intraductal carcinoma component has been identified. Metastasis to inguinal lymph nodes from adenocarcinoma of vulvar ectopic breast tissue has been observed (105). These adenocarcinomas contain secretory material similar to that of breast adenocarcinomas, including α-lactalbumin and milk fat globule protein, and may contain estrogen and progesterone receptors as well (105,148). Cystosarcoma phyllodes of ectopic vulvar breast tissue has also been described (figs. 298, 299) (134).

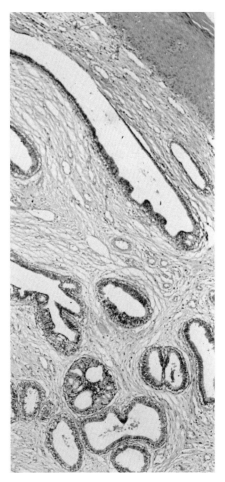

Figure 296
ECTOPIC BREAST TISSUE IN THE VULVA
The breast tissue is composed predominately of ducts, some of which are hyperplastic.

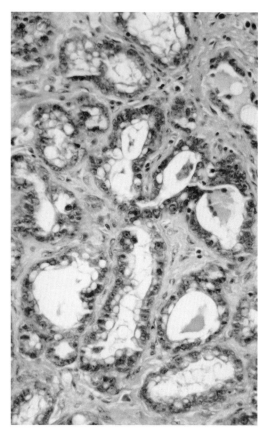

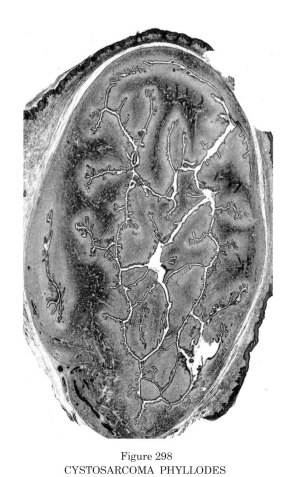

Figure 297
LACTATING BREAST TISSUE IN THE VULVA
The acini contain inspissated secretion and are lined by vacuolated epithelium.

Figure 298
CYSTOSARCOMA PHYLLODES
IN ECTOPIC BREAST TISSUE
The tumor is well circumscribed, has a leaf-like papillary growth, and elevates the overlying surface epithelium and superficial dermis.

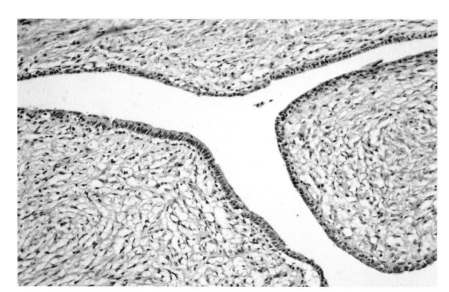

Figure 299
CYSTOSARCOMA
PHYLLODES IN
ECTOPIC BREAST TISSUE
Relatively bland epithelium covers a highly cellular and somewhat myxoid stromal component.

Metastatic carcinoma may be difficult to exclude, but if breast tissue or in situ carcinoma is also evident, the lesion is a primary carcinoma of ectopic breast tissue. Unlike carcinomas arising in ectopic breast tissue, metastatic carcinomas to the vulva are not associated with adjacent breast tissue and are usually larger (97,131).

Ectopic breast tissue within the vulva may need to be excised if it results in a symptomatic mass when the patient is not pregnant. The development of a malignant tumor within ectopic breast tissue requires a radical surgical operation, either total vulvectomy or radical wide local excision and inguinal-femoral lymphadenectomy.

Carcinomas of Sweat Gland Origin

Carcinomas of sweat glands account for less than 1 percent of all vulvar cancers. Wick et al. (156) have described ductal eccrine adenocarcinoma, eccrine porocarcinoma, and clear cell hidradenocarcinoma of the vulva. A number of vulvar apocrine carcinomas have been associated with vulvar Paget disease (134). Apocrine carcinoma is composed of tumor cells with the distinctive eosinophilic granular cytoplasm of the cells of origin, and may be associated with apocrine decapitation type secretion. The tumor may have solid, glandular, or papillary areas. Nuclear pleomorphism and hyperchromasia are present.

Other Adenocarcinomas

Rare adenocarcinomas of the vulva may arise from Skene glands (151) or ectopic cloacal tissue (153).

BENIGN MESENCHYMAL TUMORS

These tumors are not specific for the vulva, occurring more often in other sites. Brief descriptions follow; for more detailed discussions, the reader is referred to other references on soft tissue tumors.

Lipoma/Fibrolipoma

A lipoma is a benign tumor composed of mature adipocytes. When the tumor contains prominent fibroblasts and collagen, it is termed a fibrolipoma.

Lipomas of the vulva are rare and are typically encountered in adults, usually presenting as soft, circumscribed masses of variable size in the labium majus. They grow slowly and may present with hemorrhagic infarction or surface ulceration. On microscopic examination, lipomas are composed of mature adipocytes supported by fibrovascular tissue. Adipocytes contain S-100 antigen (180). Pleomorphic and spindle cell variants of vulvar lipoma, as well as malignant change, have not been reported to date. Adipose tissue may be seen within the dermis in nevus lipomatous superficialis (see fig. 331). In contrast to a lipoma, the adipose tissue in nevus lipomatous superficialis is limited to the superficial dermis and distinct from the underlying subcutaneous fat.

Hemangioma

Hemangiomas are benign tumors composed of blood vessels. Hemangiomas of the vulva may occur at any age, but specific types are usually confined to either the very young or old patient. Clinically significant hemangiomas are rare in the vulva (170). Hemangiomas generally regress spontaneously and therefore require no treatment; bleeding or symptoms related to ulceration or trauma may require therapy (170).

Capillary Hemangioma (Strawberry Hemangioma, Juvenile Hemangioma). This form of hemangioma is most commonly encountered in infants and young children. It presents as a soft red to violaceous, slightly raised, well-demarcated lesion. Usually it does not exceed 1 cm in diameter. It occasionally bleeds due to ulceration or trauma. The clinical appearance of this lesion is usually sufficiently typical to make biopsy unnecessary. Because it usually regresses spontaneously, therapy is rarely necessary. Microscopic examination discloses a well-circumscribed mass composed of a dense aggregate of capillaries.

Cavernous Hemangioma. Cavernous hemangiomas are rare on the vulva. They are typically deeper, more complex, and larger than capillary hemangiomas. Pelvic involvement by hemangiomas may be a concurrent finding (183). Biopsy is not indicated unless ulceration or other clinical features suggest malignancy. Cavernous hemangioma of the clitoris may mimic clitoral hypertrophy (176), raising the question of the adrenogenital syndrome in a young child.

Acquired Hemangioma. Vulvar acquired hemangioma of adults typically occurs in older women and is relatively common, although rarely biopsied. It usually presents as multiple, 1 to 3 mm, purple to red, asymptomatic papules on the lateral aspects of the labia majora. On microscopic examination the mass is well-circumscribed and is composed of aggregated capillaries, some of which may be dilated.

Differential Diagnosis. The differential diagnosis of hemangiomas includes angiokeratoma, pyogenic granuloma, bacterial angiomatosis, hemangiopericytoma, angiosarcoma, and Kaposi sarcoma (165,166,180). Angiokeratomas are warty or polypoid lesions characterized by an acanthotic, slightly hyperkeratotic epidermis overlying dilated capillary spaces. Pyogenic granuloma is superficial, resembles granulation tissue, and has a distinctive collarette of elevated epithelium around it. Bacterial angiomatosis containing the *Rochalimaea henselae* bacteria within the lesion that can be identified by a Warthin-Starry stain (165,185a). Hemangiopericytomas are solid vascular tumors, with a distinctive perivascular pericyte proliferation, demonstrated by a reticulin stain. Kaposi sarcoma is a malignant vascular tumor that has distinctive slit-like spaces containing red blood cells surrounded by malignant spindle cells.

Angiokeratoma

Angiokeratomas are commonly identified on the vulva of women of childbearing age and tend to be warty or polypoid. They are usually slightly larger than acquired hemangiomas and may occur as solitary or multiple lesions. Histological examination reveals superficial vascular channels that lie adjacent to the basal cells of the overlying epithelium (fig. 300). The epithelium is often acanthotic and hyperkeratotic (162,172). Angiokeratomas do not require therapy unless they become symptomatic.

Pyogenic Granuloma

Pyogenic granuloma is a solitary, rapidly growing, raised vascular lesion considered to be exuberant granulation tissue with features of a benign neoplasm. It is rare on the vulva, usually occurring during gestation. Microscopic examination shows a lobulated capillary hemangioma composed of multiple small endothelial-lined vessels. A prominent inflammatory cell infiltrate may be seen, especially near the surface, when ulceration or secondary infection is present. The

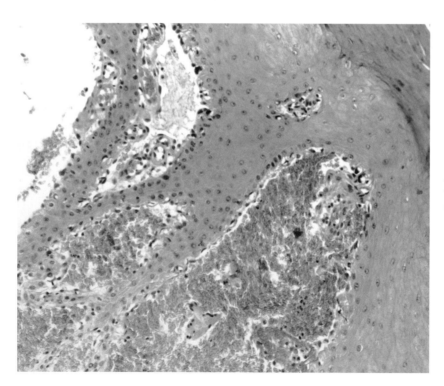

Figure 300
ANGIOKERATOMA
Prominent dilated blood-filled vessels are present immediately below the overlying, slightly thickened parakeratotic epithelium.

surface epithelium may proliferate with downward growth forming a "collarette" around the lesion. Excisional biopsy is therapeutic.

Lymphangioma

Lymphangiomas of the vulva are rare; they may be congenital or acquired. When congenital they may be associated with lymphangiomas of the lower extremities. Congenital lymphangiomas may be large and cavernous with deep lymphatic involvement (173). Acquired vulvar lymphangioma may occur after pelvic radiation therapy (191).

Lymphangiomas are composed of variably-sized endothelial-lined spaces that contain lymph and generally lack a muscular wall (fig. 301). Delicate fibrous connective tissue supports

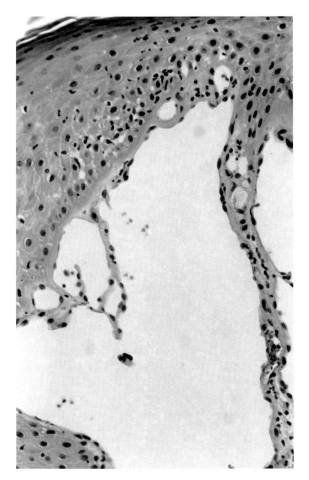

Figure 301
LYMPHANGIOMA
Lymphatic spaces of various sizes lie beneath the squamous epithelium.

the endothelial-lined spaces. Hemangiomas (see above) are the main lesion in the differential diagnosis of lymphangiomas.

Surgical excision is applicable in selected cases, but no type of treatment is uniformly effective. Late local recurrence is not uncommon because of the difficulty of complete resection. Secondary infection is a serious complication.

Fibroma

The fibroma is a relatively rare benign tumor of the vulva. It usually arises from the deeper fibrous tissue of the introitus, the perineal body, or the round ligament. Although fibromas may become very large, they rarely exceed 8 cm in diameter. Infarction or hemorrhage may be associated with pain and rapid enlargement of the tumor. The overlying skin is not attached to the fibroma and is usually similar in appearance to the adjacent vulvar skin. Malignant transformation is rare.

Histologic features include fibrocytes arranged in parallel and interlacing bundles. Cystic, hemorrhagic, hyaline, and myxomatous changes may be observed (180). The differential diagnosis includes a number of benign tumors and tumor-like lesions including fibroepithelial polyp, aggressive desmoid tumor (177), nodular fasciitis (169,180,182), leiomyoma dermatofibroma (174) or fibrous histiocytoma, neurofibroma, Schwannoma, and postoperative spindle cell nodule (184). Treatment is local excision.

Leiomyoma

Leiomyomas of the vulva arise from smooth muscle of blood vessels, erectile tissue, and erector pili muscles. Solitary leiomyomas rarely exceed 7 cm in diameter. Although considered the most common of the soft tissue neoplasms of the vulva, the tumors are relatively rare.

Microscopic Findings. Microscopically the tumor is composed of interlacing fascicles of smooth muscle (fig. 302). The smooth muscle cells have prominent eosinophilic cytoplasm with poorly defined cell borders. The nuclei are oval with rounded rather than pointed poles. A number of associated microscopic changes have been observed in vulvar leiomyomas including a myxoid change in pregnancy (174,188).

The smooth muscle cells of a leiomyoma are immunoreactive for desmin, myosin, and actin and are distinguished from rhabdomyoma in that they do not contain myoglobin. Epithelioid leiomyoma of the vulva has been reported (fig. 303) (161). The major differential diagnosis of leiomyoma is leiomyosarcoma, which can be distinguished by its cellular atypia, a mitotic rate of more than 5 mitotic figures per 10 high-power fields and an infiltrative growth pattern (188). Therapy for primary or recurrent vulvar leiomyoma is wide local excision because leiomyosarcoma cannot be excluded until multiple sections of the tumor are studied microscopically (188) (see Leiomyosarcoma).

Granular Cell Tumor

Approximately 7 percent of all granular cell tumors occur in the vulva. This is a tumor of peripheral nerve sheath origin which is usually benign. However, regional and pulmonary metastases from a malignant granular cell tumor that was ultimately fatal were reported in a 32-year-old woman (181).

These tumors may arise in the vulva of children or adults and present as painless subcutaneous nodules. They usually are under 3 cm in diameter (163,179). They may occur on the mons pubis or in the labia majora or clitoris. In the latter location they may mimic clitoral hypertrophy (167,190). Priapism of the crus of the clitoris has been reported secondary to a locally aggressive granular cell tumor (187). Granular cell tumors, when all sites are included, are multiple in 10 to 15 percent of cases (180).

Microscopic examination reveals a nonencapsulated mass with an infiltrative margin; perineural involvement may occur (180). The tumor cells are large and polyhedral, with abundant eosinophilic granular cytoplasm. The cell borders are indistinct and groups of cells are often separated by a small amount of hyalinized stroma (figs. 304, 325).

The nuclei are small and uniform. No unique morphologic features were found in the granular cell tumor with pulmonary metastasis (181). In approximately 25 percent of the cases the overlying epithelium exhibits pseudoepitheliomatous hyperplasia, which may mimic squamous cell carcinoma if the biopsy is not sufficiently deep to include the underlying granular cell tumor (see fig. 325) (190).

The cells of the granular cell tumor are immunoreactive for S-100 antigen, myelin basic proteins

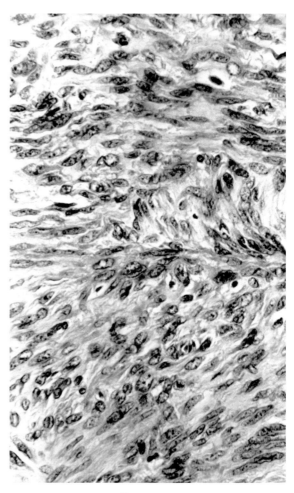

Figure 302
LEIOMYOMA
The tumor is composed of spindle cells arranged in swirling and interlacing patterns.

PO and P2, lectin, and carcinoembryonic antigen (180,185). The differential diagnosis includes superficially invasive squamous cell carcinoma, metastatic carcinoma, and xanthogranulomatous inflammation. A positive mucin stain may help distinguish metastatic carcinoma although the bland, small uniform nuclei of the granular cells are usually quite distinct from metastatic carcinoma cells. Xanthogranulomatous inflammation differs in the more variable size of the histiocytes, an absence of prominent cytoplasmic granules, the presence of scattered inflammatory cells, and an absence of S-100 positivity. The treatment of choice for granular cell tumors, primary and recurrent, is wide local excision.

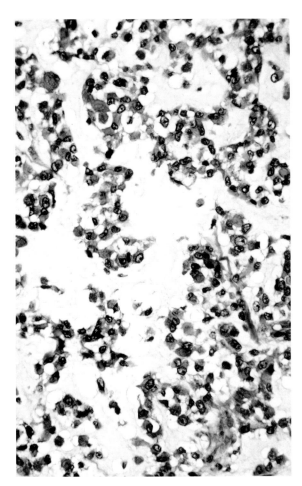

Figure 303
EPITHELIOID LEIOMYOMA
This tumor is composed of rounded smooth muscle cells.

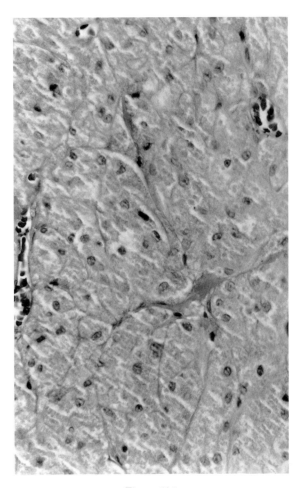

Figure 304
GRANULAR CELL TUMOR
The tumor cells have abundant granular cytoplasm and relatively small uniform nuclei. A delicate fibrovascular stroma separates groups of tumor cells.

Neurofibroma

Definition. A benign tumor of nerve sheath origin, which may be solitary or multiple and is associated with the inherited disorder von Recklinghausen disease.

General Features. Nearly half of the neurofibromas arising within the vulva occur in women with von Recklinghausen neurofibromatosis. The tumors are polyclonal in origin when associated with von Recklinghausen disease, whereas neurofibromas from normal individuals are monoclonal. Eighteen percent of women with neurofibromatosis have neurofibromas of the vulva (168,186). These painless tumors are rare before puberty, but rapid growth may occur thereafter. Growth at puberty may be related to the presence of estrogen and progesterone receptors in the tumors (164). The tumors usually do not exceed 3 cm in diameter, but may attain a diameter of 25 cm (189).

Microscopic Findings. On microscopic examination neurofibromas are composed of spindle-shaped cells arranged in bundles that, when cut on the long axis, exhibit a distinctive wave-like whorled appearance. The cells have indistinct cell borders and may be associated with strands of collagen and mast cells. The nuclei are usually small with somewhat pointed poles and may have a wavy appearance. Occasionally, large bizarre hyperchromatic nuclei are encountered. This feature is referred to as *ancient change* and is not an indication of malignant transformation (180).

Neurofibromas that involve the skin are not encapsulated and may infiltrate the dermis and the underlying fat. The presence of even 1 mitotic figure per 10 high-power fields is considered sufficient evidence for the diagnosis of a neurofibrosarcoma (180).

Differential Diagnosis. The differential diagnosis includes aggressive angiomyxoma, malignant schwannoma, fibroma, and fibrous histiocytoma. Aggressive angiomyxomas have clustered arteries within a myxoid stroma and are poorly circumscribed. Malignant schwannomas are highly cellular with a high mitotic count. In addition, nuclear palisading is distinctive and heterologous elements may be found. Neurofibromas are immunoreactive for S-100 antigen, whereas fibromas lack S-100 immunoreactivity, as do fibrous histiocy-tomas, which are rich in α-1-antichymotrypsin.

Small vulvar neurofibromas associated with neurofibromatosis do not require treatment. Enlarging or symptomatic tumors are surgically excised (168). Although neurofibromas are benign, malignant transformation occasionally occurs in von Recklinghausen disease.

Schwannoma (Neurilemmoma)

Schwannomas of the vulva are usually solitary and encapsulated, and may involve the clitoris, mimicking clitoral hypertrophy (171). They characteristically exhibit both cellular and hypocellular areas. The cellular (Antoni type A) areas contain spindle cells with elongated or oval nuclei that are palisaded and often have a wavy appearance. Mitotic figures are usually rare, but may be observed in low numbers within the cellular areas. The cytoplasm is fibrillar with poorly defined cell borders. Verocay bodies are commonly observed in these areas and form as a result of alignment of the nuclei in rows separated by acellular zones. The hypocellular (Antoni type B) areas may contain spindle cells, small cells with hyperchromatic nuclei, and histiocytes filled with lipid vacuoles. Collagen fibers and mast cells are also usually seen. The hypocellular areas are typically myxomatous and occasionally cystic. Schwannomas must be differentiated from leiomyomas. Like neurofibromas, schwannomas contain S-100 protein and lack desmin (see Malignant Schwannoma).

Glomus Tumor

The glomus tumor presents as a painful solitary tumor, usually less than 4 cm in diameter. It may cause severe introital dyspareunia (175,178) with pain characteristically localized to the tumor nodule.

On microscopic examination glomus tumors are composed of epithelioid-appearing cells, which may be of smooth muscle or pericyte origin, and are arranged in lobules about vascular channels. The surrounding hyalinized stroma contains mast cells as well as identifiable nerve elements.

Fibrous Histiocytoma

This benign tumor of fibrohistiocytic origin has also been referred to as dermatofibroma, subepidermal nodular fibrosis, histiocytoma, or sclerosing hemangioma, but the term fibrous histiocytoma is preferred. This neoplasm is rare on the vulva and presents as a solitary pigmented subcutaneous nodule. Microscopically, the cells are arranged in a distinctive storiform pattern (fig. 305). Variable degrees of cellularity and collagenization occur. Mitotic activity is low or absent. Histiocytes, lymphocytes, and giant cells may be seen. This tumor is immunoreactive for α-1-antichymotrypsin (180).

Rhabdomyoma

Rhabdomyomas rarely occur in the vulva. They are usually polypoid and unencapsulated (fig. 306), and are composed of mature striated muscle cells (fig. 307).

MALIGNANT MESENCHYMAL TUMORS

As with the benign mesenchymal tumors, most of the malignant mesenchymal tumors involving the vulva occur more frequently at other sites. A brief discussion of these tumors follows. For a more complete discussion, the reader is referred to the referenced articles or to a comprehensive reference on soft tissue tumors.

Embryonal Rhabdomyosarcoma (Sarcoma Botryoides)

Definition. A malignant rhabdomyoblastic neoplasm which tends to grow in a distinctive polypoid manner.

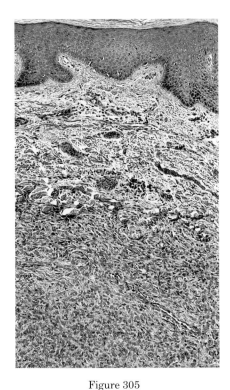

Figure 305
FIBROUS HISTIOCYTOMA
The tumor is composed of relatively uniformly shaped cells. It blends with and is confined to the dermis.

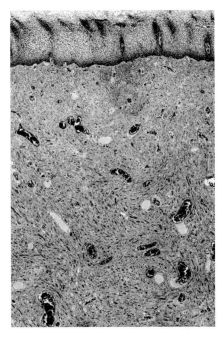

Figure 306
RHABDOMYOMA
The tumor is within the dermis, contains numerous moderately large vessels, and is composed of interlacing spindle-shaped cells.

General Features. Embryonal rhabdomyosarcoma is almost always encountered in infants and children and is rare in the vulva and vagina beyond 10 years of age. It usually arises from the labial or perineal area and presents with bleeding due to ulceration (201). Rhabdomyosarcoma of the vagina may involve the labia minora, in which case the tumor is classified as vaginal in origin. Rhabdomyosarcomas arising in the vulva are often of the alveolar rather than the embryonal type (202).

Gross Findings. Sarcoma botryoides may appear as a polypoid mass simulating a bunch of grapes although this appearance is more common for those arising in the vagina (see Tumors of the Vagina). In the vulva, the tumor presents as a solid mass.

Microscopic Findings. In the polypoid form, the tumor is covered by a thin layer of epithelium overlying edematous or myxoid hypercellular tissue, with a richly cellular subepithelial (cambium) layer. The tumor cells may invade the epithelium singly or in small groups. The round to spindle-shaped rhabdomyoblasts have prominent, dense,

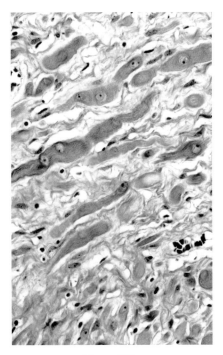

Figure 307
RHABDOMYOMA
Multinucleated mature striated muscle cells are seen within a fibrous stroma.

221

eosinophilic cytoplasm and relatively large, pleomorphic, and hyperchromatic nuclei. In addition, there are undifferentiated spindle-shaped cells with small nuclei and dense chromatin. In the vulva, the rhabdomyoblasts may occur in groups and may be associated with a prominent foamy histiocytic infiltrate that can obscure the typical histopathologic features (226). Cross striations are seen in less than 15 percent of cases (219). The myxoid areas may contain small round to spindle-shaped cells with small nuclei that lack nuclear atypia. Cystic degeneration may occur within the myxoid areas, resulting in a microcystic appearance (202).

Immunohistochemical Findings. The cytoplasm of the tumor cells can be immunoreactive for myoglobin, actin, myosin, desmin, and vimentin. Of these antigens, only myoglobin is specific for skeletal muscle but it is not always demonstrable (203). Actin and desmin are usually detectable but may also be absent.

Ultrastructural Findings. Electron microscopy can be of value in identifying cross striations in rhabdomyoblasts. Only 41 percent of tumors in one series contained both actin and myosin filaments, whereas actin filaments were identified in all the cases studied (219).

Clinical Behavior and Treatment. The tumor invades locally with late metastasis to regional lymph nodes, lungs, and distant sites. Recent therapeutic approaches have combined conservative surgery and chemotherapy. The overall 5-year survival has been reported to range from 25 to 50 percent (201,202), but results are improving with modern chemotherapy.

Aggressive Angiomyxoma

Although placed in the malignant category, it should be emphasized that this neoplasm is locally infiltrative but not malignant in the true sense. It is not a sarcoma. The tumor is composed of myofibroblastic cells, prominent blood vessels, and myxoid intercellular material. This tumor is rare and presents as a large mass that may mimic a Bartholin cyst. It may extend paravaginally into the pelvic floor or buttocks.

On gross examination the tumor has a uniform, soft, myxoid consistency and an ill-defined margin, although it may appear partially encapsulated. Microscopically, the tumor contains numerous blood vessels, particularly capillaries and medium-sized arteries with a thick muscle layer. The bulk of the tumor is composed of fibroblasts and myofibroblasts, which are spindle-shaped to stellate, with relatively small uniform nuclei containing dense chromatin (fig. 308). Mitotic figures and nuclear pleomorphism are absent. The tissue surrounding the cells appears myxoid in some areas and densely collagenous elsewhere. Epithelial elements have been described in aggressive angiomyxomas, with mucin-secreting columnar cells forming small glandular structures. Focally, cells are immunoreactive for muscle actin. The tumor does not contain cells that stain for carcinoembryonic antigen or keratin and only the endothelium of the blood vessels reacts with factor VIII–related antibodies (198).

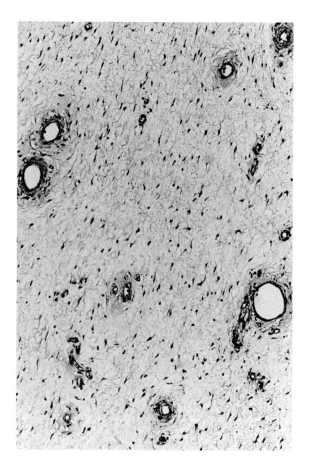

Figure 308
AGGRESSIVE ANGIOMYXOMA
The tumor is composed of myxoid stroma with prominent blood vessels of variable size. The vessels are typically clustered in some areas. (Courtesy of Dr. Philip Clement, Vancouver, British Columbia, Canada.)

The prominent arborizing small arteries distinguish aggressive angiomyxoma from intramuscular myxoma. The tumor entraps fat, but the absence of lipoblasts distinguishes it from liposarcoma. Neural elements may also be entrapped within the tumor, but the tumor lacks S-100 antigen, which is expected in a neurofibroma or schwannoma. The myxoid features may suggest myxoid malignant fibrous histiocytoma (MFH). Myxoid MFH may have a local infiltrative pattern similar to aggressive angiomyxoma. In contrast to aggressive angiomyxoma, myxoid MFH has both acellular myxoid areas rich in mucopolysaccharides and more cellular areas composed of spindle-shaped cells arranged in a storiform pattern. In addi-

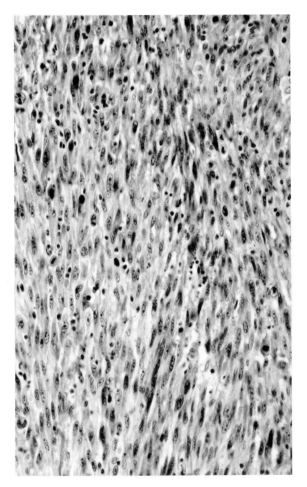

Figure 309
LEIOMYOSARCOMA
The tumor is composed of spindle-shaped cells with oval nuclei and prominent cytoplasm.

tion, the myxoid MFH has multinucleated giant cells, pleomorphic giant tumor cells, histiocytic cells with foamy cytoplasm, and inflammatory cells consisting mainly of lymphocytes. Immunohistochemical studies demonstrate reactivity with α-1-antichymotrypsin and α-1-antitrypsin.

The treatment of choice is wide local excision. Lymphadenectomy is not indicated. Local recurrence has been observed in approximately half the reported cases. Most recurrences occur within 3 to 4 years after excision; however, recurrence has been described as late as 14 years postoperatively (196,225). Successful reexcision of recurrences has been reported.

Leiomyosarcoma

General Features. Leiomyosarcoma of the vulva occurs predominantly in women of reproductive age but may also occur in postmenopausal women up to 66 years of age (227). Although rare, it is the most common sarcoma of the vulva (204). It arises in the labium majus, the Bartholin gland area, the clitoris, and the labium minus in decreasing order of frequency. It is usually 5 cm in diameter or larger when diagnosed. The clinical manifestations include pain and rapid growth.

Microscopic Findings. Microscopically, the tumor is composed of interlacing bundles of spindle-shaped cells with eosinophilic cytoplasm (figs. 309–311). When the cells are sectioned at right angles to their long axis, a perinuclear halo can usually be seen. Epithelioid varieties of leiomyosarcoma have been described in the vulva (227). Leiomyosarcomas can be distinguished from leiomyomas by differences in size, type of margin, cytological atypia, and mitotic activity. No single feature definitively establishes the diagnosis of sarcoma except for recurrence or metastasis. Leiomyosarcomas usually have mitotic counts exceeding 10 per 10 high-power fields (204). Smooth muscle tumors with infiltrative borders that have a mitotic rate exceeding 5 per 10 high-power fields have a higher rate of recurrence than tumors that are well circumscribed. Neoplasms that are 5 cm or greater in diameter also have a higher rate of recurrence than those less than 5 cm in diameter (204). A diagnosis of leiomyosarcoma is made if there is nuclear atypia and pleomorphism associated with a mitotic count greater than 5 per 10 high-power fields. If the tumor has no atypia, or only a slight

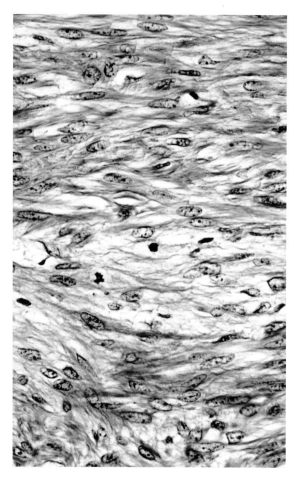

Figure 310
LEIOMYOSARCOMA
Mitotic figures are present; one of which is abnormal. The nuclei are pleomorphic and hyperchromatic.

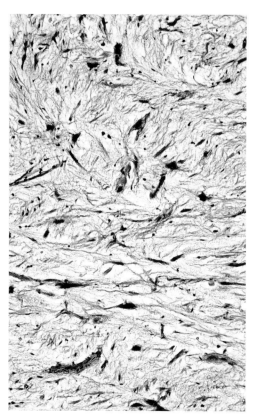

Figure 311
MYXOID LEIOMYOSARCOMA
The tumor is composed of cells with pleomorphic nuclei and a prominent myxoid stroma. Mitotic figures are rare. Adjacent smooth muscle elements, not pictured, and appropriate immuoperoxidase studies, assist in identifying tumors arising in smooth muscle.

degree of it, but has a diameter exceeding 5 cm, an infiltrative margin, and a mitotic figure count of 5 per 10 high-power fields or higher, the risk of recurrence is uncertain. It should be emphasized, however, that a rare variant, myxoid leiomyosarcoma (fig. 311) may have low mitotic counts but still behave in a malignant fashion. The immunohistochemical findings are the same as those for leiomyomas.

Clinical Behavior and Treatment. Leiomyosarcoma of the vulva tends to recur locally and the growth pattern is highly variable. Pulmonary, hepatic, and other distant metastases may occur (192,204,205). Wide local excision, or vulvectomy, is the initial treatment of choice if the tumor is confined to the vulva (192).

Dermatofibrosarcoma Protuberans

Definition. A cutaneous tumor of low-grade malignancy which has fibrohistiocytic features.

General Features. This tumor, which is relatively rare in the vulva, typically presents in young or middle-aged adults as a subcutaneous nodule. It tends to grow slowly but may exhibit rapid growth during pregnancy. Satellite nodules and metastasis may occur in advanced cases (fig. 312).

Gross Findings. These tumors average 5 cm in diameter, and often the overlying surface epithelium is pigmented or ulcerated.

Microscopic Findings. The tumor diffusely infiltrates the dermis and may invade the epidermis with resultant ulceration (214). Invasion of the subcutaneous fat may be seen. Satellite nodules may be present.

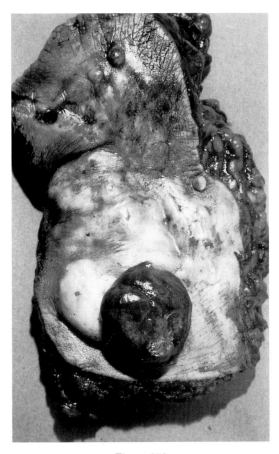

Figure 312
DERMATOFIBROSARCOMA
PROTUBERANS
A large, nodular mass and multiple small satellite nodules are evident.

The fibroblast-like cells are arranged in a distinctive storiform pattern, which is most readily apparent near the center of the tumor. Peripherally the cells may appear bland and relatively uniform, but centrally some nuclear pleomorphism and atypia with moderate numbers of mitotic figures may be evident.

Clinical Behavior and Treatment. Wide local excision is the treatment of choice. Local recurrence, regional and distant lymph node involvement, and pulmonary metastasis rarely occur.

Malignant Fibrous Histiocytoma

Definition. A malignant neoplasm that arises from histiocytes that have undergone fibroblastic differentiation.

General Features. This tumor, although rare on the vulva, is the second most common sarcoma in this site (204). It usually presents as a large solitary mass in middle-aged women (211,228).

Gross Findings. Malignant fibrous histiocytoma (MFH) is typically a solid tumor which is white to yellow on section. Areas of necrosis and focal hemorrhage may be seen.

Microscopic Findings. MFH is characterized by infiltrative growth and marked nuclear pleomorphism with giant cells and multinucleated cells. Cells with large nuclei containing multiple prominent nucleoli and abundant eosinophilic cytoplasm are admixed with smaller round to spindle-shaped cells with moderate nuclear pleomorphism. Mitotic figures are usually present and commonly atypical. The spindle cells may be arranged in a storiform pattern or in interlacing bundles.

Subtypes. The most commonly described variants are an inflammatory type, which contains many acute inflammatory cells; a giant cell variant (giant cell tumor of soft parts), which contains giant cells with osteoclast-like features but no osteoid or bone; a myxoid variant containing a prominent hypocellular myxoid component; and an angiomatoid variant containing prominent blood vessels and blood-filled spaces (212,233,234).

Immunohistochemical Findings. The cells of MFH usually contain α-1-antitrypsin and α-1-antichymotrypsin, one or both of which can be identified in approximately 80 percent of cases (216).

Clinical Behavior and Treatment. Characteristically, MFH is locally invasive. Involvement of the underlying fascia increases the risk of local or distant metastasis (204,233). The treatment is wide local excision or radical vulvectomy. Lymphadenectomy is reserved for those cases with clinical evidence of regional node involvement. Postoperative radiotherapy is believed of value in reducing local recurrence. An insufficient number of cases have been described in the vulva to permit a definitive statement about the prognosis, but approximately half of the patients reported have had recurrences or died of metastatic disease.

Epithelioid Sarcoma

This sarcoma, which is composed of large rounded cells resembling squamous epithelial cells, is rare in the vulva, arising in the labia majora and subclitoral areas (206,210,222,231). The tumor usually originates in the reticular dermis, but may arise in deeper soft tissue.

The tumor has a granuloma-like appearance, with nodules composed of epithelial-appearing tumor cells and areas of necrosis (fig. 313). The tumor cells have eosinophilic cytoplasm and moderately pleomorphic nuclei. Metaplastic bone and cartilage may be present. The most difficult differential diagnosis is with squamous cell carcinoma and malignant rhabdoid tumor. In contrast to squamous cell carcinoma, epithelioid sarcoma lacks keratinization, intracellular bridges, and an intraepithelial component. The differential features of malignant rhabdoid tumor are summarized below.

Immunohistochemical studies have identified cytokeratin within these tumors. The immunoreactivity is similar to that of synovial sarcoma, supporting a common origin of the two tumors (199). The presence of cytokeratin distinguishes these tumors from histiocytic and inflammatory conditions (214,218).

The treatment is wide excision with regional lymphadenectomy and local radiation therapy. The tumor may recur locally, but it rarely metastasizes to distant sites (221).

Malignant Rhabdoid Tumor

This is a rare soft tissue malignant neoplasm of uncertain origin. It has been reported presenting as a labial subcutaneous mass, resembling a Bartholin abscess, in young women of reproductive age (221).

Gross Findings. The tumor is typically multinodular and firm, with poorly defined margins. It is found deep within the subcutaneous tissue. In the vulva the tumor may be under 2 cm in diameter, however, there are insufficient cases in this site to determine the size range.

Microscopic Findings. The tumor may be solid or have an alveolar growth pattern. It contains lobulated aggregates of cells that invade the subcutaneous tissue and dermis, often in a finger-like pattern (figs. 314, 315). Areas of hemorrhage within the stroma may give an angiomatoid appearance. The tumor cells are large and polygonal, with eccentric vesicular nuclei and prominent nucleoli. The nuclei are pleomorphic and mitoses are common. The cytoplasm is eosinophilic, resembling that of rhabdomyoblasts or squamous carci-

noma. Eosinophilic cytoplasmic inclusions are present, some of which indent the nucleus and give the cells a signet-ring appearance. Electron microscopy demonstrates that these inclusions are composed of intermediate filaments.

Immunohistochemical Findings. Immunohistochemical findings are essentially the same as those found in epithelioid sarcoma. Both tumors are immunoreactive for cytokeratin (AE 1/3, MAK 6, CAM 5.2) and epithelial membrane antigen. They both may also contain human milk fat globulin-2 and CEA. Actin may be weakly immunoreactive or absent and desmin and S-100 antigen are absent (221).

Differential Diagnosis. Distinction between epithelioid sarcoma and malignant rhabdoid tumor depends on light microscopic identification of the lobulated architecture of the rhabdoid

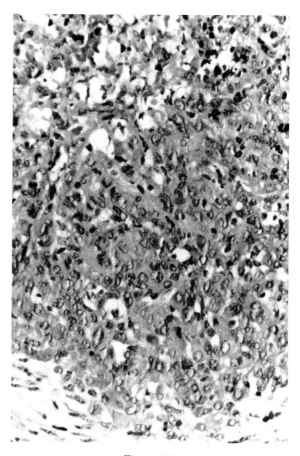

Figure 313
EPITHELIOID SARCOMA
The tumor is composed of loosely cohesive, round, epithelial-like cells. (Courtesy of Dr. T. Perrone, St. Louis, MO.)

tumor, the absence of necrosis, and the granulomatous appearance of epithelioid sarcoma. The typical large tumor cells, containing cytoplasmic inclusions and pleomorphic nuclei, are not present in epithelioid sarcoma. Electron microscopy does not assist in the differential diagnosis unless the character of cytoplasmic inclusions is in question, then the presence or absence of intermediate filaments within the inclusions can be determined (221).

The distinction is important regarding therapy because epithelioid sarcomas are relatively indolent and can be treated by wide local extended excision, whereas malignant rhabdoid tumors are aggressive and may metastasize. Although only a few cases have been reported, extended wide local excision to the fascia, or total vulvectomy, with bilateral inguinal-femoral lymphadenectomy, appears to be the initial surgical procedure of choice.

Malignant Schwannoma

Malignant schwannomas have been reported to involve the labia minora, labia majora, and other vulvar sites. They occur almost exclusively in women of reproductive age. Approximately half of the patients also have neurofibromas or von Recklinghausen disease (204,205,213,230). On gross examination these tumors have a homogeneous fibrous-appearing cut surface. A nerve trunk may be attached to the tumor.

Malignant schwannomas are highly cellular with numerous mitotic figures. Although the tumor may be predominantly fibrohistiocytic, nuclear palisading is usually present. Heterologous elements including cartilage, glandular epithelium,

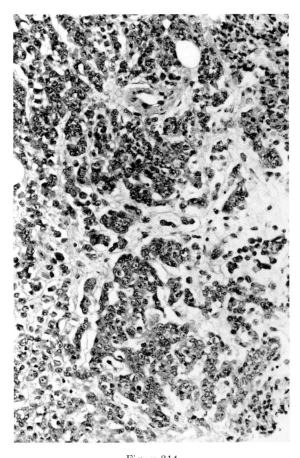

Figure 314
MALIGNANT RHABDOID TUMOR
Cords and nests of cells growing in a finger-like pattern. (Courtesy of Dr. T. Perrone, St. Louis, MO.)

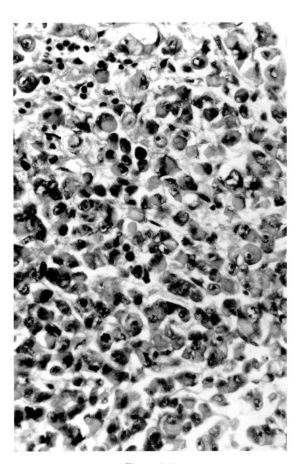

Figure 315
MALIGNANT RHABDOID TUMOR
The tumor cells are large and polygonal with prominent eosinophilic cytoplasm. Nuclei are eccentric and vesicular with prominent nucleoli. Eosinophilic cytoplasmic inclusions are present, indenting some nuclei. (Courtesy of Dr. T. Perrone, St. Louis, MO.)

and striated muscle may be found. The tumor is immunoreactive for S-100 protein in approximately half the cases (235). Electron microscopy may be helpful in establishing the diagnosis (214,229). Branching nontapered cytoplasmic processes of the spindle-shaped cells contain microtubules. The basal lamina may be poorly formed and collagen may be present in the adjacent matrix.

Therapy is wide local excision including the fascia. Regional lymphadenectomy is of little value and radiotherapy is thought to be ineffective (230). Although the prognosis cannot be determined accurately because of the limited number of reported cases, pulmonary metastasis has occurred in some patients.

Angiosarcoma

Angiosarcomas occur in the vulva as deep red masses with infiltrative margins (204). Perianal angiosarcomas have been described after pelvic radiotherapy (215). Angiosarcomas are composed of variable-sized slit-like vessels that extensively anastomose. The tumor cells have enlarged, pleomorphic, hyperchromatic nuclei with mitotic activity. In poorly differentiated areas the tumor may appear solid. Factor VIII and *Ulex europaeus* lectin antigen can be demonstrated in the tumor cells immunohistochemically (209,217). These antigens may not be demonstrable in poorly differentiated tumors.

Kaposi Sarcoma

Kaposi sarcoma has been described in the vulva of an elderly woman after radiation therapy (214). The tumor typically presents as one or more violaceous skin nodules. Microscopic examination reveals a spindle cell proliferation with slit-like spaces containing red blood cells. The spaces usually interconnect. Many of the neoplastic cells of Kaposi sarcomas are immunoreactive for factor VIII and *Ulex europaeus* lectin antigen. Desmin has also been reported in the tumor cells (194,195). Kaposi sarcoma must be distinguished from bacillary angiomatosis, which may have a clinical presentation and morphologic features similar to Kaposi sarcoma, but a Warthin-Starry stain demonstrates bacteria within bacillary angiomatosis (200). The bacteria has been characterized and named *Rochalimaea henselae* (185a).

Hemangiopericytoma

Hemangiopericytoma is a rare primary tumor of the vulva (204,223,236). It is composed of small, relatively uniform, spindle-shaped pericytes associated with a complex capillary component. The vessels have a stellate or staghorn arrangement. Reticulin stains demonstrate that the tumor cells lie external to the vascular spaces and are individually invested by fibrils. Significant cellular atypia is unusual. Hemangiopericytomas may resemble monophasic synovial sarcomas or angiosarcomas.

Electron microscopy and immunohistochemical studies are valuable in assisting in the diagnosis. The pericytes in these tumors do not contain factor VIII, cytokeratins, or S-100 antigen (214). Benign hemangiopericytomas tend to be small, have a mitotic count of less than 4 per 10 high-power fields, and lack areas of necrosis or hemorrhage (214). A malignant vulvar hemangiopericytoma has been reported to have metastasized to the femur (223).

Liposarcoma

Liposarcoma is rare on the vulva (207). Well-differentiated liposarcomas are composed of neoplastic adipocytes, some of which contain atypical nuclei arranged in poorly defined lobules (207,208). Myxoid liposarcomas are myxoid sarcomas containing lipoblasts and supported by a "chicken wire" vascular framework (197). The tumor cell nuclei are uniform in size and shape. The round cell liposarcoma is cellular, and the cytoplasm of most of the cells is eosinophilic. Some liposarcomas are immunoreactive for S-100 antigen.

Alveolar Soft-Part Sarcoma

Alveolar soft-part sarcoma is composed of loosely arranged groups of epithelial-like cells with prominent granular eosinophilic cytoplasm arranged in an alveolar pattern (224). The tumor cells have relatively uniform round nuclei, with only rare mitotic figures. Within the cytoplasm, highly characteristic groups of PAS-positive, diastase-resistant, rod-shaped crystalline structures can be found. The specific cell of origin of alveolar soft-part sarcoma is uncertain, although striated muscle-related antigens have been demonstrated in some cases (193,220).

MISCELLANEOUS TUMORS

Benign Melanocytic Tumors

Congenital Melanocytic Nevus. Congenital nevi are classified as "small" if they are under 2 cm in diameter, "medium" if 2 to 10 cm in diameter, and "large" if over 10 cm in diameter. Most of them are small, usually under 0.4 cm in diameter. Large nevi can involve large areas of the body (e.g. "garment" or "bathing suit" nevi), and are associated with an increased risk of developing into malignant melanoma with advancing age (256). Small congenital nevi do not carry a similar risk (263).

Common Acquired Melanocytic Nevus. Vulvar nevi are relatively uncommon, occurring in 2.3 percent of women in one series (264a). Acquired nevi appear in early childhood and continue to develop into early adulthood. These lesions are most often junctional, but may be compound or intradermal (dermal); the distinction is based upon the location of the melanocytes. On microscopic examination junctional nevi typically have dendritic nevus cells aggregated within intradermal nests or within the dermal epidermal junction. They are usually confined to the basal and parabasal epithelium. Typical dendritic melanocytes are often seen in the adjacent normal epithelium. The compound nevus has features of a junctional nevus but also has epithelioid, or less commonly spindle-type nevus cells within the papillary or reticular dermis. The nevus cells may be aggregated or individually surrounded by fibrous tissue within the dermis. A dermal nevus, like a compound nevus, has nevus cells within the dermis. Dermal nevi are completely confined to the dermis, and the junctional component is absent. Within nevi, dendritic and spindle-type nevus cells often have melanin pigment, whereas epithelioid nevus cells are usually not pigmented.

Lentigo simplex is a lesion which presents as a flat pigmented area on the vulva, usually under 0.5 cm in diameter. It is regarded by some as an early stage in the development of a junctional nevus. Microscopic examination of lentigo simplex reveals a focal increase in melanocytes and melanin pigment in the basal layer. There is usually elongation of the rete ridges, but no melanocytic junctional cell nests.

Whereas lentigo simplex refers to a small lesion, *melanosis vulvae* describes a large pigmented area on the vulva. Microscopically, it is indistinguishable from lentigo simplex (268).

Cellular Blue Nevus. Cellular blue nevus is a congenital nevus that, although rare on the vulva, has been described on the hymen (266). The cellular blue nevus is composed of spindle-type nevus cells that are aggregated within the dermis and surrounded by fibrous tissue. They may locally infiltrate superficial peripheral nerves.

Atypical Vulvar Nevus. The so-called atypical vulvar nevus has many clinical and histopathologic features in common with acquired dysplastic nevi. They occur in young women ranging from 20 to 30 years of age. Although not considered specifically as dysplastic by some authors, or associated with dysplastic nevi in other sites, they demonstrate prominent variable-sized junctional melanocytic nests. Although some features of atypical vulvar nevus may suggest a diagnosis of melanoma, the lesion is small, well circumscribed, and lacks pagetoid spread, necrosis, or mitotic activity in the dermis (245,249).

Dysplastic Melanocytic Nevus. Dysplastic melanocytic nevi are most often seen in young women of reproductive age. Rare on the vulva, they present as pigmented, elevated lesions greater than 0.5 cm in diameter with irregular borders. Microscopic examination reveals large epithelioid or spindle-shaped nevus cells with nuclear pleomorphism and prominent nucleoli. The nevus cells are clustered in intraepithelial nests and are present in skin appendages, including hair shafts and the ducts of sweat glands (249,265). They often have a low-power microscopic appearance of a large junctional nevus, with a dermal component that has spindle- or epithelioid-type nevus cells in nests or isolated within the papillary and reticular dermis. Three features distinguish a dysplastic nevus from melanoma: 1) symmetrical growth, which is evident on microscopic examination of a full cross-section of the nevus. This can be determined by visualizing a line drawn perpendicular to the surface of the center of the nevus. The halves should be mirror images of each other; 2) the presence of the most atypical cells in the superficial levels of the nevus, with smaller, and more uniform cells in the deeper areas; 3) pagetoid spread of single melanocytes with little or no

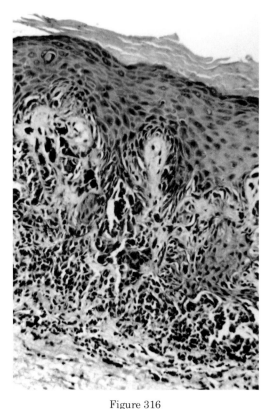

Figure 316
DYSPLASTIC NEVUS
Many junctional melanocytes are seen, some of which are in clusters. There is minimal pagetoid spread.

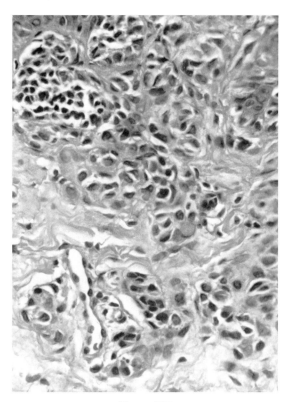

Figure 317
DYSPLASTIC NEVUS
Many melanocytes are seen in the junctional, basal, and parabasal areas. These cells are larger and have greater nuclear pleomorphism than the adjacent keratinocytes.

involvement of the upper one third of the epithelium (figs. 316, 317) (237,242,263,265). Besides malignant melanoma, a lesion of the dysplastic nevus syndrome should be included in the differential diagnosis. Individuals with dysplastic nevus syndrome have multiple large nevi, usually over 0.5 cm in diameter, which may be found on the vulva and on the trunk and extremities. Individuals with dysplastic nevus syndrome have a high risk of subsequent malignant melanoma, whereas women with isolated atypical nevi of the vulva do not.

Malignant Melanoma

General Features. Melanomas account for approximately 9 percent of all malignant tumors of the vulva, occurring predominantly in white women, with the highest frequency in the sixth and seventh decades; approximately one third occur in women under 50 years of age. A vulvar mass is the most common presentation although pruritus and bleeding are also frequent. In some cases the melanoma has arisen from a preexisting benign or atypical pigmented lesion (246, 258,259,272). Melanomas occur on the clitoris, labia minora, and labia majora with approximately equal frequency (252). The mass is usually slightly elevated or nodular and may be pigmented or nonpigmented (fig. 318). Pigmented epithelium may be seen adjacent to the mass and satellite nodules may be present. Clinically, malignant melanoma may resemble melanosis vulva, nevi, pigmented VIN or if nonpigmented, squamous cell carcinoma.

Microscopic Findings. Vulvar melanomas are of three distinct histopathologic types: *superficial spreading melanoma* (fig. 319), *nodular melanoma* (fig. 320) and *acral lentiginous melanoma* (figs. 321, 322) (239,257,264). The relative frequency of these types differs in various reports. Acral lentiginous melanoma was the most common type identified in one series, accounting for 10 of the 16 cases (63 percent); nodular melanoma accounted for 3 of 16 (18.6 percent) (239). In another series of 14 patients who died of vulvar melanoma, 65 percent had nodular melanoma, 21 percent had superficial spreading melanoma, and 14 percent had acral lentiginous melanoma (254). Some of this variation may relate to differences in the criteria used to distinguish superficial spreading melanoma from nodular melanoma. Superficial spreading melanoma can usually be differentiated from nodular melanoma by evaluating the adjacent epithelium. If the radial growth of a melanoma or atypical melanocytes involves four or more adjacent rete ridges, the tumor should be classified as superficial spreading melanoma (fig. 323) (263). Acral lentiginous melanomas have both vertical growth, as is seen in nodular melanoma, and radial growth, as is seen in superficial spreading melanoma. Atypical melanocytes can usually be identified within the epithelium adjacent to acral lentiginous and superficial spreading melanomas.

Malignant melanomas may consist predominantly of epithelioid, dendritic (nevoid), or spindle cell types, either pure or mixed, within a given tumor. The cells may contain no melanin or variable amounts, ranging from minimal to very large quantities. The histopathologic features vary considerably and certain features can be correlated with the subtype of the melanoma.

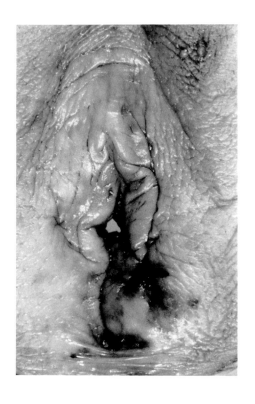

Figure 318
NODULAR MELANOMA
A nodular, partially pigmented mass in the inferior labia majora with extension into the vagina.

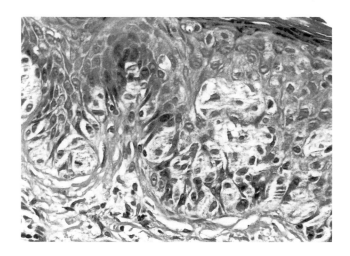

Figure 319
SUPERFICIAL
SPREADING MELANOMA
Many clear cells (atypical melanocytes) are present within the epidermis, some of which are clustered in nests. There is some pagetoid growth. (Courtesy of Dr. F. Mack Sexton, Charlotte, NC.)

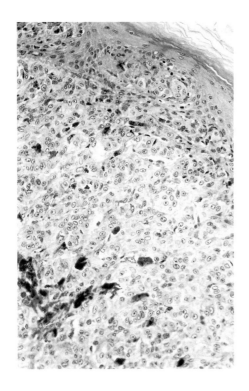

Figure 320
NODULAR MELANOMA
A nodular tumor in a superficial location. The tumor is highly cellular, moderately pleomorphic, and contains some pigment.

Within the invasive area of a superficial spreading melanoma, the malignant melanocytic cells are usually large and have relatively uniform nuclei with prominent nucleoli. Similar melanocytic cells can be found within the adjacent epithelium, representing the radial growth phase of the tumor. Junctional melanocytes are numerous and distributed within the epithelium in a pagetoid distribution. In nodular melanomas an intraepithelial component may be present in addition to an invasive component, but without an adjacent radial growth phase. The cells of nodular melanomas may be polygonal (epithelioid) or spindle shaped. The polygonal cells contain abundant eosinophilic cytoplasm, large nuclei, and prominent nucleoli. The dendritic cells have tapering cytoplasmic extensions resembling nerve cells and show moderate nuclear pleomorphism. Spindle cells have smaller, oval nuclei and may be arranged in sheets or bundles.

Acral lentiginous melanomas of the vulva most commonly arise within the vestibule. They may show little or no pagetoid spread and are characterized by spindle cells within the junctional zone with extension into the adjacent dermis in a diffuse pattern (see fig. 321). The spindle cells are uniform with little nuclear pleomorphism. Within the subepithelial tissue the tumor cells usually evoke a desmoplastic response.

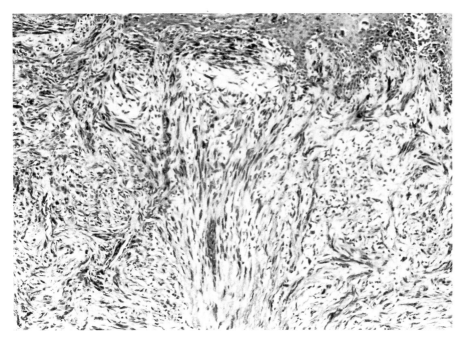

Figure 321
ACRAL
LENTIGINOUS
MELANOMA
The tumor is composed of spindle-shaped melanocytes separated by collagen. There is minimal pagetoid spread.

Both the level of invasion of a malignant melanoma, and its thickness have prognostic significance (241). The Clark classification of cutaneous melanomas into five levels of invasion is well accepted and can be applied to most melanomas of the vulva, with the exception of those arising within mucocutaneous areas. This system has been modified somewhat to accommodate vulvar melanomas (fig. 324) (246). A level I melanoma is a melanoma in situ; level II melanoma extends into the superficial papillary dermis; level III melanoma fills and expands the papillary dermis; level IV melanoma invades the reticular dermis; and level V melanoma invades beyond the reticular dermis into fat or other deeper tissues. Thickness measurements for cutaneous malignant melanomas as proposed by Breslow (241) require measurement from the deep border

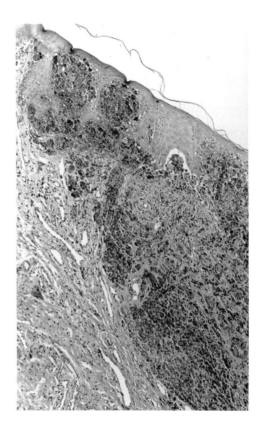

Figure 323
SUPERFICIAL SPREADING MELANOMA

This malignant melanoma shows superficial spread with vertical growth. Prominent junctional activity is seen adjacent to the vertical growth. The junctional activity fills the papillary dermis and partially obliterates the rete ridges.

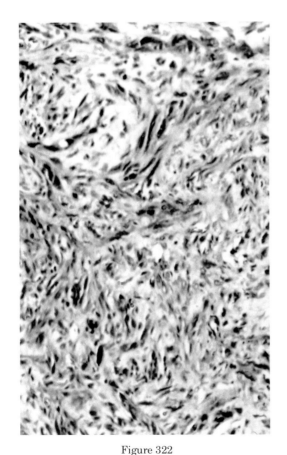

Figure 322
ACRAL LENTIGINOUS MELANOMA

The spindle cells are hyperchromatic and haphazardly arranged.

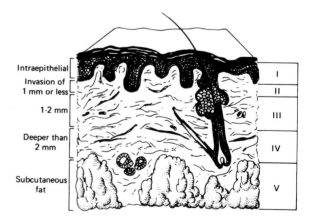

Figure 324
MALIGNANT MELANOMA MEASUREMENT

Methods of measurement of malignant melanoma of the vulva are shown here. (Fig. 2 from Chung AF, et al. Malignant melanoma of the vulva. Obstet Gynecol 1975;45:638–46.)

of the granular layer of the overlying epithelium to the deepest point of tumor invasion. If a lesion is less than 0.76 mm in thickness, it has little or no metastatic potential. Correlations between the thickness and the level of a vulvar melanoma can be made (246). Level I melanomas have no measurable thickness. In one study it was observed that level II melanomas had a thickness of 1 mm or less, level III melanomas had a thickness exceeding 1 mm up to 2 mm, and level IV melanomas had a thickness exceeding 2 mm but did not involve subcutaneous fat or adjacent deeper structures (246).

Differential Diagnosis. Superficial spreading malignant melanoma must be distinguished from Paget disease, VIN, and dysplastic nevi (265). The resemblance to Paget disease is greatest in cases of superficial spreading melanoma. The cells of Paget disease are usually larger, have more cytoplasm, and are clustered with occasional gland formation. Some of the cells almost always contain mucin. Immunohistochemical studies to distinguish these include studies for CEA , S-100 protein, HMB-45, and cytokeratins. Paget disease is immunoreactive for CEA whereas melanomas are not (260,261). Melanomas usually are immunoreactive for S-100 protein and HMB-45, whereas the non-melanocytic tumors are negative (250). Melanin stains are not of value because Paget cells may contain melanin pigment, and amelanotic melanomas do not contain detectable melanin. Melanomas do not contain cytokeratins 54-kD, which are identified in Paget cells. Electron microscopy is of value in this differential diagnosis in that melanoma cells contain melanosomes and other cytoplasmic ultrastructural features which are not present in Paget cells.

Squamous cell carcinomas with tumor giant cells, or those predominantly composed of spindle cells, may resemble malignant melanoma. In these, more typical squamous cell carcinoma may be identifiable adjacent to the giant cell or spindle cell component. Immunohistochemical studies are of value in the differential diagnosis (271). Spindle cell tumors of soft tissue origin, large cell lymphomas, and metastatic tumors including choriocarcinoma, may be included in the differential diagnosis. In these cases, review of the clinical history and physical and radiologic findings, as well as thorough sectioning of the submitted tissue and a panel of immunoperoxidase tests, will usually provide sufficient evidence to permit an accurate diagnosis. The immunoperoxidase panel should include a spectrum of antibodies, including epithelial markers (e.g., AE1/3, 54-kD, EMA), hematopoietic markers (e.g. leukocyte common antigen [LCA]), muscle markers (e.g., desmin, actin), fibrohistiocytic markers (e.g., α-1-antitrypsin, α-1-antichymotrypsin), neural and neuroendocrine tumor markers (e.g., S-100, chromogranin, synaptophysin), common adenocarcinoma markers (e.g., CEA), and melanoma markers (e.g., HMB-45, S-100).

It should be emphasized that when faced with a poorly differentiated vulvar tumor that defies classification on initial microscopic examination, melanoma should be placed first on the list of the differential diagnosis.

Treatment. The usual treatment for vulvar melanomas with a thickness of 0.75 mm or less is wide local excision with a 2-cm circumferential and deep margin. Melanomas of greater thickness are treated by wide excision to the fascia or partial or total vulvectomy. Depending on the size of the tumor, the surgical procedure may include bilateral inguinal lymphadenectomy (272). Radical vulvectomy does not appear to improve survival when compared to radical local excision with bilateral groin lymphadenectomy (267).

Prognosis. Factors that adversely influence survival include a tumor thickness exceeding 2 mm, Clark level V, a mitotic count exceeding 10 per mm^2, surface ulceration, and a minimal or absent inflammatory reaction (254,272). Vascular space invasion and tumor necrosis are also associated with a poorer prognosis and are more commonly seen with large melanomas (263). No recurrences of vulvar melanoma have been observed when the thickness was 0.75 mm or less (262,272). An excellent prognosis has been associated with melanomas at Clark level II or less, and those with a thickness of 1.49 mm or less. A tumor volume of less than 100 mm^3 also correlates with an excellent prognosis (238).

Vulvar melanomas may recur locally, or in the cervix, urethra, vagina, or rectum (264). Distant metastasis may be the first sign of recurrence. Metastases to the lungs, brain, urinary bladder, bone marrow, and abdominal wall have all been observed (254). The prognosis after recurrence is guarded, with a 5-year survival of only 5 percent (264).

Malignant Lymphoma

Primary malignant lymphoma of the vulva is rare, although the vulva is second only to the cervix as a primary site of lymphoma in the female genital tract (244,251). Vulvar malignant lymphoma usually occurs in women of reproductive age and presents as a mass, that may have an erythematous surface.

The lymphoma is usually of the diffuse, large cell type. It typically has a deep pushing border and seldom infiltrates the overlying epithelium (251). The dermal border may be associated with a desmoplastic stromal response, with small isolated groups of neoplastic cells surrounded by fibrous tissue within the deeper adjacent dermis. The cells are monomorphic, unlike those of an inflammatory infiltrate; phagocytosis is absent (273).

Tumors of Germ Cell Type

Yolk Sac Tumor (Endodermal Sinus Tumor). The yolk sac tumor is a rare primary tumor in the vulva, arising in the clitoris or in the labia (243,248,255,270). The patients have ranged in age from 22 months to 26 years.

Microscopic examination characteristically reveals a reticular pattern with irregular spaces lined by primitive epithelial cells; some of the spaces contain single papillae with a central vessel (Schiller-Duval bodies); PAS-positive globules are common. Alpha-fetoprotein is a marker of the tumor. It is detected in the tumor cells by immunohistochemical staining and is elevated in the serum.

To date, only one patient, a 2-year-old girl with clitoral yolk sac tumor, has survived. The other three patients have died of recurrent tumor. The current therapy is wide local excision with combination chemotherapy of the type used to treat analogous tumors in the ovary and vagina.

Neuroectodermal Tumors

Merkel Cell Tumor. Merkel cell tumors are rare in the vulva, usually presenting as an intradermal nodule or nodules in older women (240,247,253). The overlying surface may be erythematous. The tumor may be associated with VIN or invasive squamous cell carcinoma (240,269). Merkel cell tumors have three subtypes; the trabecular or carcinoid-like, the intermediate, and the small cell (oat cell–like) types.

The Merkel cell tumor lies within the dermis and is composed of relatively uniform small cells containing nuclei with a characteristic punctate chromatin pattern, high mitotic activity, and little cytoplasm. The tumor is infiltrative and vascular space invasion is common.

The tumor cells are immunoreactive for neuroendocrine markers such as neuron-specific enolase (NSE), synaptophysin, and chromogranin (260). Tumor cells are also focally immunoreactive for low–molecular-weight keratin, revealing a distinctive perinuclear cytoplasmic dot. Electron microscopy reveals a dense core and membrane-bound neurosecretory granules, which have been associated with ACTH production in one case (253). These findings distinguish this tumor from lymphoma, basal cell carcinoma, and poorly differentiated squamous cell carcinoma, but do not exclude a metastatic tumor with neuroendocrine features. Lymphoma shows LCA reactivity, which is absent in Merkel cell tumor. Metastatic small cell carcinoma of cervical origin is associated with an evident cervical lesion or a history of one.

Merkel cell tumors commonly metastasize to regional lymph nodes with subsequent distant metastasis often occurring within a year of diagnosis. The treatment is usually radical wide local excision with lymphadenectomy and chemotherapy.

SECONDARY TUMORS

Metastatic tumors to the vulva may occur at any site as single or multiple intradermal or subcutaneous masses. The metastases usually present within the labia majora and in some cases in the Bartholin gland (274,276). Metastatic tumor in the vulva was identified concurrently with the diagnosis of the primary tumor in 27 percent of the cases in one series (274), but it usually presents within 18 months of the initial diagnosis. The primary site is usually elsewhere in the genital tract with the cervix being the most common (274), followed by the endometrium and ovary. Metastatic squamous cell carcinomas from the cervix typically involve the dermal capillaries without involvement of the overlying epithelium, whereas metastatic adenocarcinomas more characteristically involve both the dermis and overlying epithelium, and are often ulcerated (274). Metastasis from remote sites outside of the genital tract, such as the breast, kidney (274,276, 278), stomach (97), and lung may also occur. In addition, gestational choriocarcinoma, malignant melanoma, and neuroblastoma have been reported to metastasize to the vulva (274,280).

Tumors may also involve the vulva secondarily by direct extension from the vagina, urethra, urinary bladder, or rectum. Urethral carcinomas account for less than 1 percent of carcinomas involving the female genital tract and are usually encountered in elderly women (277). The majority arise in the distal urethra and are squamous cell carcinomas, but some are transitional cell carcinomas (275,277,279). The survival rate for patients with urethral carcinoma is poor, ranging between 22 and 27 percent, probably due to the relatively high rate of metastasis to the inguinal or pelvic nodes, which occurs in 20 to 50 percent of the cases (275, 277,279).

Metastatic tumor involving the vulva is associated with a poor prognosis, with few patients surviving over one year after the diagnosis. Accordingly, radical operations are not indicated.

TUMOR-LIKE LESIONS

Pseudoepitheliomatous Hyperplasia

Pseudoepitheliomatous hyperplasia (PEH) is an epidermal reactive proliferative process which, although benign, morphologically mimics squamous cell carcinoma. PEH has been identified in approximately 50 percent of cases of granular cell tumor of the vulva (298). However, it has also been associated with over 30 diseases that involve the skin (285).

Microscopically, PEH is characterized by a proliferation of squamous cells resulting in downgrowth by rete pegs into the underlying papillary dermis (fig. 325). The proliferating squamous cells have bland nuclei and mitotic figures are sparse. Nonetheless, because of the marked downward growth of the rete pegs, sectioning leads to the appearance of irregularly-shaped nests of epithelium in the stroma that can be confused with squamous cell carcinoma. It may not always be possible to distinguish PEH from squamous cell carcinoma, if the biopsy does not demonstrate the underlying causative or associated process (298). Besides identifying the underlying process, additional findings that are of value in distinguishing PEH from squamous

Figure 325
PSEUDOEPITHELIOMATOUS
HYPERPLASIA WITH
UNDERLYING GRANULAR
CELL TUMOR
The hyperplastic epithelium forms irregular nests with keratin pearls. A granular cell tumor (right side of field) composed of uniform cells with abundant cytoplasm and relatively small uniform nuclei lies immediately beneath the lesion.

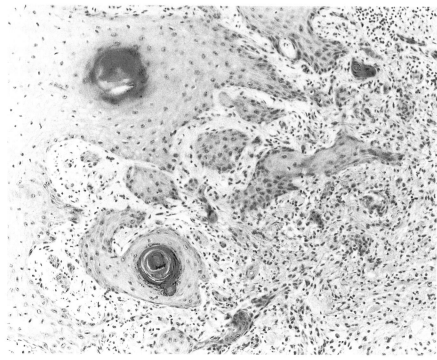

cell carcinoma include the absence of nuclear enlargement, pleomorphism, and hyperchromasia. Prominent enlarged nucleoli or abnormal mitotic figures are also not present in PEH (298). In addition, PEH is confined to the papillary dermis and there is little, or no, cellular necrosis (285). These related findings are not as reliable as the absence of nuclear atypia or the presence of an associated process, such as a granular cell tumor (298). An adequate deep biopsy is essential in establishing the diagnosis of PEH because it not only permits more thorough evaluation of the epithelial changes, but also reveals the underlying process responsible for the PEH.

Endometriosis and Decidua

Endometriosis of the vulva usually involves an episiotomy site or other area of trauma. It is most commonly found in the vestibule, presenting as a bluish to red cyst or nodule or as a deep subcutaneous mass. The presence of endometrial glands and stroma, or endometrial glands with surrounding hemofuscin or hemosiderin-laden macrophages and blood are characteristic. In pregnancy, or after progestin therapy, endometriosis may appear only as decidual tissue, with stromal cells containing pale amphophilic cytoplasm sometimes associated with macrophages filled with altered blood pigment. Clear cell adenocarcinoma has been described arising from endometriosis of the canal of Nuck adjacent to the right labium majus (292). The differential diagnosis includes metastatic adenocarcinoma and hidradenoma, neither of which has endometrial stroma. Treatment of a localized mass is excisional biopsy. Hormonal therapy may be of benefit in advanced cases.

Langerhans Cell Histiocytosis (Histiocytosis X Including Eosinophilic Granuloma)

Histiocytosis X includes three clinical forms: *Letterer-Siwe disease, Hand-Schüller-Christian disease (the chronic progressive form),* and *eosinophilic granuloma* (the benign localized form) (284). Among these clinical forms eosinophilic granuloma has been well documented to involve the vulva (297,299). Eosinophilic granuloma (benign localized Langerhans cell histiocytosis) is a benign localized proliferation of histiocytes of Langerhans cell type. It can present as a local-

ized cutaneous pigmented papule or nodule, which may be ulcerated. The lesion occurs predominantly in children between 5 and 13 years of age, but also may be found in young women (284,299). Systemic symptoms are rare but regional lymph nodes may be involved. Microscopic examination reveals localized histiocytes of Langerhans cell type with associated eosinophils, granulocytes, lymphocytes, and plasma cells (fig. 326). Foci of necrosis surrounded by an acute inflammatory infiltrate may be present. The histiocytes are immunoreactive for S-100.

Benign Xanthogranuloma

Benign xanthogranuloma, currently classified within the nonhistiocytosis X group, is a benign self-limited histiocytosis which is seen most commonly in infants or newborns. It is

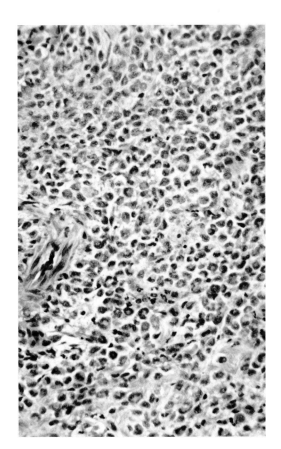

Figure 326
EOSINOPHILIC GRANULOMA
The lesion has a histiocytic Langerhans cell element intermixed with inflammatory cells, which include many eosinophils.

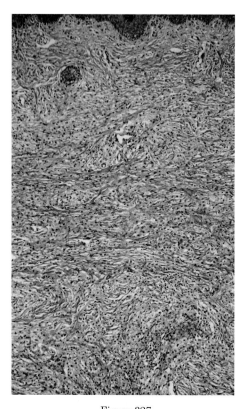

Figure 327
BENIGN XANTHOGRANULOMA
This nodule is composed predominantly of histiocytes, fibroblasts, and collagen fibers.

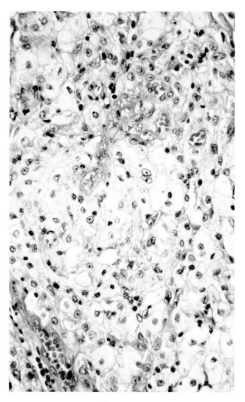

Figure 328
BENIGN XANTHOGRANULOMA
Lipid-laden histiocytes are evident in this figure.

manifested in the genital area by multiple yellow to yellow-brown papules, plaques, or nodules. The eyes, as well as other cutaneous and visceral sites, may also be involved. Xanthogranuloma may occur as a solitary lesion in adults.

On microscopic examination the early lesions consist predominantly of histiocytes with little or no lipid. Older lesions are composed of histiocytes, most of which contain lipid intermixed with fibroblasts. Touton giant cells, foreign-body giant cells, eosinophils, neutrophils, and plasma cells are usually present in mature lesions (figs. 327, 328).

Verruciform Xanthoma

Verruciform xanthoma is a benign superficial cutaneous and papillomatous lesion that has been reported on the vulva in women of reproductive age (295). The xanthomas may be single or multiple, and may range in diameter from less than 2 mm to over 10 mm; a 15-mm periclitoral

verruciform xanthoma has been reported (295). It results from an accumulation of lipid-laden histiocytes within the papillary dermis, and is occasionally associated with hyperlipidemia. Verruciform xanthoma is rare on the vulva. However, because of its papular appearance, it may clinically be misinterpreted as condyloma acuminatum, carcinoma, or VIN (295).

On microscopic examination the epithelial surface is focally elevated with some degree of acanthosis. The papillary dermis is filled with lipid-laden histiocytes (figs. 329, 330).

Desmoid Tumor (Extra-abdominal Fibromatosis, Aggressive Fibromatosis)

The desmoid tumor is a benign, locally infiltrative, fibromatous process originating in muscle-related connective tissue and adjacent fascia. It occurs rarely in the vulva (288). The peak age incidence is at approximately 30 years. Localized pain may be associated with advanced growth.

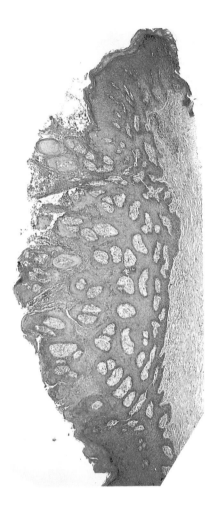

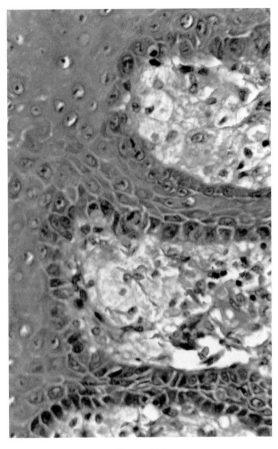

Figure 330
VERRUCIFORM XANTHOMA
Lipid-laden histiocytes are present within the papillary dermis.

Figure 329
VERRUCIFORM XANTHOMA
This papillomatous growth is characterized by proliferating acanthotic epithelium enclosing cellular areas of the papillary dermis.

Multiple desmoid tumors, involving more than one anatomical site, have been described.

Microscopically, the lesion is characterized by uniform cells that lack atypia and show no more than rare mitotic activity. A mitotic count of 1 mitotic figure per 10 high-power fields or more, with nuclear atypia and pleomorphism, suggests fibrosarcoma. Muscle involvement may result in atrophy. Atypical changes associated with atrophy of myocytes include nuclear pleomorphism. Chronic inflammation, small hemorrhagic foci, and calcification may occur.

Sclerosing Lipogranuloma

This lesion, which is generally secondary to the injection of oily material, may involve the external genitalia. In the vulva it presents as a discrete subcutaneous mass (287). On microscopic examination the lesion is composed of globules of fat engulfed by histiocytes and multinucleated giant cells, with a variably hyalinized fibrous stroma. Regional lymph nodes may be enlarged and contain lipid-laden histiocytes.

Nodular Fasciitis

This is a benign solitary, subcutaneous lesion composed of spindle-shaped cells of myofibroblastic origin. This rare vulvar lesion is typically highly vascular, may undergo a local myxoid change, and may have a mitotic count as high as 8 per 10 high-power fields (289,290,291).

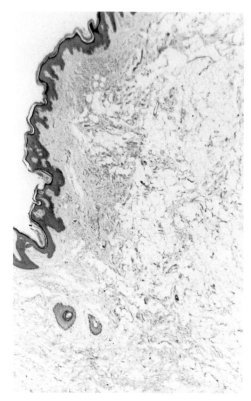

Figure 331
NEVUS LIPOMATOUS SUPERFICIALIS
The fat tissue is within the dermis. The overlying epithelium and superficial dermis is elevated from the normal adjacent epithelium seen in the upper left corner. (Courtesy of Dr. David Dolson, Gainesville, FL.)

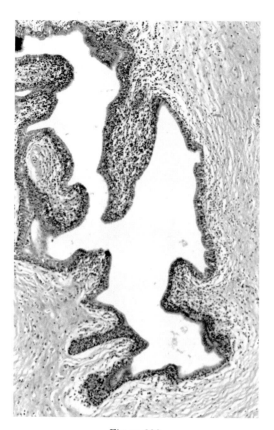

Figure 332
BARTHOLIN DUCT CYST
The cyst is lined by flattened transitional type epithelium.

Nevus Lipomatosis Superficialis

This congenital superficial connective tissue hamartoma is usually found on the medial aspects of the thigh or buttock, and is occasionally found on the vulva. Clinically, nevus lipomatosis superficialis is plaque-like or sessile, and soft on palpation. On gross examination, the mass is covered by normal-appearing skin. On microscopic examination, the lesion is composed of mature fat confined within the superficial dermis, and distinct from the underlying subcutaneous fat (fig. 331). No other hamartomatous elements are associated with this nevus.

Crohn Disease

Crohn disease of the vulva typically presents as slit-like nonhealing ulcers that characteristically follow the natural folds of the skin. In addition to the vulva, the inguinal and perianal areas may be involved. These ulcers may communicate with anal, rectal, or small intestinal fistulae. In some cases vulvar ulcers may precede intestinal symptoms of Crohn disease.

Microscopically, Crohn disease is characterized by a noncaseating granulomatous reaction without detectable causative organisms such as acid-fast bacilli, other bacteria, or fungi.

Cysts

Bartholin Duct Cyst. Bartholin duct cysts are caused by obstruction of the duct of the gland with distal distension of the duct (figs. 332, 333). Most have a squamous lining.

Mucinous Cyst. Mucinous cysts are typically found within the vestibule and may be solitary or multiple. Most arise from the minor vestibular glands. The cyst is lined by mucinous epithelium that is strongly stained by mucicarmine and alcian blue (fig. 334). Focal squamous metaplasia of the cyst lining may occur (293). No

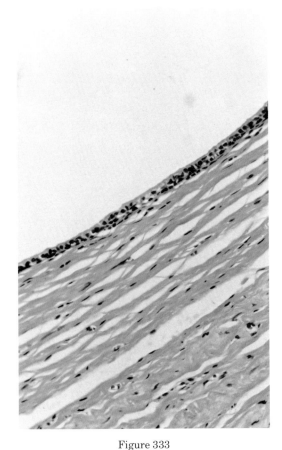

Figure 333
DILATED BARTHOLIN DUCT
The Bartholin duct is dilated and surrounded by a moderate chronic inflammatory infiltrate.

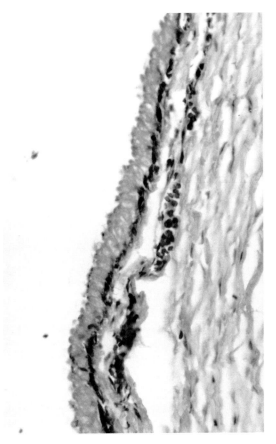

Figure 334
MUCINOUS CYST
Mucinous epithelium lines the cyst.

myoepithelial cell layer or outer smooth muscle layer is present (283,293,294). Similar cysts lined by columnar epithelium have been described following 5-fluorouracil therapy of the vagina and vulvar vestibule for condyloma acuminatum, supporting evidence that such cysts can be acquired (281). Excisional biopsy is therapeutic.

Epidermal Inclusion (Keratinous) Cyst. Epidermal inclusion cysts may occur in infants, children, and adults. They are characteristically superficial, range in size from 2 to 5 mm, and involve the labia majora and the lateral portions of the labia minora. They are usually multiple (286).

The cysts contain cheesy to grumous yellow-white keratinous debris. They are lined by stratified squamous cornified epithelium, which has a granular layer and is immunoreactive for high–molecular-weight keratin. In some cases the epithelial lining is markedly flattened (fig. 335). The cysts may be adjacent to sebaceous glands within the vulva. They do not require surgical excision unless there is secondary infection, rapid enlargement, or symptoms.

Mesonephric-Like Cyst. Since the mesonephric ducts do not descend to the vulvar anlage during embryologic development, these cysts are referred to as mesonephric-like. The cyst is usually solitary and superficial, presenting as a blue-violet to dark red cystic mass, which is thin-walled and contains clear fluid. Microscopic examination reveals a single layer of low cuboidal to columnar nonciliated epithelium, which may be flattened as a result of pressure of the cyst contents. A smooth muscle layer is characteristically present beneath the basement membrane of the epithelium. Surgical excision is therapeutic.

241

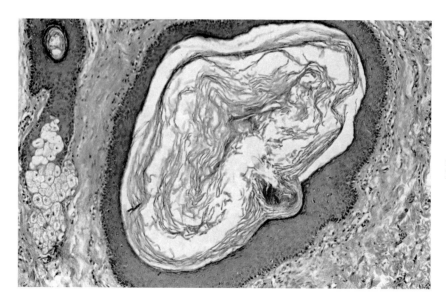

Figure 335
KERATINOUS CYST
The epithelial lining is stratified squamous epithelium and the
lumen contains keratin debris.

Ciliated Cyst. Ciliated cysts are rare in the vulva. The epithelial lining of the cyst consists of columnar cells which include ciliated and secretory cells similar to those of tuboendometrial-type epithelium (fig. 336) (282,294). No muscle layer is present. The origin of the ciliated cyst is uncertain. Although it has been postulated that the ciliated cyst results from a developmental abnormality of the müllerian duct there is no evidence that müllerian ducts contribute to formation of the vulva (283). Ciliated columnar cells in vaginal and vulvar epithelium have been observed following laser and 5-fluorouracil therapy (281,296). In one study these changes were designated *vulvar adenosis* (296). The ciliated cyst can be distinguished from endometriosis because of the absence of endometrial stroma. Surgical excision is therapeutic.

Mesothelial Cyst (Cyst of the Canal of Nuck). This cyst is typically located at the superior and lateral aspect of a labium majus at the level of the insertion of the round ligament. In approximately one third of the cases it is associated with an inguinal hernia. The cyst is thin-walled, and lined by flattened mesothelial cells. It varies in size and may exceed 5 cm in diameter. A large cyst may mimic an inguinal hernia clinically. Treatment is surgical excision.

Periurethral Cyst. Periurethral cysts are found just lateral to the urethral meatus and are lined by transitional epithelium (fig. 337). They may arise from the ducts of Skene glands. Surgical excision is therapeutic.

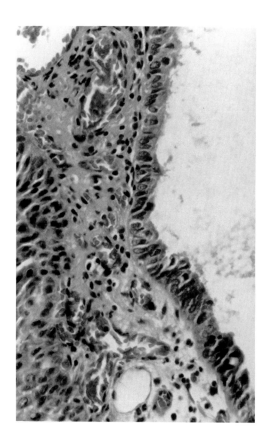

Figure 336
CILIATED CYST
The cyst contains ciliated cells and has some features of tuboendometrial-type epithelium, but there is no adjacent endometrial stroma. The overlying vestibular surface epithelium is seen at the left. Mild chronic inflammation is seen within the vestibular submucosa.

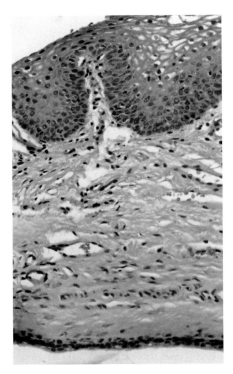

Figure 337
PERIURETHRAL CYST (SKENE GLAND CYST)
The cyst lies immediately beneath the squamous epithelium. It is lined by flattened transitional-type epithelium.

OTHER EPITHELIAL DISORDERS OF SKIN AND MUCOSA

Lichen Sclerosus
(Formerly Lichen
Sclerosus et Atrophicus)

Definition. A dermatosis of unknown etiology characterized by progressive thinning of the epithelium, subepithelial edema with fibrin deposition, and an underlying zone of chronic inflammation within the dermis.

General Features. Lichen sclerosus is the most common dermatosis of the vulva. It may occur at any age, but is most common in women of reproductive age or older. The disease may also effect the trunk and extremities when it involves the anogenital area. It may be limited to the vulva or involve the vulva and perianal area in a symmetric "butterfly" pattern.

Patients with lichen sclerosus may have a family history of the disorder, and have a higher than expected rate of autoimmune disease (307). In 15 to 30 percent of cases of vulvar invasive squamous cell carcinoma, lichen sclerosus can be found adjacent to the carcinoma (305,311).

Gross Findings. The vulvar lesions are usually pale white, depigmented, flat plaque-like areas. In advanced cases the skin has a wrinkled, parchment-like appearance. Areas of ecchymosis and excoriation, secondary to scratching, are often present. In severe cases formation of bullae and ulceration may be seen. With long-standing disease shrinkage of the labia minora, majora, and frenulum may occur, associated with agglutination of the labia and stenosis of the vaginal introitus.

Microscopic Findings. Microscopic examination reveals thinning of the epithelium with loss of rete ridges and a paucity of melanocytes. These findings become more pronounced as the disease progresses (figs. 338, 339) (306,307). Hyperkeratosis and follicular plugging are highly variable, but may be marked. Immediately beneath the epithelium, there is marked edema and fibrin deposition, and below the zone of edema there is an inflammatory infiltrate, which may be band-like, composed predominantly of lymphocytes accompanied by other chronic inflammatory cells. The epithelium may be separated from the basement membrane resulting in a focal subepithelial vacuolar change. This is a useful feature in the distinction of lichen sclerosus from localized scleroderma (309). In severe cases the subepithelial vacuolar change may progress to the formation of bullae. Extravasated blood within the superficial dermis is a common finding. Lichen sclerosus may be associated with squamous cell hyperplasia. When this occurs both diagnoses should be given.

Immunohistochemical Findings. Fibrin has been detected within the subepithelial dermis with the use of immunofluorescence techniques (301). Complement (C3) and IgM have also been identified within this edematous area (302,303). The presence of these substances may reflect reactive, rather than primary accumulation because they have also been found within areas of superficial trauma in otherwise normal skin (308). Immunohistochemistry is not helpful diagnostically.

Differential Diagnosis. The differential diagnosis includes lichen planus and morphea (localized scleroderma). Lichen planus may resemble lichen sclerosus microscopically. In one of its several phases, lichen planus has a distinctive lichenoid chronic inflammatory infiltrate, involving the basal layer of the epithelium, the adjacent

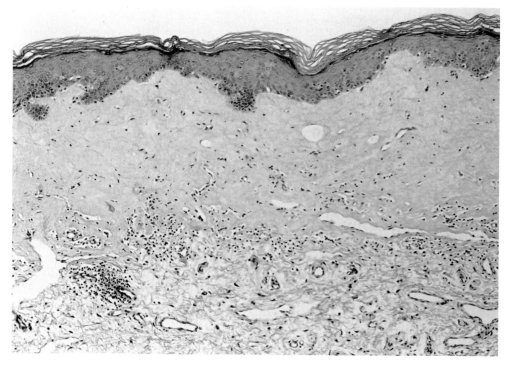

Figure 338
LICHEN SCLEROSUS
The epithelium is markedly thinned with loss of rete ridges. Below the epithelium the dermis is moderately edematous and hypocellular with small isolated blood vessels. Deeper to this area chronic inflammatory cells are seen above the more normal deeper dermis.

superficial dermis, and preserved rete ridges. The prominent dermal edema of lichen sclerosus is not present. Morphea is characterized by epithelial thinning, loss of rete ridges, and collagenization of the dermis. The collagenization is deeper than seen in lichen sclerosus and may extend around the eccrine gland ducts. The subepithelial edema of lichen sclerosus is typically absent in morphea. A deep inflammatory cell infiltrate may be seen in both processes. In lichen sclerosus, however, it is more band-like and not localized to the advancing edge of the lesion, as seen in the early phases of morphea. Vascular changes, including perivascular lymphocytic infiltrates and subsequent fibrosis are characteristic of morphea, but absent in lichen sclerosus (309).

Clinical Behavior and Treatment. Squamous cell carcinoma develops in 1 to 3 percent of women with vulvar lichen sclerosus (305,307). In children with the disease some regression of symptoms and physical findings often follows menarche, however, the disease often persists.

There is no completely effective treatment for lichen sclerosus. The most commonly used therapy in adults is the topical administration of 2 percent testosterone propionate, but topical administration of either progesterone or corticosteroids has also been used.

Squamous Cell Hyperplasia (Formerly Hyperplastic Dystrophy)

Definition. An epithelial disorder characterized by acanthosis and variable hyperkeratosis without atypia, significant associated inflammation, or evidence of a specific dermatosis.

General Features. This lesion is a relatively common disorder, but not as common as lichen sclerosus.

Gross Findings. Squamous cell hyperplasia usually appears as a discrete white lesion, reflecting the presence of epithelial thickening and edema or hyperkeratosis. The lesion is plaque-like and seldom extensive. A dark red to violet color may be observed if hyperkeratosis and prominent acanthosis. Hyperkeratosis and parakeratosis are usually present and epithelial edema (spongiosis) may be present (figs. 340, 341). The epithelial cells mature and there is no nuclear atypia. Abnormal mitotic figures are not present. Mild dermal inflammation may be seen, but it is not conspicuous unless there is associated excoriation or infection. Multiple biopsies are recommended to exclude foci of VIN. Should lichen sclerosus be found in adjacent epithelium, the diagnosis should be lichen sclerosus with adjacent squamous cell hyperplasia instead of mixed dystrophy (304,310).

Differential Diagnosis. The differential diagnosis includes monilia and HPV infection. If evidence of either of these infections is found, squamous cell hyperplasia should not be diagnosed. Also included in the differential diagnosis is lichen simplex chronicus (chronic neurodermatitis). Like squamous cell hyperplasia, lichen simplex chronicus has prominent acanthosis, and may have marked elongation and widening of the rete ridges. Hyperkeratosis and parakeratosis may also be found in both. Lichen simplex chronicus is distinguished from squamous cell hyperplasia by the presence of a superficial dermal chronic lymphocytic inflammatory infiltrate. The inflammation may be perivascular, and extend into the epidermis (exocytosis). In addition, dense collagenization of the dermis immediately beneath the epidermal dermal junction may also be seen. These findings are found in lichen simplex chronicus and distinguish it from squamous cell hyperplasia. White sponge nevus has been described on the vulva and, although rare, may be included in the differential diagnosis (300).

Clinical Behavior and Treatment. The prognosis is usually good and most patients respond within 1 month to topical corticosteroid treatment. Local contact irritant factors or associated vaginitis may be contributing factors and should also be treated.

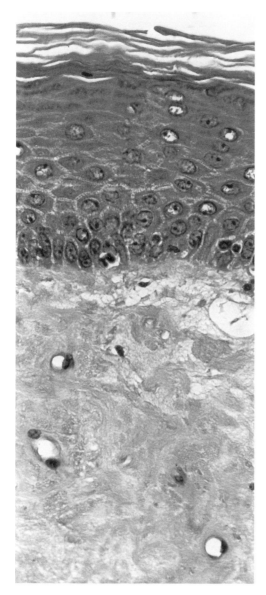

Figure 339
LICHEN SCLEROSUS
The subepithelial dermis is edematous and hypocellular and contains a few small vessels. There is no squamous hyperplasia or dysplasia.

edema are lacking or if scratching causes areas of excoriation. Unlike lichen sclerosus, squamous cell hyperplasia is rarely symmetric. Fissures may form, especially when the lesion involves the fourchette or perineal body.

Microscopic Findings. The microscopic appearance is that of a hyperplastic epithelium with

Other Dermatoses

(See differential diagnosis under Lichen Sclerosus and Squamous Cell Hyperplasia.) The dermatoses that appear in other areas of the body may involve the vulva as well. The reader is referred to appropriate textbooks and references for descriptions of these lesions.

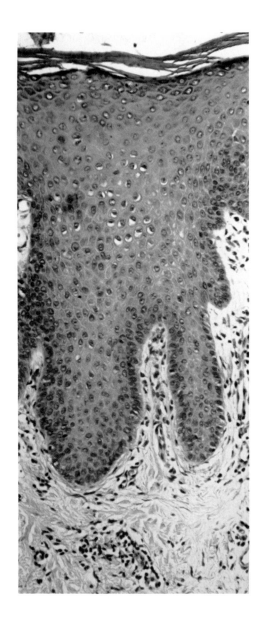

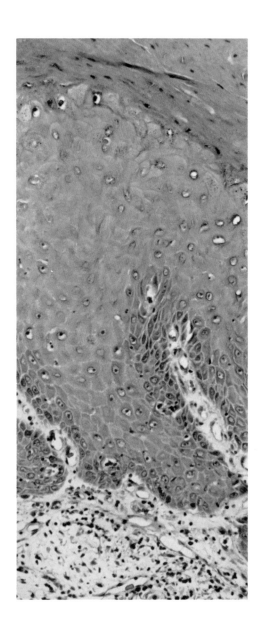

Figure 340
SQUAMOUS CELL HYPERPLASIA
Prominent acanthosis of the epithelium with slight hyperkeratosis. The perinuclear halos are artifactual, the nuclei being all displaced upward and peripherally. Unlike koilocytosis, the nuclei are not enlarged or atypical. There is a mild chronic inflammation in the dermis.

Figure 341
SQUAMOUS CELL HYPERPLASIA
The epithelium is thickened and shows surface maturation. Parakeratosis and hyperkeratosis are present. Moderate chronic inflammation is present in the dermis.

REFERENCES

General References

Balch CM, Milton GW, eds. Cutaneous melanoma. Philadelphia: Lippincott, 1985.

Elder DE, Murphy GF. Melanocytic tumors of the skin. Atlas of Tumor Pathology, 3rd Series, Fascicle 2, Washington, DC: Armed Forces Institute of Pathology, 1991.

Enzinger FM, Weiss SW. Soft tissue tumors. St. Louis: Mosby, 1988.

Friedrich EG Jr. Vulvar disease. Philadelphia: Saunders, 1983.

Fu YS, Reagan JW. Pathology of the uterine cervix, vagina and vulva: major problems in pathology; Vol 21. Philadelphia: Saunders, 1989.

Kaufman RH, Friedrich EG Jr, Gardner HL. Benign diseases of the vulva and vagina. 3rd ed. Chicago: Year Book Medical Publishers, 1989.

Lever WF, Schaumburg-Lever G. Histopathology of the skin. 7th ed. Philadelphia: Lippincott, 1990.

Murphy GF, Elder DE. Atlas of Tumor Pathology, 3rd Series, Fascicle 1, Washington, DC: Armed Forces Institute of Pathology, 1991.

Reed RJ. Neoplasms of the skin. In: Silverberg SG, ed. Principles and practice of surgical pathology. 2nd ed. New York: Churchill Livingstone, 1990:193–254.

Ridley CM, ed. The vulva. New York: Churchill Livingstone, 1988.

Rosai J, ed. Ackerman's surgical pathology. 7th ed. St. Louis: Mosby, 1989.

Stout AP, Lattes R. Tumors of the soft tissue. Atlas of Tumor Pathology, 2nd Series, Fascicle 1. Washington, DC: Armed Forces Institute of Pathology, 1967.

True LD. Atlas of diagnostic immunohistopathology. Philadelphia: Lippincott, 1990.

Turner MLC, Marinoff SC. Dermatologic clinics-vulvar diseases. Vol 10(2). Philadelphia: WB Saunders Co, 1992.

Wilkinson EJ, ed. Pathology of the vulva and vagina. Contemporary issues in surgical pathology; Vol 9. New York: Churchill Livingstone, 1987.

Squamous Lesions

1. Abell MR. Intraepithelial carcinomas of epidermis and squamous mucosa of vulva and perineum. Surg Clin North Am 1965;45:1179–98.

2. Ackerman LV. Verrucous carcinoma of the oral cavity. Surgery 1948;23:670–8.

3. Andreasson B, Bock JE, Weberg E. Invasive cancer in the vulvar region. Acta Obstet Gynecol Scand 1982;61:113–9.

4. _____, Nyboe J. Predictive factors with reference to low risk of metastases in squamous carcinoma in the vulvar region. Gynecol Oncol 1985;21:196–206.

5. Bergeron C, Ferenczy A, Richart RM, Guralnick M. Micropapillomatosis labialis appears unrelated to human papillomavirus. Obstet Gynecol 1990;76:281–6.

6. _____, Naghashfar Z, Canaan C, Shah K, Fu Y, Ferenczy A. Human papillomavirus type 16 in intraepithelial neoplasia (bowenoid papulosis) and coexistent invasive carcinoma of the vulva. Int J Gynecol Pathol 1987;6:1–11.

7. Breen JL, Neubecker RD, Greenwald E, Gregori CA. Basal cell carcinoma of the vulva. Obstet Gynecol 1975;46:122–90.

8. Brinton LA, Nasca PC, Mallin K, Baptiste MS, Wilbanks GD, Richart RM. Case-control study of cancer of the vulva. Obstet Gynecol 1990;75:859–66.

9. Brisigotti M, Moreno A, Murcia C, Matías-Guiu X, Prat J. Verrucous carcinoma of the vulva. A clinicopathologic and immunohistochemical study of five cases. Int J Gynecol Pathol 1989;8:1–7.

10. Buscema J, Stern JL, Woodruff JD. Early invasive carcinoma of the vulva. Am J Obstet Gynecol 1981;140:563–9.

11. _____, Woodruff JD, Parmley TH, Genadry R. Carcinoma in situ of the vulva. Obstet Gynecol 1980;55:225–30.

12. Caglar H, Tamer S, Hreshchyshyn MM. Vulvar intraepithelial neoplasia. Obstet Gynecol 1982;60:346–9.

13. Campion MJ, DiPaola FM, Crozier MA, Rathrock R, Vellios F, Franklin EW. Labial micropapillomatosis human papillomavirus infection or anatomic variant. Obstet Gynecol 1992 (in press).

14. Caterson RJ, Furber J, Murray J, McCarthy W, Mahony JF, Shell AGR. Carcinoma of the vulva in two young renal allograft recipients. Transplant Proc 1984;16:559–61.

15. Chafe W, Richards A, Morgan LS, Wilkinson EJ. Unrecognized invasive carcinoma in vulvar intraepithelial neoplasia (VIN). Gynecol Oncol 1988;31:154–65.

16. Copas P, Dyer M, Comas FV, Hall DJ. Spindle cell carcinoma of the vulva. Diagn Gynecol Obstet 1982;4:235–41.

17. Crum CP, Braun LA, Shah KV, et al. Vulvar intraepithelial neoplasia. Correlation of nuclear DNA content and the presence of a human papilloma virus (HPV) structural antigen. Cancer 1982;49:468–71.

18. _____, Liskow A, Petras P, Keng WC, Frick HC II. Vulvar intraepithelial neoplasia (severe atypia and carcinoma in situ). A clinicopathologic analysis of 41 cases. Cancer 1984;54:1429–34.

19. Cruz-Jimenez PR, Abell MR. Cutaneous basal cell carcinoma of the vulva. Obstet Gynecol 1975;36:1860–8.

20. De Coninck A, Willemsen M, De Dobbeleer, Roseeuw D. Vulvar localization of epidermic acanthoma. A light- and electron-microscopic study. Dermatologica 1986;172:276–8.

21. Dennerstein GJ. The cytology of the vulva. J Obstet Gynecol Br Commonwlth 1968;75:603–9.

22. Dinh TV, Powell LC, Hanninan EV, Yang HL, Wirt DP, Yandall RB. Simultaneously occurring condylomata acuminata, carcinoma in situ and verrucous carcinoma of the vulva and carcinoma in situ of the cervix in a young woman. J Reprod Med 1988;33:510–3.

23. DiSaia PJ. Management of superficially invasive vulvar carcinoma. Clin Obstet Gynecol 1985;28:196–203.

24. _____, Creasman WT, Rich WM. An alternate approach to early cancer of the vulva. Am J Obstet Gynecol 1979;133:825–32.

25. Downey GO, Okagaki T, Ostrow RS, Clark BA, Twiggs LB, Faras AJ. Condylomatous carcinoma of the vulva with special reference to human papillomavirus DNA. Obstet Gynecol 1988;72:68–73.

26. Dudzinski MR, Askin FB, Fowler WC Jr. Giant basal cell carcinoma of the vulva. Obstet Gynecol 1984;63:57–60S.

27. Dvoretsky PM, Bonfiglio TA, Helmkamp BF, Ramsey G, Chuang C, Beecham JB. The pathology of superficially invasive, thin vulvar squamous cell carcinoma. Int J Gynecol Pathol 1984;3:331–42.

28. Ehrmann RL, Dwyer IM, Yavner BA, Hancock WW. An immunoperoxidase study of laminin and type IV collagen distribution in carcinoma of the cervix and vulva. Obstet Gynecol 1988;72:257–62.

29. FIGO news. Annual report on the results of treatment in gynecological cancer. Int J Gynecol Obstet 1989;28:189–93.

30. Franklin EW III, Rutledge FD. Prognostic factors in epidermoid carcinoma of the vulva. Obstet Gynecol 1971;37:892–901.

31. Friedrich EG Jr. Reversible vulvar atypia. A case report. Obstet Gynecol 1972;39:173–81.

32. _____, Wilkinson EJ, Fu YS. Carcinoma in situ of the vulva: a continuing challenge. Am J Obstet Gynecol 1980;136:830–43.

33. Graham JH, Helwig EB. Erythroplasia of Queyrat. A clinicopathologic and histochemical study. Cancer 1973;32:1396–414.

34. Gross G, Hagedorn M, Ikenberg H, et al. Bowenoid papulosis. Presence of human papillomavirus (HPV) structural antigens and of HPV 16 related DNA sequences. Arch Dermatol 1985;121:858–63.

35. Growdon WA, Fu YS, Lebherz TB, Rapkin A, Mason GD, Parks G. Pruritic vulvar squamous papillomatosis: evidence for human papillomavirus etiology. Obstet Gynecol 1985;66:564–8.

36. Hacker NF, Berek JS, Lagasse LD, Nieberg RK, Leuchter RS. Individualization of treatment for stage I squamous cell vulvar carcinoma. Obstet Gynecol 1984;63(2): 155–62.

37. _____, Nieberg RK, Berek JS, et al. Superficially invasive vulvar cancer with nodal metastases. Gynecol Oncol 1983;15:65–77.

38. Hart WR, Norris HJ, Helwig EB. Relation of lichen sclerosus et atrophicus of the vulva to development of carcinoma. Obstet Gynecol 1975;45:369–77.

39. Henson D, Tarone R. An epidemiologic study of cancer of the cervix, vagina and vulva based on the third National Cancer Survey in the United States. Am J Obstet Gynecol 1977;129:525–32.

40. Iversen T, Abeler V, Aalders J. Individualized treatment of stage I carcinoma of the vulva. Obstet Gynecol 1981; 57:85–9.

41. Jacobs DM, Sandles LG, Leboit PE. Sebaceous carcinoma arising from Bowen's disease of the vulva. Arch Dermatol 1986;122:1191–3.

42. Johnson WC, Helwig EB. Adenoid squamous cell carcinoma (adenocanthoma). A clinicopathologic study of 155 patients. Cancer 1966;19:1639–50.

43. Jones RW, McLean MR. Carcinoma in situ of the vulva: a review of 31 treated and five untreated cases. Obstet Gynecol 1986;68:499–503.

44. Kabulski Z, Frankman O. Histologic malignancy grading in invasive squamous cell carcinoma of the vulva. Int J Obstet Gynecol 1978–79;16:233–7.

45. Kluzak TR, Krause FT. Condylomata, papillomas and verrucous carcinomas of the vulva and vagina. In: Wilkinson EJ, ed. Pathology of the vulva and vagina. New York: Churchill Livingstone, 1987:49–77.

46. Kneale BL. Microinvasive cancer of the vulva: report of the ISSVD Task Force, 6th World Congress. J Reprod Med 1984;29:454–6.

47. Krupp PJ, Lee FY, Bohm JW, Batson HW, Diem JE, Lemire JE. Prognostic parameters and clinical staging criteria in the epidermoid carcinoma of the vulva. Obstet Gynecol 1975;46:84–8.

48. Kurman RJ, Potkul RK, Lancaster WD, Lewandowski G, Weck PR, Delgato G. Vulvar condylomas and squamous vestibular micropapilloma: differences in appearance and response to treatment. J Reprod Med 1990;35:1019–22.

49. _____, Toki T, Schiffman MH. Basaloid and warty carcinomas of the vulva. Distinctive types of squamous cell carcinoma frequently associated with human papillomavirus. Am J Surg Pathol (in press).

50. Kurzl RG, Messerer D, Baltzer J, Lohe KJ, Zander J. Vulvar carcinoma: a clinical, histologic and morphometric study of 197 patients with squamous cell carcinoma of the vulva. J Reprod Med 1986;31:980.

51. Lasser A, Cornog JL, Morris JM. Adenoid squamous cell carcinoma of the vulva. Cancer 1974;33:224–7.

52. LiVolsi VA, Brooks JJ. Soft tissue tumors of the vulva. In: Wilkinson EJ, ed. Pathology of the vulva and vagina: contemporary issues in surgical pathology; Vol 9. New York: Churchill Livingstone, 1987:209–38.

53. Lupulescu A, Mehregan AH, Rahbari H, et al. Venereal warts vs Bowen disease. A histologic and ultrastructural study of 5 cases. JAMA 1977;237:2520–2.

54. Magrina JF, Webb MJ, Gaffey TA, Symmonds RE. Stage I squamous cell cancer of the vulva. Am J Obstet Gynecol 1979;134:453–9.

55. Merino MJ, LiVolsi VA, Schwartz PE, Rudnicki J. Adenoid basal cell carcinoma of the vulva. Int J Gynecol Pathol 1982;1:299–306.

56. Mucitelli DR, Charles EZ, Kraus FT. Vulvovaginal polyps. Histologic appearance, ultrastructure, immunocytochemical characteristics, and clinicopathologic correlations. Int J Gynecol Pathol 1990;9:20–40.

57. Nadji M, Ganjei P. The application of immunoperoxidase techniques in the evaluation of vulvar and vaginal disease. In: Wilkinson EJ, ed. Pathology of the vulva and vagina: contemporary issues in surgical pathology; Vol 9. New York: Churchill Livingstone, 1987:239–48.

58. Nauth HF, Schilke E. Cytology of the exfoliative layer in normal and diseased vulvar skin: correlation with histology. Acta Cytol 1982;26:269–83.

59. Okagaki T, Clark BA, Zachow KR, et al. Presence of human papillomavirus in verrucous carcinoma (Ackerman) of the vagina. Immunocytochemical, ultrastructural, and DNA hybridization studies. Arch Pathol Lab Med 1984;108:567–70.

60. Oriel JD. Natural history of genital warts. Br J Vener Dis 1971;47:1–13.

61. _____, Almeida JD. Demonstration of virus particles in human genital warts. Br J Vener Dis 1970;46:37–42.

62. Park JS, Jones RW, McLean MR, et al. Possible etiologic heterogeneity of vulvar intraepithelial neoplasia. A correlation of pathologic characteristics with human papillomavirus detection by in situ hybridization and polymerase chain reaction. Cancer 1991;67:1599–607.

63. Parker RT, Duncan I, Rampone J, Creasman W. Operative management of early invasive epidermoid carcinoma of the vulva. Am J Obstet Gynecol 1975;123:349–55.

64. Patterson JW, Kao GF, Graham JH, et al. Bowenoid papulosis. A clinicopathologic study with ultrastructural observations. Cancer, 1986;57:823–36.

65. Powell LC Jr, Dinh TV, Rajaraman S, et al. Carcinoma in situ of the vulva. A clinicopathologic study of 50 cases. J Reprod Med 1986;31:808–14.

66. Rando RF, Sedlacek TV, Hunt J, Jenson AB, Kurman RJ, Lancaster WD. Verrucous carcinoma of the vulva associated with an unusual type 6 human papilloma virus. Obstet Gynecol 1986;67:70–5S.

67. Rastkar G, Okagaki T, Twiggs LB, Clark BA. Early invasive and in situ warty carcinoma of the vulva: clinical histologic and electron microscopic study with particular reference to viral association. Am J Obstet Gynecol 1982;143:814–20.

68. Rhatigan RM, Nuss RC. Keratoacanthoma of the vulva. Gynecol Oncol 1985;21:118–23.

69. Ridley CM, Frankman O, Jones ISC, Pincus S, Wilkinson EJ. New nomenclature for vulvar disease: International Society for the Study of Vulvar Disease. Hum Pathol 1989;20:495–6.

70. Ross MJ, Ehrmann RL. Histologic prognosticators in stage I squamous cell carcinoma of the vulva. Obstet Gynecol 1987;70:774–84.

71. Sedlis A, Homesley H, Bundy BN, et al. Positive groin lymph nodes in superficial squamous cell vulvar cancer. A gynecologic oncology group study. Am J Obstet Gynecol 1987:156:1159–64.

72. Sengupta BS. Carcinoma of the vulva in Jamaican women. Acta Obstet Gynecol Scand 1981;60:537–44.

73. Shafeek MA, Osman MI, Hussein MA. Carcinoma of the vulva arising in condylomata acuminata. Obstet Gynecol 1979;54:120–3.

74. Shatz P, Bergeron C, Wilkinson EJ, Arseneau J, Ferenczy A. Vulvar intraepithelial neoplasia skin appendage involvement. Obstet Gynecol 1989;74:769–74.

75. Shevchuk MM, Richart RM. DNA content of condyloma acuminatum. Cancer 1982;49:489–92.

76. Simkin RJ, Fisher BK. Basal cell epithelioma of the vulva. Obstet Gynecol 1977;49:617–9.

77. Steeper TA, Piscioli F, Rosai J. Squamous cell carcinoma with sarcoma-like stroma of the female genital tract. Clinicopathologic study of four cases. Cancer 1983;52:890–8.

78. Thomas P, Said JW, Nash G, Banks-Schegal S. Profiles of keratin proteins in basal and squamous cell carcinomas of the skin. An immunohistochemical study. Lab Invest 1984;50:36–41.

79. Toki T, Kurman RJ, Park JS, Kessis T, Daniel RW, Shah KV. Probable nonpapillomavirus etiology of squamous cell carcinoma of the vulva in older women: a clinicopathologic study using in situ hybridization and polymerase chain reaction. Int J Gynecol Pathol 1991;10:107–25.

80. Ubben K, Krzyzek R, Ostrow R, et al. Human papillomavirus DNA detected in two verrucous carcinomas. J Invest Dermatol 1979; 72:195.

81. Wade TR, Ackerman AB. The effects of resin of podophyllin on condyloma acuminatum. Amer J Dermatopathol 1984;6:109–22.

82. _____, Kopf AW, Ackerman AB. Bowenoid papulosis of the genitalia. Arch Dermatol 1979;115:30–8.

83. Walker PG, Colley NV, Grubb C, Tejerina A, Oriel JD. Abnormalities of the uterine cervix in women with vulva warts. A preliminary communication. Br J Vener Dis 1983;59:120–3.

84. Way S. Malignant disease of the vulva. Edinburgh: Churchill Livingstone, 1982.

85. Wilkinson EJ. Superficially invasive carcinoma of the vulva. In: Wilkinson EJ, ed. Pathology of the vulva and vagina: contemporary issues in surgical pathology; Vol 9. New York: Churchill Livingstone, 1987:103–17.

86. _____. Vulvar intraepithelial neoplasia and squamous cell carcinoma with emphasis on new nomenclature. Prog Reprod Urinary Tract Pathol 1990; 2:1–20.

87. _____, Croker BP, Friedrich EG Jr, Franzini DA. Two distinct pathologic types of giant cell tumor of the vulva. A report of two cases. J Reprod Med 1988;33:519–22.

88. _____, Friedrich EG Jr, Fu YS. Multicentric nature of vulvar carcinoma in situ. Obstet Gynecol 1981;58:69–74.

89. _____, Kneale B, Lynch PJ. Report of the ISSVD Terminology Committee. J Reprod Med 1986;31:973–4.

90. _____, Morgan LS, Friedrich EG Jr. Association of Franconi's anemia and squamous cell carcinoma of the lower female genital tract with condyloma acuminatum. A report of two cases. J Reprod Med 1984;29:447–53.

91. _____, Rico MJ, Pierson KK. Microinvasive carcinoma of the vulva. Int J Gynecol Pathol 1982;1:29–39.

92. Wolber RA, Talerman A, Wilkinson EJ, Clement PB. Vulvar granular cell tumors with pseudocarcinomatous hyperplasia: a comparative analysis with well-differentiated squamous carcinoma. Int J Gynecol Pathol 1991;10:59–66.

93. Woodruff JD, Julian CG, Puray T, Mermut S, Katayama P. The contemporary challenge of carcinoma in situ of the vulva. Am J Obstet Gynecol 1973;115:677–86.

94. Zaino RJ. Carcinoma of the vulva, urethra and Bartholin's gland. In: Wilkinson EJ, ed. Pathology of the vulva and vagina: contemporary issues in surgical pathology; Vol 9. New York: Churchill Livingstone, 1987:119–53.

95. _____, Husseinzadeh N, Nahhas W, Mortel R. Epithelial alterations in proximity to invasive carcinoma of the vulva. Int J Gynecol Pathol 1982;1:173–84.

Glandular Lesions

96. Abell MR. Adenocystic (pseudoadenomatous) basal cell carcinoma of vestibular glands of vulva. Am J Obstet Gynecol 1963;86:470–82.

97. Ahmed W, Beasley WH. Carcinoma of stomach with a metastasis in the clitoris. JPMA 1979;29:62–3.

98. Avinoach I, Zirkin HJ, Glezerman M. Proliferating trichilemmal tumor of the vulva. Case report and review of the literature. Int J Gynecol Pathol 1989;8:163–8.

99. Axe S, Parmley T, Woodruff JD, Hlopak B. Adenomas in minor vestibular glands. Obstet Gynecol 1986; 68:16–8.

100. Beecham CT. Paget's disease of the vulva. Recurrence in skin grafts. Obstet Gynecol 1976;47:55–8S.

101. Belcher RW. Extramammary Paget's disease. Enzyme histochemical and electron microscopic study. Arch Pathol 1972;94:59–64.

102. Brown SM, Freeman RG. Syringoma limited to the vulva. Arch Dermatol 1971;104:331.

103. Buchler DA, Sun F, Chaprevich T. A pilar tumor of the vulva. Gynecol Oncol 1978;6:479–86.

104. Chamlian DL, Taylor HB. Primary carcinoma of Bartholin's gland. A report of 24 patients. J Obstet Gynecol 1972;39:489–94.

105. Cho D, Buscema J, Rosenshein NB, et al. Primary breast cancer of the vulva. Obstet Gynecol 1985;66:79–81S.

106. Cho D, Woodruff JD. Trichoepithelioma of the vulva. A report of two cases. J Reprod Med 1988;33:317–9.

107. Copeland LJ, Sneige N, Gershenson DM, McGuffee VB, Abdul-Karim F, Rutledge FN. Bartholin gland carcinoma. Obstet Gynecol 1986;67:794–801.

108. _____, Sneige N, Gershenson DM, Saul PB, Stringer CA, Seski JC. Adenoid cystic carcinoma of Bartholin gland. Obstet Gynecol 1986;67:115–20.

109. Creasman WT, Gallager HS, Rutledge F. Paget's disease of the vulva. Gynecol Oncol 1975;3:133–48.

110. Dennerstein GJ. The cytology of the vulva. J Obstet Gynecol Br Commonwlth 1968;75:603–9.

111. Ferenczy A, Richart RM. Ultrastructure of perianal Paget's disease. Cancer 1972;29:1141–9.

112. Foushee JH, Pruitt AB Jr. Vulvar fibroadenoma from aberrant breast tissue. Report of 2 cases. Obstet Gynecol 1967;29:819–23.

113. Fowler WC Jr, Lawrence H, Edelman DA. Paravestibular tumor of the female genital tract. Am J Obstet Gynecol 1981;139:109–11.

114. Friedrich EG Jr. Vulvar vestibulitis syndrome. J Reprod Med 1987;32:110–4.

115. _____, Wilkinson EJ, Steingraeber PH, Lewis JD. Paget's disease of the vulva and carcinoma of the breast. Obstet Gynecol 1975;46:130–4.

116. Ganjei P, Giraldo KA, Lampe B, Nadji M. Vulvar Paget's disease. Is immunocytochemistry helpful in assessing the surgical margins? J Reprod Med 1990;35:1002–4.

117. Garcia JJ, Verkauf BS, Hockberg CJ, et al. Aberrant breast tissue in the vulva: a case report and review of the literature. Obstet Gynecol 1978;52:225–8.

118. Ghirardini G. Syringoma of the vulva in postmenopausal age. Diagn Gynecol Obstet 1982;4:325–6.

119. Gilks CB, Clement PB, Wood WS. Trichoblastic fibroma. A clinicopathologic study of three cases. Am J Dermatopathol 1989;11:397–402.

120. Gregori CA, Breen JL, Smith CI. Extramammary Paget's disease. Clin Obstet Gynecol 1978;21:1107–15.

121. Guerry RL, Pratt-Thomas HR. Carcinoma of supernumerary breast of vulva with bilateral mammary cancer. Cancer 1976;38:2570–4.

122. Gunn RA, Gallager HS. Vulvar Paget's disease: a topographic study. Cancer 1980;46:590–4.

123. Hart WR, Millman JB. Progression of intraepithelial Paget's disease of the vulva to invasive carcinoma. Cancer 1977;40:2333–7.

124. Hashimoto K. Hidradenoma papilliferum. An electron microscopic study. Acta Dermatol Venereol 1973;53:22–30.

125. Helwig EB, Graham JH. Anogenital (extramammary) Paget's disease. Cancer 1963;16:387–403.

126. Isaacson D, Turner ML. Localized vulvar syringomas. J Am Acad Dermatol 1979;1:352–6.

127. Johnson WC, Helwig EB. Adenoid squamous cell carcinoma (adenocanthoma). A clinicopathologic study of 155 patients. Cancer 1966;19:1639–50.

128. Kuzuya K, Matsuyama M, Nish Y, Chihara T, Suchi T. Ultrastructure of adenocarcinoma of Bartholin's gland. Cancer 1981;48:1392–8.

129. Lee SC, Roth LM, Ehrlich C, Hall JA. Extramammary Paget's disease of the vulva. A clinicopathologic study of 13 cases. Cancer 1977;39:2540–9.

130. Leuchter RS, Hacker NF, Voet RL, Berek JS, Townsend DE, Lagasse LD. Primary carcinoma of the Bartholin gland: a report of 14 cases and review of the literature. Obstet Gynecol 1982;60:361–8.

131. Mader MH, Friedrich EG Jr. Vulvar metastasis of breast carcinoma. A case report. J Reprod Med 1982;27:169–71.

132. Mazoujian G, Pinkus GS, Haagensen DE Jr. Extramammary Paget's disease: evidence for an apocrine origin. An immunoperoxidase study of gross cystic disease fluid protein-15, carcinoembryonic antigen, and keratin proteins. Am J Surg Pathol 1984;8:43–50.

133. Meeker JH, Neubecker RD, Helwig EB. Hidradenoma papilliferum. Am J Clin Pathol 1962;37:182–95.

134. Michael H, Roth L. Congenital and acquired cysts, benign and malignant skin adnexal tumors, and Paget's disease of the vulva. In: Wilkinson EJ, ed. Pathology of the vulva and vagina: contemporary issues in surgical pathology; Vol 9. New York: Churchill Livingstone, 1987:25–48.

135. Nadji M, Ganjei P. The application of immunoperoxidase techniques in the evaluation of vulvar and vaginal disease. In: Wilkinson EJ, ed. Pathology of the vulva and vagina: contemporary issues in surgical pathology; Vol 9. New York: Churchill Livingstone, 1987:239–48.

136. _____, Ganjei P, Penneys NS, Morales AR. Immunohistochemistry of vulvar neoplasms: a brief review. Int J Gynecol Pathol 1984;3:41–50.

137. _____, Morales AR, Girtanner RE, Ziegels-Weissman J, Penneys NS. Paget's disease of the skin. A unifying concept of histogenesis. Cancer 1982;50:2203–6.

138. Nagle RB, Lucas DO, McDaniel KM, et al. Paget's cells. New evidence linking mammary and extramammary Paget cells to a common phenotype. Am J Clin Pathol 1985;83:431–8.

139. Nauth HF, Schilke E. Cytology of the exfoliative layer in normal and diseased vulvar skin: correlation with histology. Acta Cytol 1982;26:269–83.

140. O'Hara MF, Page DL. Adenomas of the breast and ectopic breast under lactational influences. Hum Pathol 1985; 16:707–12.

141. Parmley TH, Woodruff JD, Julian CG. Invasive vulvar Paget's disease. Obstet Gynecol 1975;46:341–6.

142. Ramesh V, Iyengar B. Proliferating trichilemmal cysts over the vulva. Cutis 1990;45:187–9.

143. Rickert RR. Intraductal papilloma arising in supernumerary vulvar breast tissue. Obstet Gynecol 1980;55:84–7S.

144. Rorat E, Ferenczy A, Richart RM. Human Bartholin gland, duct, and duct cyst. Histochemical and ultrastructural study. Arch Pathol 1975;99:367–74.

145. _____, Wallach RC. Mixed tumors of the vulva: clinical outcome and pathology. Int J Gynecol Pathol 1984;3:323–28.

146. Roth LM, Lee SC, Ehrlich CE. Paget's disease of the vulva. A histogenetic study of five cases including ultrastructural observations and review of the literature. Am J Surg Pathol 1977;1:193–206.

147. Shah KD, Tabizadch SS, Gerber MA. Immunohistochemical distinction of Paget's disease from Bowen's disease and superficial spreading melanoma with the use of monoclonal cytokeratin antibodies. Am J Clin Pathol 1987;88:689–95.

148. Simon KE, Dutcher JP, Runowicz CD, Wiernik PH. Adenocarcinoma arising in vulvar breast tissue. Cancer 1988;62:2234–8.

149. Stapleton JJ. Extramammary Paget's disease of the vulva in a young black woman. A case report with histogenic confirmation by immunostaining. J Reprod Med 1984;29:444–6.

150. Taylor PT, Stenwig JT, Klausen H. Paget's disease of the vulva. A report of 18 cases. Gynecol Oncol 1975; 3:46–60.

151. Taylor RN, Lacey CG, Shuman MA. Adenocarcinoma of Skene's duct associated with a systemic coagulopathy. Gynecol Oncol 1985;250–6.

152. Thomas J, Majmudar B, Goreldin L. Syringoma localized to the vulva. Arch Dermatol 1979;115:95–6.

153. Tiltman AJ, Knutzen VK. Primary adenocarcinoma of the vulva originating in misplaced cloacal tissue. Obstet Gynecol 1978;51:30–33S.

154. Underwood JW, Adcock LL, Okagaki T. Adenosquamous carcinoma of skin appendages (adenoid squamous cell carcinoma, pseudoglandular squamous cell carcinoma, adenocanthoma of sweat gland of Lever) of the vulva: a clinical and ultrastructural study. Cancer 1978;42:1851–8.

155. Wheelock JB, Goplerud DR, Dunn LJ, Oates JF III. Primary carcinoma of the Bartholin gland: a report of ten cases. Obstet Gynecol 1984;63:820–4.

156. Wick MR, Goellner JR, Wolfe JT III, et al. Vulvar sweat gland carcinomas. Arch Pathol Lab Med 1985;109:43–7.

157. Woodruff JD, Richardson EH. Malignant vulvar Paget's disease. Obstet Gynecol 1957;10:10–16.

158. Woodworth H Jr, Dockerty MB, Wilson RB, Pratt JH. Papillary hidradenoma of the vulva: a clinicopathologic study of 69 cases. Am J Obstet Gynecol 1971;110:501–8.

159. Young AW, Herman EW, Tovell HMM. Syringoma of the vulva: incidence, diagnosis and cause of pruritus. Obstet Gynecol 1980;55:515–8.

160. Zaino RJ. Carcinoma of the vulva, urethra and Bartholin's gland. In: Wilkinson EJ, ed. Pathology of the vulva and vagina: contemporary issues in surgical pathology; Vol 9. New York: Churchill Livingstone, 1987:119–53.

Benign Mesenchymal Tumors

161. Aneiros J, Belträn E, Garcia del Moral R, Nogales FF Jr. Epithelioid leiomyoma of the vulva. Diagn Gynecol Obstet 1982;4:351–6.

162. Blair C. Angiokeratoma of the vulva. Br J Dermatol 1970;83:409–11.

163. Brooks GG. Granular cell myoblastoma of the vulva in a 6-year-old girl. Am J Obstet Gynecol 1985;153:897–8.

164. Chetkowski R, Sakamoto H, MacLusky N, et al. Solitary pelvic neural tumors with high steroid receptor content. Gynecol Oncol 1985;20:43–52.

165. Cockerell CJ, LeBoit PE. Bacillary angiomatosis: a newly characterized, pseudoneoplastic, infectious, cutaneous vascular disorder. J Am Acad Dermatol 1990; 22:501–12.

166. Davos I, Abell MR. Soft tissue sarcoma of vulva. Gynecol Oncol 1976;4:70–86.

167. Degefu S, Dhurandhar HN, O'Quinn AG, Fuller PN. Granular cell tumor of the clitoris in pregnancy. Gynecol Oncol 1984;19:246–51.

168. Friedrich EG Jr, Wilkinson EJ. Vulvar surgery for neurofibromatosis. Obstet Gynecol 1985;65:135–8.

169. Gaffney EF, Majmuder B, Bryan JA. Nodular fasciitis (pseudosarcomatous fasciitis) of the vulva. Int J Gynecol Pathol 1982;1:307–12.

170. Gerbie AB, Hirsch MR, Green RR. Vascular tumors of the female genital tract. Obstet Gynecol 1955;6:499–507.

171. Huang HJ, Yamabe T, Tagawa H. A solitary neurilemmoma of the clitoris. Gynecol Oncol 1983;15:103–10.

172. Imperial R, Helwig EB. Angiokeratoma of the vulva. Obstet Gynecol 1967;29:307–12.

173. Johnson TL, Kennedy AW, Segal GH. Lymphangioma circumscriptum of the vulva. A report of two cases. J Reprod Med 1991;36:808–12.

174. Katenkamp D, Stiller D. Unusual leiomyoma of the vulva with fibroma-like pattern and pseudoelastin production. Virchows Arch [A] 1980;388:361–8.

175. Katz VL, Askin FB, Bosch BD. Glomus tumor of the vulva: a case report. Obstet Gynecol 1986;67:43–5S.

176. Kaufman-Friedman K. Hemangioma of the clitoris confused with adrenogenital syndrome: case report. Plast Reconstruct Surg 1978;62:452–4.

177. Kfuri A, Rosenshein N, Dorfman H, Goldstein P. Desmoid tumor of the vulva. J Reprod Med 1981;26:272–3.

178. Kohorn EI, Merino MJ, Goldenhersh M. Vulvar pain and dyspareunia due to glomus tumor. Obstet Gynecol 1986;67:41–2S.

179. Lieb SM, Gallousis S, Freedman H. Granular cell myoblastoma of the vulva. Gynecol Oncol 1979;8:12–20.

180. LiVolsi VA, Brooks JJ. Soft tissue tumors of the vulva. In: Wilkinson EJ, ed. Pathology of the vulva and vagina: contemporary issues in surgical pathology; Vol 9. New York: Churchill Livingstone, 1987:209–38.

181. Majmudar B, Castellano PZ, Wilson RW, Siegel RJ. Granular cell tumors of the vulva. J Reprod Med 1990; 35:1008–14.

182. Meister P, Bückmann FW, Konrad E. Nodular fasciitis. Analysis of 100 cases and review of the literature. Pathol Res Pract 1978;162:133–65.

183. O'Neal MF, Ampero EG. MR demonstration of extensive pelvic involvement in vulvar hemangiomas. J Comput Assisted Tomogr 1988;12:219–21.

184. Proppe KH, Scully RE, Rosai J. Postoperative spindle cell nodules of genitourinary tract resembling sarcomas. A report of eight cases. Am J Surg Pathol 1984;8:101–8.

185. Raju GC, O'Reily AP. Immunohistochemical study of granular cell tumor. Pathology 1987;19:402–6.

185a. Reed JA, Brigati DJ, Flynn SD, et al. Immunohistochemical identification of Rochalimaea henselae in bacillary (epithelioid) angiomatosis, parenchymal bacillary peliosis, and persistent fever with bacteremia. Am J Surg Pathol 1992;16:650–7.

186. Schreiber MM. Vulvar von Recklinghausen's disease. Arch Dermatol 1963;88:320–6.

187. Slavin RE, Christie JD, Swedo J, Powell LC Jr. Locally aggressive granular cell tumor causing priapism of the crus of the clitoris. A light and ultrastructural study, with observations concerning the pathogenesis of fibrosis of the corpus cavernosum in priapism. Am J Surg Pathol 1986;10:497–507.

188. Tavassoli FA, Norris HJ. Smooth muscle tumors of the vulva. Obstet Gynecol 1979;53:213–7.

189. Venter PF, Röhm GF, Slabber CF. Giant neurofibromas of the labia. Obstet Gynecol 1981;57:128–30.

190. Wolber RA, Talerman A, Wilkinson EJ, Clement PB. Vulvar granular cell tumors with pseudocarcinomatous hyperplasia: a comparative analysis with well-differentiated squamous carcinoma. Int J Gynecol Pathol 1991;10:59–66.

191. Young AW, Wind RM, Tovell HMM. Lymphangioma of the vulva. NY State J Med 1980;80:987–9.

Malignant Mesenchymal Tumors

192. Audet-LaPointe P, Paquin F, Geurard MJ, et al. Leiomyosarcoma of the vulva. Gynecol Oncol 1980;10:350–5.

193. Auerbach H, Brooks J. Alveolar soft part sarcoma: more evidence against a myogenic origin. Lab Invest 1985;52:4A.

194. _____, Brooks J. Kaposi's sarcoma: observations and a hypothesis. Lab Invest 1985;52:4A.

195. Beckslead J, Wood G, Fletcher V. Evidence for the origin of Kaposi's sarcoma from lymphatic endothelium. Lab Invest 1985;52:6A.

196. Bëgin LR, Clement PB, Kirk ME, et al. Aggressive angiomyxoma of pelvic soft parts: a clinicopathologic study of nine cases. Hum Pathol 1985;16:621–8.

197. Brooks JJ, LiVolsi VA. Liposarcoma presenting on the vulva. Am J Obstet Gynecol 1987;156:73–5.

198. Burgdorf WH, Mukai K, Rosai J. Immunohistochemical identification of factor VIII-related antigen in endothelial cells of cutaneous lesions of alleged vascular nature. Am J Clin Pathol 1981;75:167–71.

199. Chase DR, Enzinger FM, Weiss SW, et al. Keratin in epithelioid sarcoma. An immunohistochemical study. Am J Surg Pathol 1984;8:435–41.

200. Cockerell CJ, LeBoit PE. Bacillary angiomatosis: a newly characterized, pseudoneoplastic, infectious, cutaneous vascular disorder. J Am Acad Dermatol 1990;22:501–12.

201. Copeland LJ, Gershenson DM, Saul PB, et al. Sarcoma botryoides of the female genital tract. Obstet Gynecol 1985;66:262–6.

202. _____, Sneige N, Stringer CA, et al. Alveolar rhabdomyosarcoma of the female genitalia. Cancer 1985;56:849–55.

203. Corson JM, Pinkus GS. Intracellular myoglobin: a specific marker for skeletal muscle differentiation in soft tissue sarcomas. An immunoperoxidase study. Am J Pathol 1981;103:384–9.

204. Davos I, Abell MR. Soft tissue sarcoma of vulva. Gynecol Oncol 1976;4:70–86.

205. DiSaia PJ, Rutledge F, Smith JP. Sarcoma of the vulva. Report of 12 patients. Obstet Gynecol 1971;38:1802–4.

206. Gallup DG, Abell MR, Morley GW. Epithelioid sarcoma of the vulva. Obstet Gynecol 1976;48:14–7S.

207. Genton CY, Maroni ES. Vulval liposarcoma. Arch Gynecol 1987;240:63–6.

208. Gondos B, Casey MJ. Liposarcoma of the perineum. Gynecol Oncol 1982;14:133–40.

209. Guarda LA, Ordonez NG, Smith JL Jr, Hanssen G. Immunoperoxidase localization of factor VIII in angiosarcomas. Arch Pathol Lab Med 1982;106:515–6.

210. Hall DJ, Grimes MM, Goplerud DR. Epithelioid sarcoma of the vulva. Gynecol Oncol 1980;9:237–46.

211. Hensley, GT, Friedrich EG. Malignant fibroxanthoma: a sarcoma of the vulva. Am J Obstet Gynecol 1973;116:289–91.

212. Kyriakos M, Kempson RL. Inflammatory fibrous histiocytoma, an aggressive and lethal lesion. Cancer 1976;37:1584–606.

213. Lawrence WD, Shingleton HM. Malignant schwannoma of the vulva: a light and electron microscopic study. Gynecol Oncol 1978;6:527–37.

214. LiVolsi VA, Brooks JJ. Soft tissue tumors of the vulva. In: Wilkinson EJ, ed. Pathology of the vulva and vagina: contemporary issues in surgical pathology; Vol 9. New York: Churchill Livingstone, 1987:209–38.

215. Maddox JC, Evans HL. Angiosarcoma of the skin and soft tissue. Cancer 1981;48:1907–21.

216. Meister P, Natharth W. Immunohistochemical characterization of histiocytic tumors. Diagn Histopathol 1981;4:79–87.

217. Miettinen M, Holthofer H, Lehto VP, et al. *Ulex europaeus* I lectin as a marker for tumors derived from endothelial cells. Am J Clin Pathol 1983;79:32–6.

218. _____, Virtanen I, Damjanov H. Coexpression of keratin and vimentin in epithelioid sarcoma [letter]. Am J Surg Pathol 1985;9:460–3.

219. Morales AR, Fine G, Horn RC Jr. Rhabdomyosarcoma: an ultrastructural appraisal. Pathol Annu 1972;7:81–106.

220. Mukai M, Torikata C. Histogenesis of alveolar soft part sarcoma. An immunohistochemical and biochemical study. Lab Invest 1985;52:45–6A.

221. Perrone T, Swanson PE, Twiggs L, Ulbright TM, Dehner LP. Malignant rhabdoid tumor of the vulva: is distinction from epithelioid sarcoma possible? A pathologic and immunohistochemical study. Am J Surg Pathol 1989;13:848–58.

222. Piver MS, Tsukada Y, Barlow J. Epithelioid sarcoma of the vulva. Obstet Gynecol 1972;40:839–42.

223. Reymond RD, Hazra TA, Edlow DW, et al. Haemangiopericytoma of the vulva with metastasis to bone 14 years later. Br J Radiol 1972;45:765–8.

224. Shen JT, D'Ablaing G, Morrow CP. Alveolar soft part sarcoma of the vulva: report of first case and review of literature. Gynecol Oncol 1982;13:120–8.

225. Steeper TA, Rosai J. Aggressive angiomyxoma of the female pelvis and perineum. Report of nine cases of a distinctive type of gynecologic soft-tissue neoplasm. Am J Surg Pathol 1983;7:463–75.

226. Talerman A. Sarcoma botryoides presenting as a polyp of the labium majus. Cancer 1973;32:994–9.

227. Tavassoli FA, Norris HJ. Smooth muscle tumors of the vulva. Obstet Gynecol 1979;53:213–7.

228. Taylor RN, Bottles K, Miller TR, et al. Malignant fibrous histiocytoma of the vulva. Obstet Gynecol 1985;66:145–8.

229. Taxy JB, Battifora H, Trujillo Y, et al. Electron microscopy in the diagnosis of malignant schwannoma. Cancer 1981;48:1381–91.

230. Terada KY, Schmidt RW, Roberts JA. Malignant schwannoma of the vulva. A case report. J Reprod Med 1988;33:969–72.

231. Ulbright TM, Brokaw SA, Stehman FB, et al. Epithelioid sarcoma of the vulva. Evidence suggesting a more aggressive behavior than extra genital epithelioid sarcoma. Cancer 1983;52:1462–9.

232. Venter PF, Röhm GF, Slabber CF. Giant neurofibromas of the labia. Obstet Gynecol 1981;57:128–30.

233. Weiss SW, Enzinger FM. Malignant fibrous histiocytoma, an analysis of 200 cases. Cancer 1978;41:2250–66.

234. _____, Enzinger FM. Myxoid variant of malignant fibrous histiocytoma. Cancer 1977;39:1672–85.

235. _____, Langloss JM, Enzinger FM. Value of S-100 protein in the diagnosis of soft tissue tumors with particular reference to benign and malignant Schwann cell tumor. Lab Invest 1983;49:299–308.

236. ZaKut H, Lotan M, Lipnilsky M. Vulvar hemangiopericytoma. A case report and review of previous cases. Acta Obstet Gynecol Scand 1985;64:619–21.

Miscellaneous Tumors

237. Ackerman AB, Mihara I. Dysplasia, dysplastic melanocytes, dysplastic nevi, the dysplastic nevus syndrome, and the relation between dysplastic nevi and malignant melanomas. Hum Pathol 1985;16:87–91.

238. Beller U, Demopoulos RI, Beckman EM. Vulvovaginal melanoma. A clinicopathologic study. J Reprod Med 1986;31:315–9.

239. Benda JA, Platz CE, Anderson B. Malignant melanoma of the vulva: a clinical-pathologic review of 16 cases. Int J Gynecol Pathol 1986;5:202–16.

240. Bottles K, Lacey CG, Goldberg J, et al. Merkel cell carcinoma of the vulva. Obstet Gynecol 1984;63:61–5S.

241. Breslow A. Tumor thickness, level of invasion and node dissection in stage I cutaneous melanoma. Ann Surg 1975;182:572–5.

242. Brodell RT, Santa Cruz D. Borderline and atypical melanocytic lesions. Semin Diagn Pathol 1985;2:63–86.

243. Castaldo TW, Petrilli ES, Ballon SC, et al. Endodermal sinus of the clitoris. Gynecol Oncol 1980;9:376–80.

244. Chorlton I, Karnei RF Jr, King FM, et al. Primary malignant reticuloendothelial disease involving the vagina, cervix and corpus uteri. Obstet Gynecol 1974;44:735–48.

245. Christensen WN, Friedman KJ, Woodruff JD, Hood AF. Histologic characteristics of vulvar nevocellular nevi. J Cutan Pathol 1987;14(2):87–91.

246. Chung AF, Woodruff JM, Lewis JL Jr. Malignant melanoma of the vulva: a report of 44 cases. Obstet Gynecol 1975;45:638–46.

247. Copeland LJ, Cleary K, Sneige N, Edwards CL. Neuroendocrine (Merkel cell) carcinoma of the vulva: a case report and review of the literature. Gynecol Oncol 1985;22:367–78.

248. Dudley AG, Young RH, Lawrence WD, et al. Endodermal sinus tumor of the vulva in an infant. Obstet Gynecol 1983;61:76–9S.

249. Friedman RJ, Ackerman AB. Difficulties in the histologic diagnosis of melanocytic nevi on the vulvae of premenopausal women. In: Ackerman AB, ed. Pathology of malignant melanoma. New York: Masson, 1981:119–27.

250. Glasgow BJ, Wen DR, Al-Jitawi S, Cochran AJ. Antibody to S-100 protein aids the separation of pagetoid melanoma from mammary and extramammary Paget's disease. J Cutan Pathol 1987;14:223–6.

251. Harris NL, Scully RE. Malignant lymphoma and granulocytic sarcoma of the uterus and vagina. Cancer 1984;53:2530–45.

252. Hulagu C, Erez S. Juvenile melanoma of clitoris. J Obstet Gynaecol Br Commw 1973;80:89–91.

253. Husseinzadeh N, Whesseler T, Newman N, Shbaro I, Ho P. Neuroendocrine (Merkel cell) carcinoma of the vulva. Gynecol Oncol 1988;29:105–12.

254. Johnson TL, Kumar NB, White CD. Prognostic features of vulvar melanoma: a clinicopathologic analysis. Int J Gynecol Pathol 1986;5:110–8.

255. Krishnamurthy SC, Sampat MB. Endodermal sinus (yolk sac) tumor of the vulva in a pregnant female. Gynecol Oncol 1981;11:379–82.

256. Mark GJ, Mihm MC, Liteplo MG, et al. Congenital melanocytic nevi of the small and garment type. Hum Pathol 1973;4:395–418.

257. Mihm MC Jr, Clark WH Jr, From L. The clinical diagnosis, classification and histogenetic concepts of the early stages of cutaneous malignant melanomas. N Engl J Med 1971;284:1078–82.

258. Morgan L, Joslyn P, Chafe W, Ferguson K. A report on 18 cases of primary malignant melanoma of the vulva. Colposcopy Gynecol Laser Surg 1988;4:161–70.

259. Morrow CP, Rutledge F. Melanoma of the vulva. Obstet Gynecol 1972;39:745–52.

260. Nadji M, Ganjei P. The application of immunoperoxidase techniques in the evaluation of vulvar and vaginal disease. In: Wilkinson EJ, ed. Pathology of the vulva and vagina: contemporary issues in surgical pathology; Vol 9. New York: Churchill Livingstone, 1987:239–48.

261. _____, Ganjei P, Penneys NS, Morales AR. Immunohistochemistry of vulvar neoplasms: a brief review. Int J Gynecol Pathol 1984;3:41–50.

262. Phillips GL, Twiggs LB, Okagaki T. Vulvar melanoma: a microstaging study. Gynecol Oncol 1982;14:80–8.

263. Pierson KK. Malignant melanomas and pigmented lesions of the vulva. In: Wilkinson EJ, ed. Pathology of the vulva and vagina: contemporary issues in surgical pathology; Vol 9. New York: Churchill Livingstone, 1987:155–79.

264. Podratz KC, Gaffey TA, Symmonds RE, Johansen KL, O'Brien PC. Melanoma of the vulva: an update. Gynecol Oncol 1983;16:153–68.

264a. Rock B, Hood AF, Rock JA. Prospective study of vulvar nevi. J Am Acad Dermatol 1990;22:104–6.

265. Rhodes AR, Mihm MC Jr, Weinstock MA. Dysplastic melanocytic nevi. A reproducible histologic definition emphasizing cellular morphology. Mod Pathol 1989; 2:306–19.

266. Rodriguez HA, Ackerman LV. Cellular blue nevus. Clinicopathologic study of forty-five cases. Cancer 1968;21:393–405.

267. Sondergaard K, Schou G. Survival with primary cutaneous malignant melanoma evaluated from 2012 cases. A multivariate regression analysis. Virchows Arch [A] 1985;406:179–95.

268. Sison-Torre EQ, Ackerman AB. Melanosis of the vulva: a clinical simulator of malignant melanoma. Am J Dermatopathol 1985;7:51–60.

269. Tang CK, Toker C, Nedwich A, et al. Unusual cutaneous carcinoma with features of small cell (oat cell) and squamous cell carcinomas. A variant of Merkel cell neoplasm. Am J Dermatopathol 1982;4:537–48.

270. Ungerleider RS, Donaldson SS, Warnke RA, et al. Endodermal sinus tumor. The Stanford experience and the first reported case arising in the vulva. Cancer 1978;41:1627–34.

271. Wilkinson EJ, Croker BP, Friedrich EG Jr, Franzini DA. Two distinct pathologic types of giant cell tumor of the vulva. A report of two cases. J Reprod Med 1988;33:519–22.

272. Woolcott RJ, Henry RJ, Houghton CR. Malignant melanoma of the vulva. Australian experience. J Reprod Med 1988;33:699–702.

273. Young RH, Harris NL, Scully RE. Lymphoma-like lesions of the lower female genital tract: a report of 16 cases. Int J Gynecol Pathol 1985;4:289–99.

Secondary Tumors

274. Dehner LP. Metastatic and secondary tumors of the vulva. Obstet Gynecol 1973;42:47–57.

275. Grabstald H. Proceedings: Tumors of the urethra in men and women. Cancer 1973;32:1236–55.

276. Leiman G, Markowitz S, Veiga-Ferreira MM, Margolius KA. Renal adenocarcinoma presenting with bilateral metastases to Bartholin's glands: primary diagnosis by aspiration cytology. Diagn Cytopathol 1986;2:252–5.

277. Levine RL. Urethral cancer. Cancer 1980;45:1965–72.

278. Mader MH, Friedrich EG Jr. Vulvar metastasis of breast carcinoma. A case report. J Reprod Med 1982;27:169–71.

279. Mayer R, Fowler JE Jr, Clayton M. Localized urethral cancer in women. Cancer 1987;60:1548–51.

280. Pierson KK. Malignant melanomas and pigmented lesions of the vulva. In: Wilkinson EJ, ed. Pathology of the vulva and vagina: contemporary issues in surgical pathology; Vol 9. New York: Churchill Livingstone, 1987:155–79.

Tumor-Like Lesions

281. Dungar C, Wilkinson EJ. Vaginal mucinosis: a columnar cell metaplasia associated with topical 5-fluorouracil therapy. J Reprod Med (in press).

282. Farmer ER, Helwig EB. Cutaneous ciliated cysts. Arch Dermatol 1978;114:70–3.

283. Friedrich EG Jr, Wilkinson EJ. Mucous cysts of the vulvar vestibule. Obstet Gynecol 1973;42:407–14.

284. Gianotti F, Caputo R. Histiocytic syndromes: a review. J Am Acad Dermatol 1985;13:383–404.

285. Grunwald MH, Lee JY, Ackerman AB. Pseudocarcinomatous hyperplasia. Am J Dermatopathol 1988;10:95–103.

286. Junaid TA, Thomas SM. Cysts of the vulva and vagina: a comparative study. Int J Gynecol Obstet 1981;19:239–43.

287. Kempson RL, Sherman AI. Sclerosing lipogranuloma of the vulva. Am J Obstet Gynecol 1968;101:854–6.

288. Kfuri A, Rosenshein N, Dorfman H, Goldstein P. Desmoid tumor of the vulva. J Reprod Med 1981;26:272–3.

289. LiVolsi VA, Brooks JJ. Nodular fasciitis of the vulva. A report of two cases. Obstet Gynecol 1987;69:513–6.

290. _____, Brooks JJ. Soft tissue tumors of the vulva. In: Wilkinson EJ, ed. Pathology of the vulva and vagina: contemporary issues in surgical pathology; Vol 9. New York: Churchill Livingstone, 1987:209–38.

291. Meister P, Bückmann FW, Konrad E. Nodular fasciitis. Analysis of 100 cases and review of the literature. Pathol Res Pract 1978;162:133–65.

292. Mesko JD, Gates H, McDonald TW, Youmans R, Lewis J. Clear cell ("mesonephroid") adenocarcinoma of the vulva arising in endometriosis: a case report. Gynecol Oncol 1988;29:385–91.

293. Pyka RE, Wilkinson EJ, Friedrich EG Jr, Croker BP. The histopathology of vulvar vestibulitis syndrome. Int J Gynecol Pathol 1988;7:249–57.

294. Robboy SJ, Ross JS, Prat J, Keh PC, Welch WR. Urogenital sinus origin of mucinous and ciliated cysts of the vulva. Obstet Gynecol 1978;51:347–51.

295. Santa Cruz DJ, Martin SA. Verruciform xanthoma of the vulva. Report of two cases. Am J Clin Pathol 1979;71:224–8.

296. Sedlacek TV, Riva JM, Magen AB, Mangan CE, Cunnane MF. Vaginal and vulvar adenosis. An unexpected side effect of CO_2 laser vaporization. J Reprod Med 1990;35:995–1001.

297. Thomas R, Barnhill D, Bibro M, Hoskins W, Hambidge W. Histiocytosis X in gynecology. A case presentation and review of the literature. Obstet Gynecol 1986;67:46–9S.

298. Wolber RA, Talerman A, Wilkinson EJ, Clement PB. Vulvar granular cell tumors with pseudocarcinomatous hyperplasia: a comparative analysis with well-differentiated squamous carcinoma. Int J Gynecol Pathol 1991;10:59–66.

299. Zinkham WH. Multifocal eosinophilic granuloma. Natural history, etiology and management. Am J Med 1976;60:457–63.

Other Epithelial Disorders of Skin and Mucosa

300. Büchholz F, Schubert C, Lehmann-Willenbrock E. White sponge nevus of the vulva. Int J Gynecol Obstet 1985;23:505–7.

301. Bushkell LL, Friedrich EG, Jordon RE. An appraisal of routine direct immunofluorescence in vulvar disorders. Acta Dermatol Venereol (Stockholm) 1981;61:157–61.

302. Dickie RJ, Horne CHW, Sutherland HW, Bewsher PD, Stankler L. Direct evidence of localized immunological damage in vulvar lichen sclerosus et atrophicus. J Clin Pathol 1982; 35:1395–7.

303. Frances C, Wechler J, Meimon G, Labat RJ, Grimaud J, Hewitt J. Investigation of intercellular matrix macromolecules involved in lichen sclerosus. Arch Dermatol Venereol (Stockholm) 1983;63:483–90.

304. Friedrich EG Jr. International Society for the Study of Vulvar Disease. New nomenclature for vulvar disease: Report of the Committee on Terminology. Obstet Gynecol 1976;47:122–4.

305. Hart WR, Norris HJ, Helwig EB. Relation of lichen sclerosus et atrophicus of the vulva to development of carcinoma. Obstet Gynecol 1975;45:369–77.

306. Mann PR, Cowan MA. Ultrastructural changes in four cases of lichen sclerosus et atrophicus. Br J Dermatol 1973;89:223–31.

307. Meyrick Thomas RH, Ridley CM, MacGibbon DH, Black MM. Lichen sclerosus et atrophicus and autoimmunity: a study of 350 women. Brit J Dermatol 1988;118:41–6.

308. Miller RA, Griffiths WAD. Experimentally induced complement and immunoglobulin deposition along the basement membrane zone (BMZ) and in dermal blood vessels. Br J Dermatol 1982;106:275–9.

309. Patterson JA, Ackerman AB. Lichen sclerosus et atrophicus is not related to morphea. A clinical and histological study of 24 patients in whom both conditions were reported to be present simultaneously. Am J Dermatopathol 1984; 6:323–35.

310. Ridley CM, Frankman O, Jones ISC, Pincus S, Wilkinson EJ. New nomenclature for vulvar disease: International Society for the Study of Vulvar Disease. Hum Pathol 1989;20:495–6.

311. Zaino RJ, Husseinzadeh N, Nahhas W, Mortel R. Epithelial alterations in proximity to invasive carcinoma of the vulva. Int J Gynecol Pathol 1982;1:173–84.

✧ ✧ ✧